T0221187

breathe, baby, breathe!

NEONATAL INTENSIVE CARE, PREMATURITY, AND COMPLICATED PREGNANCIES

Every year in the United States, 12 per cent of all births are preterm births, 5 per cent of all babies need help to breathe at birth, and 3 per cent of neonates are born with at least one severe malformation. Many of these babies are hospitalized in a neonatal intensive care unit. Annie Janvier and her husband, Keith Barrington, are both paediatricians who specialize in the care of these sick babies and are internationally known for their research in this area. In 2005, when their daughter Violette was born extremely prematurely, four months before her due date, they faced the situation "from the other side" as parents. Despite knowing the scientific facts, they knew nothing about the experience itself. *"Knowing how a respirator works did not help me be the mother of a baby on a respirator,"* writes Annie. She did not know how to navigate the guilt, uncertainty, fears, predictions of providers, and responses of friends and family. In a society obsessed with goals, performance, efficiency, and high percentages, she discovered that the daily lack of control that new parents of sick babies face changes their lives. And that, for physician parents, it also changes the way they practice medicine.

Most of the articles and books written about premature babies and neonatal intensive care units examine the technological and medical aspects of neonatology. *Breathe, Baby, Breathe!*, however, is written in the voice of a parent-doctor and tells the story of Violette and her parents alongside the stories of other fragile babies and their families with different journeys and different outcomes. With the story of Violette at the core of the book, the interwoven stories and empirical articles provide essential insights into the medical world of premature birth. This original and clever blend of narrative and evidence provides a new, experiential view of the way forward during a parental crisis.

ANNIE JANVIER, MD, PHD, is a professor of Pediatrics and Clinical Ethics at the University of Montreal and a neonatologist, clinical ethicist, and researcher at CHU Sainte-Justine.

PHYLLIS ARONOFF and HOWARD SCOTT won the 2018 Governor General's Literary Award for their translation of *Descent into Night* by Edem Awumey.

breathe, baby, breathe!

NEONATAL INTENSIVE CARE, PREMATURITY, AND COMPLICATED PREGNANCIES

Annie Janvier, MD, PhD

Translated by Phyllis Aronoff and Howard Scott

UNIVERSITY OF TORONTO PRESS
Toronto Buffalo London

© University of Toronto Press 2020
Toronto Buffalo London
utorontopress.com

ISBN 978-1-4875-0401-4 (cloth)   ISBN 978-1-4875-1927-8 (EPUB)
ISBN 978-1-4875-2306-0 (paper)   ISBN 978-1-4875-1926-1 (PDF)

Library and Archives Canada Cataloguing in Publication

Title: Breathe, baby, breathe! Neonatal intensive care, prematurity, and complicated
    pregnancies / Annie Janvier; translated by Phyllis Aronoff and Howard Scott.
Other titles: Respire, bébé, respire! English
Names: Janvier, Annie, author. | Aronoff, Phyllis, 1945– translator. | Scott, Howard,
    1952– translator.
Description: Translation of: Respire, bébé, respire! | Includes bibliographical
    references.
Identifiers: Canadiana 20190173556 | ISBN 9781487504014 (cloth) |
    ISBN 9781487523060 (paper)
Subjects: LCSH: Janvier, Annie. | LCSH: Janvier, Annie – Family. | LCSH: Premature
    infants – Care. | LCSH: Premature labor. | LCSH: Neonatologists – Biography. |
    LCSH: Premature infants – Biography.
Classification: LCC RJ250.J3613 2019 | DDC 618.92/011–dc23

Ornaments used for journal articles and medical updates: iStock.com/JoyTasa and
iStock.com/bubaone

University of Toronto Press acknowledges the financial assistance to its publishing
program of the Canada Council for the Arts and the Ontario Arts Council, an agency
of the Government of Ontario.

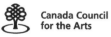

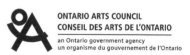

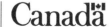

For Debbie and Lorraine, and

for Sophie and Gene,

who cared for Violette and our family

and knew that, when she was at her sickest, so were we

––––––––––––––

Making the decision to have a child – it is momentous. It is to decide forever to have your heart go walking around outside your body.

Elizabeth Stone

Contents

Part 2: The Delivery and the First Days

Part 3: The NICU

Part 4: Progress and Setbacks

Part 5: Coming Home

Part 6: Neonatology Information for Parents, Families, Clinicians, and All Those Who Care about Babies

Foreword

John D. Lantos and William Meadow

On the day her baby Violette was born, Annie Janvier felt no joy. Instead, she writes, "I did not feel pain, sad emotions. I felt nothing – such a big black hole, a void. I was empty; nothing had any meaning. I learned the definition of nothing, of meaninglessness, the meaning of meaninglessness."

Violette was born extremely prematurely. She had less than a 50 per cent chance of surviving. If she survived, she might have chronic physical and cognitive problems.

Annie, and her husband, Keith Barrington, are neonatologists. They had spent their professional lives taking care of extremely premature babies and talking to stressed-out parents about the decisions that they faced. They were both very good at what they did. But having a preemie of their own changed the way that they thought about parents and doctors in the neonatal intensive care unit (NICU). This book recreates Janvier's experience. It tells what she learned. It shows how painful those lessons were. Most importantly, it led her to change the way she interacted with parents and to do research on doctor-patient communication that would help other doctors be better at guiding parents through the emotionally treacherous minefield of the NICU experience.

This book is not a how-to guide about neonatal practice. Although written by experts in the field, it is not a neonatology textbook. Instead, it is a book written by a mother who is in pain, a mother who is uncertain, terrified, hopeful, miserable, angry, and mystified. Those emotions are surprising because we think that knowledge helps. We think that we help parents by informing them of the facts. This book makes us rethink that presumption.

Before Violette was born, Annie and Keith knew all the facts. But they didn't understand just how inadequate those facts were in the face overwhelming emotions. "Being a parent in the NICU changed me," she writes. "I hit bottom. I learned how easy it is to fall, and how fast it can happen."

Janvier came to understand how much she didn't know, even when she thought she knew a lot. As a doctor, she had written the information sheet for parents whose babies were admitted to the NICU. The information was mostly facts about the baby's chances for survival and about the possible long-term complications associated with prematurity. She once thought that such information was crucial. As a parent, she sees how wrong she was. As she writes, she thought "that knowing the bad things that could happen would help parents." Yet she and Keith "had all the necessary knowledge ... but in fact we knew nothing, nothing at all."

Instead of statistics about the baby's outcomes, she wanted information about her own survival and her family's survival. She wanted someone to tell her that, at the end of all the pain, there was a possibility of joy and happiness. She wanted acknowledgment of the guilt she felt about having gone into premature labor and brought her baby into the nightmare world of the NICU rather than the dream world of a warm and loving snuggle. She writes, "Parents are, of course, concerned about the child's development and the likelihood of death. But they also ask themselves all kinds of other questions. How can I be a parent in the NICU? What does the NICU look like? Who will be able to come to see my baby? How can I be a parent to a disabled child? What will happen to my family? What will happen to the other children? Who can visit my baby and when? What about nursing the baby? How do we include family and friends? What will my baby look like?"

The heart of the book is a beautiful, raw, funny, frightening, insightful, bawdy, profane, profound, and very personal memoir. Janvier describes how all her knowledge and experience meant little when she went into labour at 23 weeks. At that moment, she was as confused and vulnerable as any other mother in labour. "It's dark and I'm scared ... I can't believe

all this is happening to us!" "I felt as if I were in an Almodovar film –
woman *really* on the verge of a nervous breakdown."

The descriptions of being in the labour ward pull no punches in
recounting what Janvier felt like to be helpless, bloated, and constipated,
trying to move her bowels without triggering uterine contractions. "I
didn't want to stay on my back in the hospital, choking on every mouthful of food, pissing in my hair, and getting 'deconstipated,' all for a dead
baby or, worse, I thought at the time, for a disabled baby."

She writes about her fears and her doubts when she first saw her tiny
daughter. "I'd like to be put under general anaesthetic and wake up in
six months. Hopeless. Despair. Despair. I'm devastated. I'm going crazy
imagining all the horrible scenarios in which Violette is injured, dies,
has even more complications."

She writes about despair: "A knot of stress, pain, and despair is choking me. I have to repeat to myself that one day, everything will be fine
and I'll no longer feel the way I feel now. I read last year in an article that
when you smile, you feel better, because the muscles you use to smile
send messages to the brain telling it that you're happy. I try, but it doesn't
work. I see my reflection on my computer screen and it's pathetic. My
smile is empty."

She addresses a diary entry to Violette: "Dear Violette, I don't know
where to start ... You are on the respirator, and I am so scared. Scared to
lose you, scared to try to save you too hard. Scared of wanting too much
and ending up more hurt. Scared of loving you too much and ending up
empty, filled up with air and loss and guilt and nothing."

She addresses much of the book to other mothers. She writes, "Mothers, it's perfectly normal to occasionally have selfish or negative thoughts
that you can't share with anyone."

Parents who have had a critically ill child know how profoundly iso-
lating it can be. Aleksandar Hemon said it felt like they were in an aquarium, separated by glass walls from the rest of the world. "I could see
out, the people outside could see me, but we were living and breathing
in entirely different environments."[1] Janvier describes that isolation and
about how it leads her to understand that the most important thing that
doctors and nurses can offer is companionship on this lonely journey.
She tries to break the aquarium glass, to reach out to other parents (and
their doctors and nurses) and to tell them, "You are not alone."

The competent and compassionate doctors who were caring for Violette were friends and colleagues of Annie and Keith. Even they didn't know what to say. One wrote about talking to them right after Violette was born, "What does one say? Congratulations? Hardly. Sorry? Hardly ... I felt extremely sorry for both of them ... 'Things will be OK' is what I recall saying. There was no evidence whatsoever to support this statement."

As it turns out, there is some evidence that, for many people, things are OK in the end. This evidence is also presented in this book.

But the lessons Annie learned are equally applicable to situations in which babies do and don't survive. Janvier has become intolerant of health professionals who presume to understand what parents need without asking them. She warns her colleagues that they can never understand parents' hopes and fears and goals without letting the parents explain what they believe. She rejects the idea that doctors have to tell parents about all the possible bad outcomes in order for parents to make an informed decision. Instead, she suggests, they must also tell parents about the possibilities for good outcomes, for redemption, for lights at the ends of tunnels. "These health professionals see only handicaps and suffering; they don't understand the positive changes ... They have only negative conversations about the future of premature babies."

Her insights have led her to do groundbreaking research that has changed the way that doctors counsel parents. Some of that work is included in this book.

The book is written in many different voices – some more objective, some grittier, some scientific or clinical. There are excerpts from cold, objective, and jargon-filled medical records. There are chapters that she wrote long after her daughter was discharged from the NICU. There are scientific papers, studies that Janvier and her colleagues wrote over the years, trying to better understand the experiences that parents have and the ways that doctors can help them.

The most heart-wrenching passages are those that she wrote in a diary while she was in hospitalized in premature labour and when her daughter Violette was in the NICU. They are filled with the anguish, the doubt, the self-loathing, and the anger that she felt, day-by-day, as she rode the emotional roller coaster. She had nobody to talk to about those feelings. Instead, she kept these diary entries in a file on her computer called "Toxic Shit."

The book ends with a recognition of the ways in which such experiences irrevocably change every parent. People "rewrite chapters of the book of their life." They adjust their hopes and try to accept the prospect of a life completely different from the one they had dreamed. There is no way around the despair, anger, and fear. The only way is to go through them.

There are many books out today about the experience of illness. Literary scholars even have a name for them – "pathographies." Anne Hunsaker Hawkins is a scholar of pathographies. She has noted that the act of writing about serious illness can facilitate recovery. "Writing about an illness experience is a kind of psychic rebuilding ... a testimony to the capacity to transform [the experience of being seriously ill] in ways that heal."[2] This book not only helped Dr Janvier heal herself. It also will help others heal.

She ends with a message of hope. With help, people do get through. And sometimes, they come out on the other side with more compassion. "My heart bled for a long time but, since it has healed, it is twice as big as before. The world is no longer the same. My coffee tastes better than most people's, and the sun shines brighter for me than for others."

Ultimately, then, this book is about the transformative power of love. That love was apparent in the ways Annie and Keith helped each through a very dark time in their lives. It is about how both had uncompromising love for Violette and how that love helped Violette survive and thrive. Love was the energy that transformed Janvier's suffering into scholarship and education and new understandings that can help other parents and doctors who face similar situations. It is a book that can be both hard to read and hard to put down.

Acknowledgments

I wish to thank my children (my prince, my microflower, and my caramel baby) and James, who keep me real and regularly remind me of the value of life, and place in perspective the stress of clinical work, on-call duties, articles, (rejected) grants, research, conferences, publications, and the disintegration of one's physical attributes.

I thank my husband, my love, soulmate, and fellow brain, for his love and support in good times and bad. Who always believed in Violette and loved her unconditionally from before she was born and when she was at her best and her worst, who literally saved her life. Keith, thank you for standing strong when I was falling apart, for being the guard dog of our sick child, and for having the sensitivity to let me get my head above water before crashing momentarily.

I thank my parents, who were constant examples of integrity for me. They did everything to stress what is fair and what should be done, without bothering too much about the rules of diplomacy. I thank my sisters and brother, my emotional safety net. My father showed us how to deal with hard times and seize all the happiness life offers us. When he saw me tormenting myself with my studies and making endless lists and plans, he would often remind me that life is what goes on while you're writing your Post-it notes.

I want to thank all those who cared for Violette when she was in the hospital. Thank you to all the nurses of the Royal Victoria Hospital

NICU who took care of my family, especially Debbie and Lorraine, Violette's primary nurses, her "second moms." A big thank you to all our neonatologist colleagues who took care of her, particularly Daniel Faucher and Diana Willis, and very special thanks to Sophie Nadeau and Gene Dempsey. Sophie, I will never be able to thank you enough for the excellent care you gave her. Gene, I will always be grateful for your first intubations in less than twenty seconds, and I'll never forget the incredible composure with which you installed a central venous catheter on 22 June, a day that will always be etched in our memories. Thank you to Lucie, my obstetrician, for being my Adalat pusher and for convincing me to accept a catheter. Thank you to the obstetrics nurses, thank you for calling Violette by her name, thank you for emptying my urine bag, thank you for all the times when you took care of my shit, literally.

Catherine, thank you for your support, your humour, and your gummy bears. Annabelle, thank you for your example: your record for forced bed-rest and your experience as an expert NICU mom are an inspiration and a source of courage for all of us. Jean, thank you for the hours of games.

I want to thank Élise Couture, who cared for Violette in the neonatal clinic and who recommended her sister as a babysitter. Marjolaine was a gift from heaven. She took care of our kids while we were taking care of sick babies. Marjolaine is also Violette's second mom! It's hard to sum up what she represents for me: a combination of sister-confidant-organizer-governess-witness-friend and Maman no. 2 to my kids. Without her support, we wouldn't be the family we are.

Thank you to the kids' school, École Laurier, an excellent school that helps children and their families grow and that adapts to their specific characteristics. A thousand thank yous to the staff and the wonderful teachers, with special thanks to Diane, Anne-Marie, Édith, Ariane, Marie-Josée, Julie, and Mélissa.

Thank you to my great friends and mentors John Lantos and Bill Meadow, who read the first drafts of this book in English and gave me their valuable opinions. I will always be grateful for your support throughout my career. Thank you, Barbara, my co–researcher-mom-collaborator, you expanded my horizons and made me a better doctor. Thank you, Martha, for suggesting the University of Toronto Press for the English version of this book. Thank you to Saroj Saigal and Peter

Ubel, who are doing research essential to our medical practice, research that goes beyond statistics and numbers, research on life. I thank Antoine Payot, my ethics "boss," friend, and colleague, for reading certain chapters of this book and giving me his opinion, and supporting me in my project. Ginette, the driving force of Préma-Québec, thank you, too, for your contribution, for your careful reading; thank you for supporting the cause year after year with energy and conviction, thank you for talking to so many parents, thank you for teaching me things.

Jean-François, thank you for reading this from beginning to end several times, for convincing me that it was "damn good," for giving me a boot in the ass to make it work.

Finally, I'd like to thank all the families I've had the privilege of knowing in the NICU over the years. I admire your inexhaustible love, your sincere words, your combative realism, your incredible resilience. You've taught me a great deal about life and death. You've strengthened my belief in the values I hold dearest. You've helped me deal better with adversity and see seeing things more clearly: health and sickness, the quality of life, family ties, relationships with others, uncertainty, and the immense joys of the simple life. Thanks to you, the normal irritants of life seem trivial to me, and the little pleasures take on their full importance.

You will always be my inspiration.

My Plastic in Your Baby

Woken from deep sleep
"The asphyxia for cooling has arrived"
Disoriented in the overheated call room
Antiseptic smell on my hands
Brain-fog quickly vanishing
Body sticking to the synthetic mattress

The wush-wush of the respirator
Ocean sounds
Chest up and down
Waves of hope
Naked on a cold blanket
Quiet
An oxygen and nitric-oxide-pink baby
Pure
Perfect like the smooth stone angel sculptures in museums

Surgical mask, heating lamp, fog in my glasses
Prepping of the lines
Needles on syringes, rising clear bubbles
Spiral of disinfectant around his umbilicus
Scalpel neatly cutting the cord

Opaque snake of life
Two small muscular arteries
Tweezers dilating
The large vein waiting, it's gaping mouth open
And reality sinks in
The enormity of what I am doing
Sticking plastic in perfection

This is your baby under the blue sterile fields
Your treasure with his perfect silk skin
Ready to be instrumented
The baby they removed from you
After sticking a tube down your throat
Taking over your body
Tiny tubes in his great vessels
Crawling under his heart
Where your fed him inside you
The privilege to meet your boy
The tragedy of meeting him before you
While you are crying in your room
Alone
Awake after the Caesarean surgery, bleeding
Empty

Red hot blood removed slowly
Condensation in the tubes
I am entrusted with your son's life
Fragility under fluorescent lights
Plastic in perfection
Drops in my glasses
Tears

Introduction

In 2008, while clearing files from my work computer before changing universities, I came across a file called "Toxic Shit." In it, I found texts I'd written during one of the darkest periods of my life: the birth of my daughter and the time she spent in the neonatal intensive care unit (NICU).

Keith, my husband, and I are both neonatologists – both doctors for sick babies, or "broken babies," as our kids say. We take care of babies who are beginning their lives in neonatal intensive care. It's a field of medicine marked by distress, hope, death, and also indescribable joy when parents leave the hospital holding their baby in their arms, their beautiful baby. Keith and I love our work and the babies we care for.

Violette was born on 22 May 2005, at 24 weeks' gestation. In the delivery room, she weighed only 670 grams (less than 1.5 pounds). She was transferred to the NICU, where Keith and I both worked. Her hospital stay was complicated. The doctors and nurses were a little afraid of this pair of parents: we know every test, every bit of clinical information, and every treatment. Nothing could escape our scrutiny, and they feared we would be pitiless judges of their slightest actions. We had all the medical knowledge, certainly, but in fact we knew nothing, nothing at all. When Violette was sick, so were we. When she was one month old, we had to plan her funeral. I was completely empty. I learned the meaning of devastation, annihilation, emotional void.

I've always liked talking with the parents of my little patients. Throughout my career, I've spoken to them about things I've rarely spoken about with my own family or best friends: the meaning of life, death, faith; whether to embrace religion, reject it, or continue to ignore it; the fears, the guilt, the uncertainty. And it was these parents who helped me become a mother when I found myself at Violette's bedside. Their stories took on a new meaning. Nothing to do with the scientific or academic knowledge I had mastered so well. It was no longer a matter of theoretical knowledge, nor of that automatic action-reaction mechanism that governed me as a doctor. It was the complete opposite. Seeing your child in critical condition, her life hanging by a thread (and some tubes!), has nothing to do with knowing and controlling. It's about letting go, waiting, hoping, no longer being in control, compartmentalizing your brain. This isn't really me at all. I am a highly organized overachiever control freak. The words of those parents came back to me in relation to what I was experiencing, and I repeated them out loud. Those parents essentially saved me from drowning. Their stories taught me that I wasn't crazy, incompetent, or a bad parent.

Before Violette's birth, I had seen many parents who were, like me, tottering through the unit, hunched over, their eyes dull, dazed from hearing bad news again and again, wondering if it all would end some day. Parents who were afraid of calling because they didn't want to hear bad news; parents who were plunged into anxiety every time the phone rang. Parents who felt guilty for not calling. Parents who were praying for the cruel uncertainty to end, for the train to finally be put back on the tracks toward a familiar destination. Parents who were doubting, who were wondering how to cope with it all, when they weren't tempted to simply throw themselves off the train. Yet, in spite of their exhaustion, those parents always found strength somewhere.

This book is not a thesis explaining the scientific aspects of neonatology and intensive care for babies. There are lots of books on the properties of oxygen, on respirators, on all the catastrophes that can strike little babies and on what doctors do to care for them. The internet is full of statistics, and it has thousands of scientific articles on sick babies. I've written quite a few myself. I knew all the science. But knowing how a respirator works didn't help me be the mom of a baby on a respirator. This is a book about patience, becoming a parent, resilience, and transformation. These are stories of courageous families, and this is also my story.

This book was first published in French, but I first wrote it in English. Not because my English is better than my French – French is my first language. But I simply couldn't write it in my mother tongue. In English, it's easier for me to step back and look at my life as if I were flying over it in an airplane. From above, you can see the bomb damage, but not so much the suffering of the victims. The birth of my daughter was the bomb that fell on my family.

My story was translated into French; I couldn't have done it myself. Then it underwent cosmetic surgery by the publisher, Éditions Québec Amérique (*merci*, Marie-Noëlle Gagnon). After some words of encouragement from doctors, ethicists, researchers, and, above all, parents and families, here is the English version of the book, adapted and retranslated.

This book is intended for anyone who is interested in sick babies, neonatology, and prematurity, but who is looking for an alternative to statistics and rational explanations. It is also intended for parents and the families who are doing their best to support them. Professionals in paediatrics and obstetrics, residents, and medical students will learn how to cultivate their empathy with their patients and families dealing with high-risk pregnancies and sick babies. Ethicists and academics who are drawn to narrative will also find something of interest. Because, sometimes, in order to truly understand, one story is worth more than dozens of scientific chapters. Finally, this book is intended for anyone interested in the phenomenon of birth, in the complexity of families, and in the challenges of paediatrics and birth.

My experience has given me a new perspective on life, that precious gift that doesn't come with an instruction manual. That is what I'm sharing with you in this book.

We are often stronger than we think. Even in our darkest moments

How to Read This Book

Although the idea of this book sprouted from the "Toxic Shit" folder in my computer, I did not want it to be only about our story. For this reason, this volume has different types of chapters. The "Dear Computer" chapters are from my "Toxic Shit" folder. They are diary-style chapters, written to my computer, with many curses deleted. They usually start with "Dear Computer" and are written in the present tense. A few chapters are letters written to Keith, Violette, and even nature! These usually start with "Dear Keith," "Dear Violette," or "Dear the-person-I-am-speaking-to." These chapters were written while my daughter was in the neonatal intensive care unit. Other chapters are more academic. "Expert chapters" communicate in my physician, ethicist, or researcher voice. These may tell the story of other families I have met who inspired me and taught me something. They also speak about medicine, paediatrics, families, and ethics, and examine these subjects with a scientific or ethical lens. Many of these chapters have been published in academic journals, and the references for these articles are included at the back of the book; some are written with other academics and/or parents. The book ends with practical recommendations and information for parents, families, providers, and researchers.

Scattered throughout the text excerpts from Violette's chart. These speak about her respiratory system, the IVs, the fluids, the nutrition, the ID, the neuro status – nothing one can easily explain. The NICU is a strange place where there are formulas, numbers, and science. If you are not a neonatal provider, it is likely that you will not understand the content of these chart excerpts. These excerpts are here to demonstrate the clash between the medical jargon and the human side of the NICU. The mother of a premature baby wrote me to thank me for my book. She had some kind of revelation reading these "jargon lines":

> I liked the bits in medical jargon, they are like Chinese, just like when I heard them talk about my baby. Exactly like that. I did not know my baby, was trying to be a parent, the way you explained. And then it clicked and I realized, like you wrote, that it was OK if there were a lot of things I did not understand. I did not have to understand anything. If you understood that jargon and were lost, then it is OK if I was lost too. I mean now I can understand the machines, but what is happening to me, I cannot make sense of it. I will ride the wave one day at a time.

On the other hand, you will find that I generally tell – in a simple parental language – what is happening to Violette in the chapters that follow these excerpts. For those who are interested, you will find a list of common abbreviations that we use in the neonatal world at the end of the book. They are often called "the three-letter words" by parents!

Warning for parents who have a sick baby in the NICU at the moment: Although the majority of parents like you find the diary entries beneficial, because they may translate your feelings in words, many still find them too hard to read. On the other hand, parents have all told me that the book was beneficial for their friends and families and others who wanted to help them, but often "*didn't quite get it.*" For parents who find the diary entries too raw, many parents gave me the advice to tell you to jump to the practical recommendations at the end of the book.

part one

LABOUR AND PRENATAL COUNSELLING

The "Perfect Pregnancy" Is a Scam

When I had Axel, pregnancy lost all its romanticism for me. He was my first child, but not Keith's. James, his first son, had been living with us since 2003; he had moved in with us a year after we got together, when he was 14 years old. We were delighted to tell him he was going to have a little brother.

I was a paediatrician specializing in neonatology, and I cared for premature babies every day. Keith was chief of the NICU. We were a loving couple and had decided to have children, and we wanted a lot of them. At the time, I was 29 years old. I was a former athlete, an endorphin and adrenalin junkie.

I had my first contractions at 23 weeks, in the middle of a Canadian Paediatric Society conference in Calgary. The contractions began while I was giving a podium presentation. Pain swept over me in waves, and I could barely breathe. I thought I was having violent intestinal cramps. The next fifteen minutes felt like an hour. I attributed it to stage fright and thought I should consider giving up public speaking, and yet I had always felt comfortable at a podium.

As I listened to the other presentations, I found myself short of breath and doubled over with pain every five minutes, and Francine, a colleague, suggested I might be having contractions. "Me? Oh come on!" I found the idea almost laughable. It was impossible: contractions four months too early! As a doctor, I deal every day with women who give birth prematurely, but I just couldn't imagine that I myself was going into full premature labour. The shame of it! I was at 23 weeks. In my belly, Axel weighed barely a pound. In 2005, the vast majority of babies born at 22 weeks died; at 23 weeks, most died; and at 24 weeks, about half survived. The prognosis was not very good. I replied to my colleague that I couldn't be in premature labour, that this couldn't be happening, not to me! I was physically fit, I was a paediatrician, and I was careful. And besides, I was in Calgary! I wanted to go home. I wanted to see my mother, I wanted to hide in my bed, under my bed. Maybe if I took deep breaths, the pains would stop.

Nevertheless, I went to the hospital, and the contractions finally subsided. But my cervix was dilated and my fibronectin test was positive, which meant, in medical terms, that I was at risk of giving birth within a week. The cervix is normally closed and opens up shortly before childbirth, but cervical incompetence is not rare: the cervix opens before the pregnancy has reached full term, and the baby may not stay in the uterus but instead be born prematurely. The cervix has to dilate to 10 centimetres for the baby to come out during birth. At that time I was dilated to 1 centimetre, which at 23 weeks is abnormal and worrying.

I took the first plane back to Montreal, in spite of rare residual contractions and an open cervix. On the trip, I imagined a series of catastrophic scenarios. What if I gave birth during the flight? Is there a doctor on the plane? Yes, Keith and I are baby specialists, we can take care of everything. Can the father cut the cord? Can they give us a straw to help the baby breathe, preferably the kind that bends at one end? Would someone have a little tube that we could insert in the vein of the umbilical cord? Throughout the flight, I was terrified. I talked to Axel, I told him to hang on and behave himself, that I loved him, that he had to stay quietly in his seat in spite of my uterus with its incompetent cervix.

I'd always believed I'd be a superwoman during my pregnancy. I knew pregnancy could be difficult. It was my job to know that. I knew that all women could have complications, however careful and healthy they might be. But I deluded myself with a kind of magical thinking: my pregnancy would involve waiting quietly for my baby while abstaining, like a good little girl, from drinking wine or eating raw meats or cheeses made from unpasteurized milk. I was a force of nature! I would be able to push very hard to eject the baby. It would pop right out and that would be that. I wouldn't be like those weak-kneed women I sometimes saw in my practice, the ones who moaned open-mouthed while claiming to be pushing. When you're the doctor and a fetus in distress is not coming out, it's stressful. Mothers who moan without pushing are infuriating. The tension rises in the room as the fetus's heart slows down and the doctors' hearts speed up. I saw the final push as an exercise, like in a Nike ad: "Just do it!" During my life, I have often done too many things at the same time, but I always got through everything I took on. Five hours of sleep was more than enough for me. I wanted at least four children. I would be able to push very hard and everything would go well. I was invincible.

Lucie, my obstetrician, saw me when I arrived. Yes, I was in preterm labour, and, despite the relative calm, I wasn't out of the woods. The prescription: stop working and stay in bed except to go to the toilet and wash. So there I was with my legs crossed, forbidden to walk or push anything, on my back, in my bed. A fallen superwoman. The fear, the powerlessness, and the despair were new for me.

Maybe old injuries were catching up with me. In the past, I had experienced pain and suffering. Perhaps I had a few anti-personnel mines inside me. During my first year of medical residency, my father had been diagnosed with incurable brain cancer. For eighteen months, my mother, my sisters, my brother, and I watched the slow deterioration of his body and his mind. As rational as my father was, with his doctorate in mathematics, he spent a fortune trying to find a miracle cure, from phony natural remedies to chromotherapy, acupressure, acupuncture, and candle therapy, all of which promised him eternal life. We went through very difficult times with him, but also very precious moments filled with love. At the time, I was a paediatric resident, but I learned so much about home care, neurology, radiation therapy, adult diapers, pneumonia in immunosuppressed patients, oncology … and the price of cemetery plots.

A year later, I was diagnosed with thyroid cancer, but a "good" kind, with a mortality rate of only 5 to 10 per cent. "We'll toss it in the garbage and everything will be fine," my surgeon said. "YES!" was my reply. I still had to have an operation and radiation treatments, as well as enduring hospital care that involved neither my speciality nor my patients. Two years later, fearing a return of the cancer, I had to have another quite invasive operation on my neck. I don't like hospitals much when I'm not working in them. I don't like being a patient, although I know how to keep my cool and swear only under my breath. I'd rather stay home with moderate pain than be painless in the hospital. In short, I hate hospitals. I loathe hospital beds and blue hospital gowns, and I hate hospital food. I am an impatient patient. After my last operation, I made a friend eat my jello and liquid supplements so my doctors would think I was ready to go home – even if it meant puking my guts out and enduring pain, as long as it was not in the hospital. At first, she didn't want to be my accomplice, because it wasn't good for me. "If you love me, eat that fucking jello, drink those goddamn liquids and get me out of this hellhole as fast as possible." She had no choice. And so I left the hospital in a wheelchair, more dead than alive. I was seeing stars and big black clouds, I heard buzzing in my ears, and I had a persistent metallic taste in my mouth. I was trying not to faint in my wheelchair so I could be free. Freedom! I was finally going home!

Waiting for the birth of Axel, my ticking time-bomb, meant reliving that experience, although it was very different. My body was failing again, but this time my child could suffer because of this body, because of this defective female equipment. When you're lying down, all you can do is stay calm and not move. Tell your uterus, and your baby, too, to hang on. That forced rest is torture for someone who's a maniac about action and control like me. I couldn't even cook my own meals. Before going to work, Keith would bring me my food in bed. I felt like a caged lion. The possibility of premature birth was a big black cloud over my bed, a cloud that fortunately dissipated with every additional week that Axel spent in my belly.

Besides sleeping, there's not much to do in a bed – of course, you can do other stuff, but not when your cervix is dilated and there's a risk of giving birth prematurely at any moment (which means no sex for months – you get the picture). I stayed in bed pretending to be calm and to control my emotions, focusing on my cervix. I imagined myself on a quiet lake without a ripple. When I had a contraction, a ripple would appear on the lake, then it would go back to being as smooth as a mirror – like a postcard of Switzerland with mountains cut like diamonds overlooking an unnaturally blue lake against a cloudless sky. Keith was frustrated; he would have liked to have had unilateral sexual relations more often. I was irritated by the very idea that he wanted me to pleasure him. "Sex. Are you kidding? That's what got us into this mess!"

So during my first pregnancy, I was on my back for eleven weeks, during which time I had contractions whenever I moved a little too much or had to get up to go to the bathroom. My cervix was gradually dilating. At 28 weeks, I was 4 centimetres dilated; 5 centimetres at 30 weeks. I left my "bed rest" at 35 weeks, thinking – and hoping – that I would give birth, that I would finally meet Axel. While it's not ideal to give birth five weeks before term, there's usually no risk. But I didn't give birth.

I weighed 125 pounds before my pregnancy, 140 when I took to my bed, and 200 when I got back on my feet. I had imagined my pregnant self as a super-Amazon, and here I was, a beached whale. I hated those glamorous women as thin as toothpicks who put on only 15 pounds, who just developed a nice little baby bump shaped like an olive, a cherry tomato, or bocconcini, and who kept their firm little butts: appetizer-toothpick women. Swollen like a balloon, I couldn't even walk anymore. My feet hurt, and carpal tunnel syndrome severely limited my wrist movements. During my bed rest, my old sports injuries came back to haunt me: a slipped disc, back pain and sciatica, and old toe fractures, although they were healed, returned like horrible demons. My swollen feet no longer fit in any of my shoes. I could wear only cheap flip-flops. But I couldn't stand to stay home any longer, talking to myself. It was summer, and Keith was personally fulfilling almost all my professional obligations. I went back to work, days only and with a reduced patient load. At 36 weeks, big black spots appeared in my right eye. I was diagnosed with a vitreous detachment, "sometimes associated with pregnancy." I had to close that eye to see properly. At any moment, I would start slapping myself on the right cheek to shoo away the imaginary insects or birds that were coming at me, before realizing that they were only floaters moving in my eye. I looked like a woman possessed. As a result of keeping my right eye closed, I started having migraines. What a nasty business pregnancy is! I continued to silently curse the appetizer-toothpick Amazons in the waiting room, where I didn't see many belugas like myself. Yes, I would have other children. But those would be adopted.

Finally, as a reward for good behaviour, my labour was induced at 37 weeks because of high blood pressure and pre-eclampsia, a serious complication of pregnancy. Completely dilated, I pushed very hard for two hours (there were witnesses!), but I still had to have an emergency

C-section, because Axel's heart was becoming weak. On top of that, the epidural wasn't completely effective, which was confirmed by the intense pain.

When I woke up, addled with drugs, I saw Keith, a big smile on his lips, holding a strange baby in his arms. I was outraged. How dare he bring another baby here while I was giving birth to ours? You bastard! Go put that baby back in the nursery where it belongs! Then I fell asleep again, and then woke up again, still convinced that Keith was lovingly holding somebody else's baby in his arms. But that wasn't all! There were two huge seals in my bed, and I shouted for someone to get them out. "Les phoques, les phoques!" I yelled in French. In the fog I was in, I had mistaken my swollen legs for phocids, but all the anglophone nurses heard was "Fuck! Fuck!" They must have thought I was pretty vulgar. They still tease me about that incident.

When I came to my senses, I saw Axel, with the horizontal fold above his nose, his soft skin, and his perfect toes, and I fell madly in love. MY BABY! MY LITTLE BOY! My crease-nose! The words "I'm a mother, I have a son, I'm a mom now" echoed in my head like an incantation. At the same time, I was frightened by the responsibility and the power I had over that little creature that had come out of my body. I also realized that I couldn't move my left arm at all. The large tendon in my rotator cuff, which holds the shoulder stable, had been torn while I was pushing, because I was hanging on to the sides of the bed like crazy, pushing with all my might so I would *not* have to have a C-section. As an added bonus, the pain in my left shoulder was unbearable.

When I got home with Axel, I was a wreck. With only one good arm and sore wrists, I had trouble nursing, and, for the same reasons, I couldn't get relief for my hemorrhoids or even wipe my butt. Sitting on the toilet was very difficult because of my back and my feet, which I couldn't even see anymore because I was obese. Furthermore, seeing was an entirely relative concept because of the imaginary flies that obstructed my right field of vision. Axel was a little bawler who didn't sleep. He was colicky, and the six first months were really difficult. He was an adorable baby with very pale skin and tiny blue veins in his eyelids. He would fall asleep every night to a Norah Jones record; usually it was at the eleventh song ("Nightingale"), after spitting up, and imitating a smoke detector. I was full of love, but absolutely, completely drained.

I was made for parenthood, but not for pregnancy. For our next child we seriously considered adoption, but a lot of things played against us: too many debts, too old, not (yet) married, not sterile, and not in good enough health – because of my history of cancer. So we conceived, after making sure the risk of delivering preterm was acceptable. But what we didn't know was that my first pregnancy was going to be a walk in the park compared to the second one.

The rest of this book is devoted to Violette's story. Keith and I, baby doctors very much in love with each other, had to go through the trauma experienced by the parents we took care of in our practice. It was the unit where we both worked, where Keith was the chief. He was known and respected throughout the world, the chair of the Fetus and Newborn Committee of the Canadian Paediatric Society, and he knew everything there was to know about the science, even before new discoveries were published – an authority. While many "regular" doctors lag behind with respect to scientific breakthroughs, Keith is often at the forefront of them. He knows everything imaginable about the studies; he knows when they were carried out and how many babies were part of them. He calls the researchers conducting them by their nicknames and often knows their favourite foods. As for me, a doctor in neonatology and researcher in clinical ethics, I deal with difficult questions such as when end-of-life decisions should be considered for babies at high risk of death and/or disability. How should we communicate with parents in distress? How can death occur at birth, and how can comfort care improve life when its end is so close to its beginning? And many more questions. In the NICU, I was seen as a sensitive doctor who liked talking with the families. I love talking to the babies, to the parents; I enjoy clinical work; I'm fascinated by the relationships formed in the NICU. I like the human contact.

With my second pregnancy, at 23 weeks, I was dilated and bleeding. At 24 weeks, my membranes broke and my water was breaking. I lay in bed in the delivery room for ten days, from 12 to 22 May 2005. My period of bed rest during my first pregnancy – at home – was like a spa vacation compared to this one. Everything is relative.

Violette was born on 22 May 2005, at 5:21 in the morning, at 24 weeks and 5 days of pregnancy, in "OR 1" at the Royal Victoria Hospital in Montreal, Quebec, Canada. Just writing that sentence makes me cry.

You Made Your Bed …

My contractions started on May 12th in the early afternoon. Since I was supposed to leave the next day for Washington for a conference, I had been examined the day before by my obstetrician. I didn't want to have to deal with the anxiety I had experienced in Alberta before Axel's birth. My cervix was closed tight, as was confirmed by the transvaginal ultrasound, a rather odd thing – a kind of high-tech dildo is used, covered with a real condom. Since my obstetrician is a friend, transvaginal ultrasounds have often been surreal experiences. I knew very well there was nothing sexual about it, but when you unwrap the condom and unroll it over that gizmo, it does give you ideas.

That day everything was going well. In medical terms, there were no white blood cells or traces of protein in my urine. So there was no reason to worry about a possible infection. My blood pressure was good. Of course, I was too fat – I had put on 30 pounds in 23 weeks of pregnancy, which was predictable. I was not yet at the beached whale stage, but it would come. What I didn't know then was that in my second pregnancy, unlike the first one, I wouldn't have time to develop that bountiful silhouette. I would barely have a chance to reach the proportions of an elephant seal.

Because my son Axel had almost been born prematurely, this new pregnancy was making me wary and irritable. Starting at 18 weeks, I no longer took on new patients. I just did little desk jobs, and I never spent more than 40 minutes per day on my feet. I was fearful of sexual relations and light exercise, and I avoided any activity that was energetic or intense – two adjectives that are intimately linked to who I am. For the least little decision I made, I methodically listed the pros and cons, and I took an infinite number of precautions. "What should I drink today? Green mint tea, or rooibos-pomegranate? Let me see." I was moving in slow motion, like a big, oily, lethargic bubble floating in the air. I wondered if going to that conference was a good idea, but I was scheduled for two podium presentations. My obstetrician, Lucie, encouraged me to go, and so did Keith. It would be a little holiday for me, they thought. Big mistake! With what awaited me, I would have ended up on forced bed rest in Washington, spending thousands of dollars for a room with a marble floor, far from my family, from my little prince, from Lucie, from my hospital, my neonatal unit, and my nurses.

The cramps started during lunch. I thought: "This can't be. Not again! Not this time!" This was my second experience, though, and I should have known very well what was happening. But Lucie had examined me just the day before and everything had been fine! I had to pack my suitcase to leave the next day. Maybe it was stage fright; doing two presentations was a big challenge for a shapeless blob like me. Besides, the cramps were spaced out and were coming every 20 to 30 minutes, then stopped. I finally told myself they must be false labour, which occurs in normal pregnancies. I went home after picking Axel up at day care. After we got to the house, I took him to the little park a short walk away. That evening, Keith and I played Rummikub and the cramps stopped. It was our favourite game during that period. I won almost all the time, as with most of the board games I play with Keith.

My whole family is crazy about games. When my father was deteriorating because of his brain cancer, we played Settlers of Catan with him almost every night for a year. We even had two complete sets to keep the groups of players separate; we held semi-finals and then a championship. In the beginning, my father played like everyone else. After a while, he could no longer move his pieces, and he would tell us where to place them; then we had to interpret his instructions, because he was having more and more trouble expressing himself. In the end, he couldn't even sit up at the table or communicate verbally. But it was sacred; he had to be in the game and someone had to move his piece. So we strapped him to his chair back with belts, and that way he was with us. Sometimes he fell asleep, and sometimes he would win. The game was soothing for him.

That evening, I really would have liked a game of Rummikub with Keith to help me relax and chase away my dark thoughts. But my apprehensions broke my concentration, and I lost two matches out of four. It was a first in the history of our family. I packed my suitcase absent mindedly.

At two o'clock in the morning, the contractions started every five minutes. I was bleeding. Once again, the unthinkable was happening. I took a taxi to the hospital alone, carrying the suitcase I had packed for the conference I wouldn't be going to. Keith stayed with Axel.

Because of the incompetent cervix that had given me such a hard time with Axel, now Violette was also going to be born before term. My body had let me down, and I was letting my baby down. "Incompetent cervix" – I love it. Imagine how you feel when you hear "You mustn't feel guilty for giving birth prematurely – it's your incompetent cervix." No one will ever tell fathers that their child has Down syndrome because of their "incompetent sperm," or that they have problems in bed because of an "incompetent penis."

Once again, I found myself in preterm labour, on forced bed rest, because of my useless womb. Anatomically incompetent! "Bed rest." The first person who issued that injunction was probably a sarcastic male who was either heartless or drunk. All the same, it's the expression doctors use to tell mothers to lie on their backs indefinitely, immobile, as if imitating a recumbent statue could bring them divine grace. Studies have never really demonstrated the value of bed rest. But when you're bleeding, when you're having contractions, when your cervix is dilated to 4 centimetres and the membranes are coming out, if the doctor tells you to stay still, you obey. Lying down a few hours a day for a nap is a lovely luxury, but spending entire days looking at the ceiling, your body tense with stress and fear, is no fun at all.

I went into the delivery room at 23 weeks and 3 days, dilated to 4 centimetres, with membranes bulging, experiencing regular contractions. A catastrophe. Birth could occur at any moment. In 2005, in our unit, only between 25 and 50 per cent of premature babies born at that stage of pregnancy survived, with significant risks. In my hospital, I myself had written the information sheet that's given to mothers at risk of giving birth before 28 weeks. I knew what was going on very well. Reality was racing ahead. I felt as if I were in an Almodóvar film – woman *really* on the verge of a nervous breakdown. "We need to put you in the Trendelenburg position, inject you with betamethasone, give you an indomethacin suppository and intravenous antibiotics," and so on.

The Trendelenburg position is nice medical jargon for lying on an inclined bed with the legs higher than the head. In this position, it isn't easy to drink or pee – because of the force of gravity (9.8 m/sec^2) – and fluids go toward your head. I categorically refused a urinary catheter, a plastic tube inserted into the bladder that allows urine to drain without the patient having to sit up. No way they were going to stick that thing in my urethra. I'd already refused a catheter for my first operation, years earlier, when my thyroid was removed; I'd also refused it for my second operation, when there had been a possibility of a recurrence of the cancer. My opposition to the catheter was so strong that I expected them to send in a psychiatrist specializing in catheter-phobia.

But during my bed rest, refusing a catheter became my mission. If I wasn't going to have control over my birthing or over my sleep (with all the alarms constantly beeping on the speakers in the delivery room), I hoped at least to be able to decide for myself when and how I would pee. In any case, I had nothing else to do but refuse the catheter and act accordingly. I was stoical, all the more so because this wouldn't create medical problems for Violette. But the doctors enjoyed undermining my courageous resolve by constantly injecting fluids into my veins, either medications to slow down the contractions or antibiotics. Which made me a frequent pisser. I would call the nurses – who were also my friends and colleagues – to help me pee in the bedpan. I had become so fat, it was like hoisting a cetacean into a swimming pool – a job for a longshoreman. They'd have to lift the beast up on one side, then on the other, to get it onto the bedpan. Urinating in the Trendelenburg position is a sport at which I was not very talented. But at the very least, I now understood how patients feel when they have to endure this ordeal. Before that, I had found their obsession with pee and poop very childish, considering all the risks for their unborn child. My friend Annabelle won the bed-rest Olympics – she stayed in bed from the 15th to the 28th week of her pregnancy, when her son Paul was born. I remember that she too was obsessed with her excretions. I had always believed it was basically a psychosis brought about by forced bed rest, which actually can drive you crazy. Convinced that I was the strongest and that I would be able to control my sphincters, when my turn came, I felt shame. I was the worst of them all. For many days, I, Annie Janvier, had to do my business in front of everyone in a bedpan – and it was all I could do to get anything to come out. And to completely destroy my self-esteem, my colleagues were the ones taking away my shit.

The first time, Keith wasn't with me. Not certain where things stood, not knowing if I was going to give birth that day or the next day, he had left to drive Axel to my mother's house so she could look after him. So I had to manage without him. With my head down, I tried to arch my pelvis so it would be perpendicular to the bed. As with Ikea furniture, the overall design was good but the materials were not very solid. I collapsed, and that was it. What a relief, though! But a warm sensation began to spread along my back, my neck, into my hair and behind my ears. After I was completely drenched, the urine trickled onto the floor. Now I was soaked in urine, and I couldn't even take a shower, because the least movement set off my contractions and increased the bleeding. Fortunately, the bed was made of plastic, so it could be cleaned. But changing the sheets wasn't easy for the nurse with this huge mammal in the way. And wouldn't you know it, the adventure caused contractions and I started bleeding even more. I was given a fresh blue hospital gown stamped "Property of the RV hospital." Yes, I really was their thing! A half hour later, I needed to go again. I was waiting for Keith, who didn't come. I called him, on his pager, on his phone.

"Keith, please, please, come quick!"

"But I'm at your mother's house, I'm giving her an update. What's the matter? Is this it, are you about to deliver?"

"No, but I have to pee!"

"So, then, pee."

"You ignorant fool, you know very well that I use a bedpan! I need help, don't you get it? I don't want a catheter! You have to come NOW!"

"But my love, everything will be fine, that's the nurse's job – she sees that all day long, pregnant women on bedpans."

"Ohhhhhh! You're not nice. You don't understand. YOU'VE never had to piss in a bedpan. Look, men piss in a turquoise tube, that's easy! What's more, THEY don't get pregnant and they don't have periods. So come RIGHT AWAY!"

Three times I tried to pee with Keith's help, who backed me up conscientiously in all the schemes I came up with to avoid a catheter. I tried towels, the tube for men, adult diapers. Four times in ten hours, they had to change my sheets, with the contractions, the bleeding, and the tears all that caused.

I finally asked for a catheter. It was less painful than I had imagined. Women who are more docile than I am don't make a huge scene over a catheter. But if there are any craftier women who've found a way to pee in the Trendelenburg position without getting it all in their hair, please tell me how – it's really in the public interest.

And the constipation, that was something else altogether. It took me four days to decide to go on the bedpan. I just couldn't do it. When I pushed, I felt the membranes swelling, and it made me bleed. I was afraid to push. There was a super-nice, understanding nurse who came to my rescue. Keith assisted her. Obstetrics nurses, I love you! I have no problem with mustard-coloured poop, old Bud pee, or a baby's yogurt vomit. But YOU, you work with fat adults! You take care of us, without judging us, without being disgusted. With you, it's not at all humiliating to have a finger stuck up your behind to unblock your bowels. Dear nurses, you have no idea of the extent of my gratitude. As for you, my dear Keith, with everything you've seen, it's for better or for worse, till death do us part.

12 May

Violette's gestational age *in utero*: 23 weeks, 2 days

Dear Computer,

You're going to think I'm weird, but I don't know who else to talk to. I've been in the hospital only twelve hours and I haven't stopped talking to myself out loud. I also talk to Violette: I say nice things to her, to encourage her, or to encourage myself, I don't know anymore. I hum songs in my head to calm myself. Right now, I'm singing "Morgane de toi," by Renaud, a song about his daughter Lola. I think that song has come back to me because in it he is asking his daughter not to fly away. Maybe there's a message there. And maybe I just love the song. Bed rest is one hell of a forced psychoanalytic session.

The first time, with Axel, I don't remember feeling so anxious about the birth. It was a joke compared to now. That time, not everything went wrong. Right now, things are going badly. I'm extremely sensitive to everything happening around me, the least movement as well as the encouraging messages from everyone, even though I know that from a medical point of view, it doesn't mean much. I'm trying to remain optimistic with Keith and with everyone who comes to visit. My head is spinning, I have a lump in my throat, I'm lying still trying to prevent contractions, trying not to move. I'm counting my breaths. Time stands still. The day is punctuated by checks of my vital signs, administration of antibiotics, injections of betamethasone, emptying of the catheter bag, and so on.

I thought if I shared what I was feeling with you, it might help pass the time. I'd be able to spew out my rage and transfer my panic, despair, and powerlessness onto your hard disk. To put into a black box, the laptop, words that might take the pain with them and all this muck that's poisoning my soul. Then I'd be able to put the black box full of my anxieties on my bedside table. I'd look at the box from time to time and I'd know my demons were in it, but at least for a moment, they would be outside of me. This is what you learn when you do meditation: focus on your thoughts, then let them go. I'm not very good at that; sometimes it works, but usually I get nervous. I've often tried group meditation under supervision by an expert; I think about food, a book, a sick baby, the neck of the guy in front of me, the tattoo on a pretty woman, everything and nothing, and then I curse myself when the expert encourages us to acknowledge our thoughts and let them go. "Dammit, meditation stresses me!" Writing to you, my dear PC, will be my meditation. Maybe that will take away the lump in my throat, the weight on my belly, the elastic I have around my heart.

I'm lying on my back with my head down, an intravenous tube stuck in my left hand, which keeps me from moving to the right. I can't move anyway because of the urinary catheter, because it makes my bladder hurt. I need to seriously think about how I will turn on my right side. You, Computer, sitting on pillows on my right, you're showing your silly movie that I can see sideways, but now I have to turn my head the other way because my neck is starting to hurt. Turning should occupy part of my day.

Now I have a burning desire to write. I've called for help to move you to the other side. It took me an hour to convince myself that I was entitled to call a nurse for that. As a doctor, when I call a nurse, it's for something important. What kind of patient has the nerve to disturb a nurse just to move her computer? I'm in a delivery room where there are much more important problems to deal with, even if it's emptying bedpans. But since I absolutely have to unload my toxic thoughts, I manage to persuade myself that my need is of a medical nature, and that, in my capacity as patient, I have a perfect right to ask for that service. Today, it's Sandy* who's taking

---

* Names followed by an asterisk throughout the text have been changed to preserve anonymity.

care of me. She's relatively new. She's a very devoted, hard-working young woman, one of the rare nurses who don't call me Annie, but "Dr Janvier," which always embarrasses me. I have to say, Sandy is also really hot, a ten on the universal beauty scale. When she runs down the corridor to help with an emergency C-section, her muscular little behind curves exactly where it should. All the residents dream of her, with her perfect body, her freckles, her gorgeous smile, and her smooth skin. They're crazy about her. They start every shift by checking if she's working. Women who, like me, are under observation because of the risk of premature birth some-times see the residents arrive in their rooms either too early or too late, depending on Sandy's schedule. With a little ocular determination, you can make out her colourful sexy underwear through her powder blue scrubs. When she bends over me to check my intravenous, it's hard not to appreciate the perfect elegance of her bra. It's very good that Sandy works here among the beached whales, the women giving birth, and the delirious new dads. It would be dangerous if she were assigned to inten-sive care, where the cardiac patients don't need such distractions. I smile thinking what the residents would give to be nursed by Sandy.

So Sandy arrives with her angel's smile, saying, "No problem, Dr Jan-vier, call me whenever you want, that's what I'm here for." Nurses, how I love you! She asks if I want to watch another movie or if I'd prefer to read. I reply that I want to write on my laptop. She frowns.

> "Dr Janvier, you think about work too much. You should relax and let us take care of you."

> "But raising the table, putting the computer on it and plugging it in IS taking care of me! I can't do that myself. Look, all I can do is watch movies, think, talk, and maybe type on my keyboard. And what's more, I'm not 'Dr Janvier.' Please, call me Annie, Madame or Ms, but not Doctor. Do I look like a doctor now?"

> "It's true, you're here as a patient and not as a doctor. But I can't call you Annie. Ms Annie? Dr Annie? That sounds weird. And are you sure you want to work? Is that really wise?"

Even while she's reminding me that I should think only of relaxing, Sandy places my things just the way I wanted, and even helps me find the best possible posture for writing in the Trendelenburg position.

Sandy is adorable. But all this stuff about relaxation is making me agitated. Relax, Annie! Take it easy! As a matter of fact, I was going to do a series of sit-ups and jog around the delivery room to get ready to run the New York City Marathon, but, now that you've reminded me, I'm going to lie with my head down, stick an intravenous line in my arm and let my urine run into a bag on the side of my bed instead. People may think I'm here to replenish my energy, to regain my strength, as if I'd just had an operation. But it's obvious that nothing has happened! I have lots of energy; it's my thoughts that are making me sick. I'm not convalescing! The intervention will come, but that will be for my baby. I'm going to give birth, but I don't know when. I'm not a TB patient that you send to a seaside resort so they can feel the ocean breeze in their lungs. Maybe I should tell them that.

Hey, Computer! I've been typing for two hours now. I have to go slowly; there's no way I can cut and paste in my position. I type with one finger, one letter at a time, on my side. For two hours, I've been thinking of the movie *The Sea Inside*, by Alejandro Amenábar, which I saw not long ago and which is based on a true story. In it, Javier Bardem plays a quadriplegic who can't move anything but his head. He spends his days looking out the window of his room. He wants someone to help him die. His only moments of joy are when he's able to leave his body and escape through his window to fly in spirit over the sea that took his health thirty years earlier. I remember the scenes when he's flying above the forests and the sea. I would like to escape like that. On the wall in front of my bed, there's a reproduction of an unsigned painting, cheap hospital art. A flowering tree. A bubble gum pink tree against a lilac sky. I've spent so much time contemplating this image since I've been in this room that I lose myself in it. I count the flowers, the little white spots, and there are so many of them that I get a different number every time. I fly to the pink tree, examine it, and imagine the fragrance it must give off in the spring. I try to fly like the character in *The Sea Inside*, but my mind goes only as far as the washrooms. I close my eyes and imagine myself lying on the other side of the bed. I rearrange the whole room. The window is now on the right, with the pink tree behind me. But soon I hear "Narcotic keys, please!" "Keys to the desk!" and "Charge nurse desk" in the corridor and the loudspeakers, tearing me away from my escape into daydreaming.

I also think about Jean-Dominique Bauby, who wrote *The Diving Bell and the Butterfly.* He was also a quadriplegic suffering from locked-in syndrome. A prisoner of his own body, he could move only his eyelids. That was his only means of communication. He spoke with his eyelids, spelling each letter with a special code. Blinking his eyes, he told his story to a woman who wrote it one letter at a time and typed it word for word. That resulted in a great book, which they finished three days before his death.

I know I'm not really paralysed; perhaps it gives me courage to think about those exceptional individuals who were forced to stay in bed for life. I wonder if they were also told to relax and take it easy. Typing one letter at a time is nothing compared to what Bauby had to endure. But I'm not writing a book; that's a big difference. I'm just getting my toxins out onto the screen. No pressure.

Dumping of words interrupted – the doctor has just arrived.

No Bed of Roses

To all mothers forced to stay in bed,

It is completely normal to go crazy in the situation you're in. It's perfectly normal to feel guilty and wonder what you could have done to avoid this. BUT THERE'S NOTHING YOU COULD HAVE DONE! When something happens to our child, we look for the guilty party, and, more often than not, we blame ourselves. "I should have done this" and "If only I had done that." But no one is to blame in such a situation. It's just that life is sometimes cruel.

To future fathers, loved ones, and other family members: remind your partner who is languishing in bed on forced "rest" that she's amazing, that it's not her fault, and that her ordeal is not a punishment. Women who find themselves in this situation are very vulnerable. Their pregnancy dream has turned into a nightmare. They are doing their best to adapt, to review their goals, to adjust their hopes, to accept the prospect of a life completely different from the one they had dreamed of, to rewrite chapters of the book of their life. All scenarios are possible, those that lead to despair, anger, and fear, and those that bring relief. So never tell a woman who is at risk of giving birth prematurely – or, worse, the mother of a premature child – that it would have been better if she hadn't gone to work, hadn't taken part in sports, hadn't made love, hadn't eaten certain foods, hadn't said such-and-such, or hadn't listened to a particular kind of music.

Mothers, it's perfectly normal to occasionally have selfish or negative thoughts that you can't share with anyone. I remember that I didn't want to stay on my back in the hospital, choking on every mouthful of food, pissing in my hair, and getting "deconstipated," all for a dead baby or, worse, I thought at the time, for a disabled baby; but I had to go through those trials so as not to feel guilty, or to feel as little guilt as possible at any rate. I missed my son viscerally and I wondered what was going on in his child's head since his mom had left him to go to the hospital. I also wondered what neonatologist would be there for the delivery, since out of the five on the unit, two – Keith and I – couldn't do anything medically for Violette, and two were at a conference in Washington. I imagined myself personally intubating my own baby, inserting a tube in her trachea to help her breathe, if there was an emergency and no one else could do it. I would have to act quickly. Would I have the strength, the composure, the presence of mind? You have many, many hours to think all kinds of weird, crazy, incredible, happy, or guilt-inducing thoughts when you're on forced bed "rest" in a hospital.

Years after Violette's birth, I met a woman during a prenatal consultation. She was going to give birth very prematurely. She was in the same room where I had been hospitalized. I again saw the flowering tree, that framed reproduction speckled with pink, and all my memories came flooding back like a punch in the stomach. I told that woman that, no, it wasn't her hair dye that had caused her contractions. We talked about her two other children, their problems in school, their homework, the whole "Christmas tree" of catheter, intravenous pumps, drug bags, the poop that gets stuck, and the impossibility of counting the flowers in the pink tree. I had already tried, ad nauseam. To know for sure, you'd have to get up, walk over to the image, and mark them one by one. But, madame, do you think the dark pink spots flowers or leaves?

13 May

Computer,

Can you believe it? I've just been handed the sheet I wrote myself to inform parents about the statistics related to their baby's condition. In fact, you have several versions of that document on your hard drive. There's nothing in it about happiness, or the family, or the couple, or adjusting, or the capacity to deal with the uncertainty, or the stress, nor the guilt, or well-being and quality of life.

How will I manage to be a mom in the unit?

I have to go, somebody is here to see me.

Computer,

Something weird just happened. I met the neonatologist, the baby doctor.

I met the doctor I usually am. So she came to do the job I usually do: inform me of the possible outcomes for Violette and ask what we wanted to do if she came out now. Hold her in my arms and love her while she dies, or help her breathe and take her to the neonatal intensive care unit, the NICU. Of course, this neonatologist is my friend and my colleague, the best. The one you want to meet in my situation. The thing is, I am here to stay pregnant, not to deliver. My baby is NOT sick right now. We will see what will happen. Of course, I know things may not stay this way for long, and that the doctors need to know what they should do if Violette comes out. But is this necessary before we become 100 per cent certain she will come out early?

I don't think I want intensive care for her if she is going to die. She has some chance at life, but statistically she is more likely to die than to live … for another five days, then, if she stays in that long, her chances will change. And also after the steroids have had time to act. But I know this kind of thinking is crazy because we cannot be sure of exactly how old Violette is inside me, and every day, at this stage, makes a difference. I know Keith feels different; he is more optimistic than I am. She may not die. But if she dies, we will feel better if she had her chances and we tried. But we may feel worse if she went through intensive care before she died – a death in your parents' arms is better than a death in the intensive care unit. But it would be in my arms even in the NICU. If she does not die, there are still serious risks. But my body seems to always want to expel my babies at 23 weeks, so I may hold Violette in my arms while she dies and, a year later, decide to have my next 23-week baby admitted to the NICU. Fuck.

I just realized for real, now, today, that the way neonatologists talk to pregnant women is bizarre. I knew it was weird, but not this weird. I never spoke about all these possible regrets, feelings of guilt, the possibility of another preterm delivery, to pregnant women before, and yet these are the only things I am thinking about …

I am also a field experiment in my own specialty. Here I am a baby doctor. Not only a baby doctor, but one that is also a PhD student in bioethics, a field where we examine the complexities of medical decisions. And my area of study is how doctors and parents make decisions for fragile babies, which biases and values are involved. My laptop is full of PowerPoint presentations about this stuff. In fact, I am supposed to be presenting about this specific topic at the moment in Washington, at the Society for Pediatric Research. Christ, at least I am here on bed rest, not far away in Washington on bed rest.

So here I am at 23 weeks and 3 days, dilated at 4 centimetres with bulging membranes. I contract every fifteen to twenty minutes. This is bad news. Women like me usually have their babies in a matter of hours, days, but rarely weeks. The membranes that surround Violette are now in the vagina, not where they belong, and are more prone to breaking, more vulnerable to bacteria, and this is what will happen at some point. When they break, the fluid comes out, and the baby generally not long after. So I know it is just a matter of time, and statistically not weeks, before Violette comes out. Usually babies come out at 40 weeks. When they come out before 37 weeks, they are preterm. Before 28 weeks, it is called extreme prematurity. And the worst is between 22 and 25 weeks. Coming out at 23 weeks, like Violette would right now, is not a party. Right now, in 2005, preterms of that gestation have an average of survival of about 30–50 per cent, more after the steroids. If they survive, half of the children are "normal" and 25 per cent have a disability. I am the one who wrote the information sheet we give to parents at risk of delivering before 28 weeks in our hospital; I know it by heart. Jeez, I really wish I were discussing the ethics of all this in Washington after all … It now seems strangely obvious that the way I have been talking with parents over the last few years is SO incomplete, so simple, so naive. I thought informing parents about the possible outcomes for their baby was helpful. The more information, the better. That knowing the bad things that could happen would help parents. That we are mostly scared about what we do not know. That knowledge increases control and decreases anxiety. All this may be true, but it is a fragment of what helps. Keith and I know every number and possible outcome. We have a complete and detailed idea of the possible disaster tree and a good understanding of what parents face. But numbers, I realize now, do not help us. They do not erase the uncertainty about what will really happen to our baby. First, we do not know when she will be born, and then we do not know whether she will survive. Well … we do know that if we do not give her a chance, she will not. So this is certain. And if she goes to the NICU anytime within the next few days, it is more likely that she will die than live. But then, every day, the stats change. But the uncertainty continues. That is, if we decide that she goes to the NICU. So our decision is different from the decisions cancer patients make when they have to decide whether or not they want a specific type of chemotherapy. The uncertainty is similar, but they DO have cancer right now and the stats do not change every day. For Violette, every day she stays inside increases the chance she will live.

I feel like I'm drawing lottery tickets from black bags, and I do not know which one I will draw. The first bag I have to draw from is one that has only two kinds of tickets: "deliver today" and "deliver later." Today, I think I must have picked the second kind of ticket. And long as I can, I hope to keep picking this one. The second bag happens at birth: it is full of both "die" tickets and "survive" tickets. And the proportion of die and survive tickets depends upon when I will in fact squirt Violette out. A third bag is full of "normal" and "disabled" tickets, and the proportions too depend how long Violette can stay inside and what happens after she is born.

Now the bag I really want to have is one I never knew existed, full of both "you will be OK in the end" and "you will not be OK in the end" tickets. I guess you = me + my husband + my family + Violette = all of us. THIS IS WHAT I REALLY WANT TO TALK ABOUT. Not about the risks of cerebral palsy, the risk of retinopathy, the risk of PDA, the risk of hyperactivity, the risk of schooling problems, ad nauseam risks. If she is disabled, will we be OK? Will we be OK going through all this? Will we be OK, and can you tell me if we will be happy? I don't mean happy with Violette in the NICU. I know this will be really hard for her and for us, and for Axel. I mean *after*. After her death or after – during – her life as a "normal" child or as a "disabled" child? Can we be a family with a dead child, ashes in a box, or a family with an ex-preterm normal child, or a family with an ex-preterm disabled child? Do families recover? Do they adapt? How long does it take? What helps in these circumstances? Education, a loving couple to parent her, money? We have all that. But maybe it is not enough … I also have a strong extended family, resilience, love, a sense of humour. Are these better, superior to cash? Having gone through my dad's death at 23 and my cancer at 28, am I more prepared? Will I be a better mother of a dead not disabled baby? What do the scientific studies about preterm infants and their families say about that? Are families OK? Who isn't? Why? How can we predict happiness? Not disability, because I know it is not always related to happiness in families.

WHY CAN'T ANYBODY ANSWER THESE QUESTIONS?

It's all so hard to believe. I have in my hand the information sheet I give to parents to inform them of the statistics of what may happen to their baby. What do I do with this information?

The handout is empty: full of doctor numbers.

15 May, Night

Violette's gestational age: between 23 weeks and 24 weeks, 3 days

Computer,

It's dark and I'm scared. I'm alone and I'm thinking of my Keith asleep at home; my Axel in his room with the animals on the walls; my stepson, James, who must also be in bed; and Violette, in the warmth of her amniotic fluid. My scattered family. I can't believe all this is happening to us! Surely I'm going to wake up and find out that it was a bad joke or a nightmare. Why us? My stupid cervix is letting me down again. It's not like with Axel. This time, it's being a real loser.

People keep telling me that, with Axel, things didn't turn out too badly in the end, just a little scare, and that the same thing is happening again now. That I already cried wolf once. I know very well that's not true. With Axel, I didn't bleed, I wasn't dilated as much, and I didn't have my membranes coming out of my ears. Should I scream at them that the worst is yet to come? Am I tempting fate by being so pessimistic? I told them I didn't want a C-section. But Violette's head could get stuck, because she's coming bum first. And since I had one for Axel, I'd feel guilty not giving both my children the same thing. And if Violette were to be born tonight, forty-eight hours after receiving steroids to protect her lungs, what should I do? Maybe a C-section isn't a bad idea. I'd regret it my whole life if her head got stuck and she suffocated, smothered inside me. Keith wants her to go to intensive care and I'm not sure if I want to say yes or no. I can't fight with him for the death of my baby – that scares me too much; it's not possible.

And I don't really want to decide. What if I say yes, take her to the NICU? I don't know if I'm capable of it. What would it do to Axel, to my relationship with Keith, to our careers, to our lives, to all my dreams? What would remain of the life I imagined for us, with four perfect children born full-term like in a Hollywood movie with a happy ending? Everyone happy and in good health, marvellous, talented children, above average, like in Lake Wobegon,[†] where all the women are strong, all the men are good looking, and all the children are above average. I don't want my life to unfold like a French film, where the hero wins gold just before dying by falling down a staircase, and it's his demented grandmother stuck in a hospice who inherits the medal, or maybe it's somebody else, and then the credits start rolling and it's the end. They call that an open-ended story. I want a closed end, a beautiful ending, a beautiful beginning for Violette. But it's impossible for me not to imagine all kinds of catastrophic scenarios. Violette could die without going to intensive care. She could die in intensive care, despite the state-of-the-art medical interventions. In that case, at least, we won't have lost her without giving her a chance. We could live with ourselves without regrets. Or she could survive and be "normal," or survive with a disability. In either of these scenarios, we could come out of it all right, maybe after a year or two. We could also be broken by it, completely destroyed. I was broken by the death of my father, then by my cancer, then by a divorce, but I finally got back on my feet again. I'd like to be able to buy some time and not have to choose. Why are we forced to choose? I think I'll let Keith decide.

I'm still having contractions every 5 to 20 minutes. I can't sleep with this unbearable voice echoing again and again on the floor: "Narcotic keys, please," "Keys, keys, please." I feel Violette move. Maybe she knows I'm mulling over these things. I may be crazy, but she's constantly moving. I'm trying to understand what she wants. It's stupid, I know – she

---

† Lake Wobegon is a fictional town created by American author and radio personality Garrison Keillor and is the setting of his radio program, *A Prairie Home Companion.* The term "the Lake Wobegon effect" is used to express the idea that people need to believe that they are above average.

doesn't want anything, she's just there – but I try anyway. She can't be there without wanting anything.

The power of "the Eye of the Heart," which produces insight, is vastly superior to the power of thought, which produces opinions.

E.F. Schumacher

*T*he following article was written several years after I recorded my thoughts and experiences in the Toxic Shit file. Since then, neonatology has changed, but not enough. The goal of this article is to insist that life-and-death decisions are complicated and should not be reduced to one item, such as an imprecise gestational age. These decisions should be individualized and taken carefully for each patient and family.

The authors of this article all have interesting stories that probably reinforce their opinions about the complexity of life-and-death issues. The first author, Amélie Du Pont-Thibodeau, was my PhD student at the time, and she obtained her PhD with great distinction and was on the dean's honour list. She is a wonderful neonatologist and a colleague I really appreciate working with. Her mother was left to die at birth because she had a severe congenital abnormality (spina bifida). At that time in medicine, "experts" thought that a life with spina bifida was not a life worth living. Her parents took her home and cared for her, despite medical adversity. Amélie's mother wrote a great article about her life, "On the Day I Was Born ... A Testimony Saluting Her Parents' Courage and Determination," which was published in Current Problems in Pediatric and Adolescent Health Care in April 2011. She eventually became a lawyer and a mother. Amélie has a strong mind and will (like her mom). The second author is Keith, my husband. You will learn so many things about him in this book that he does not need more describing, apart the fact that he is amazing – most of the time! The third author is Barbara, an exceptional woman I met during a conference at which I presented in Seattle in 2008. In 2005, Barbara had a daughter with trisomy 13. Children with trisomy 13 typically have a short life and are disabled when they survive. Annie, the little girl, was left to die after a respiratory deterioration at several months of life. Her parents were not offered interventions to prolong her life and did not take part in the decision-making process. Barbara still does not know what she died of. Trisomy 13 and 18 are conditions that were called "incompatible with life," ones where physicians thought babies were "better off dead." With Barbara as a collaborator, we investigated the perspectives of parents who lived with these children. Parents often did not agree with clinicians: they considered the life of their children had value and enriched their life, irrespective of its length. The attitudes toward children with trisomy 13 and 18 have also changed. We now should call these conditions "life-limiting conditions," as opposed to lethal conditions that are incompatible with life.

Today, in 2019, while some policy statements of national organizations, such as the American Academy of Pediatrics, do not base life-and-death decisions on one (uncertain) factor, many unfortunately still do.

End-of-Life Decisions for Extremely Low-Gestational-Age Infants: Why Simple Rules for Complicated Decisions Should Be Avoided

Amélie Du Pont-Thibodeau, MD, PhD (Cand.), Keith J. Barrington, MBChB, Barbara Farlow, BEng, MBA, and Annie Janvier, MD, PhD†

1. INTRODUCTION

Baby Sam's Story: Mike and Julianne Caron were overjoyed to be expecting their first baby. They did not want to know if they were expecting a boy or a girl and named their baby Sam, for Samuel or Samantha. Last night, long before Sam's due date, Julianne began bleeding. She and Mike rushed to the hospital. They learned that Julianne was in labor, and the doctors told her that any interventions to save Sam would be "futile," because of the degree of prematurity. Sam would be given palliative care with the view of making Sam's short life comfortable. The doctors said that had Julianne gone into labor a week or two later, perhaps attempts could have been made to save Sam's life, but even then, the efforts would be "experimental" at best. Despite the empathy and care provided by the healthcare providers, Mike requested that his wife be transferred to a larger academic center nearby.

At the academic center, the parents were told that given Sam's prematurity, palliative care would be a very acceptable option. With interventions, doctors gave Sam a 30% chance of survival. If he/she survived, the first years would be difficult and Sam would have significant risk of long-term disability. The Carons hoped for the best but expected the worst.

Survival has improved dramatically for extremely low-gestational-age neonates (ELGANs) over the last 50 years. In most tertiary care centers, providing care to ELGANs has become commonplace. The proportion of ELGANs surviving with long-term disabilities has decreased, but since more ELGANs survive, so too have the number of children in the community living with disabilities.[1]

Decision-making for critically ill incompetent patients who are at high risk of sequelae raises three major ethical issues: whether to start life-sustaining interventions for a patient, whether life-sustaining interventions should be withdrawn when there are adverse outcomes, and who should be responsible for the decisions. Legally, physicians need a patient's consent in order to care for them. Babies, being naturally incompetent, are generally in the care of their parents who take decisions for them, a process known as "substitute consent."

Situations such as the one in which Sam's family find themselves bring to the forefront questions of futility, the best interest of the child, and quality of life. Values and experience, religious beliefs, and overall outlook on life are embedded in the decision-making process. Physicians and ethicists have written many guidelines on how to take decisions for babies like Sam. These guidelines have almost always been tailored around completed weeks of gestational age.[2] These guidelines are easy to use and avoid case-by-case in-depth analysis of ethical decision-making; however, they are patently flawed.

ELGANs have frequently been classified into three broad categories: the first consists of patients for whom interventions are determined to be beneficial; the second, for those whom interventions are futile; and the third for those who are in between. The third group is often referred to as the "Gray Zone." Traditionally, patients in the first category receive life-sustaining interventions, patients in the second category receive comfort care, and for those in the gray zone, the parents are asked to make a decision following counseling from healthcare providers. Guidelines that establish the boundaries of the zones vary, depending on where the baby is born. The determination of the borders of the gray zone is also subjective. Many guidelines identify infants born at 22 weeks of gestational age as "futile," 23 and 24 weeks as "gray zone" (or experimental), and 25 weeks as "beneficial."[3] Other guidelines deem neonates born before 25 weeks as futile.[4]

... [G]estational age estimation is imprecise.[5] Given these uncertainties, it is illogical to base life-and-death decisions only on gestational age guidelines within rigid boundaries. If one were to adhere to the recommendations, a baby born just before midnight might be denied life-sustaining interventions, but one born just after midnight would receive intensive care. Survival and long-term outcomes of ELGANs also depend on many other factors besides gestational age[6] (Table 1).

Long-term impairment (particularly neurologic or cognitive) is the concern for many healthcare providers and families of infants born extremely preterm. It must be emphasized that at all gestations, even the earliest, more than half of survivors have no impairments when examined after 2.5 years of age when evaluations are fairly predictive of the long term.[7] Also, among the surviving ElGANs born before 26 weeks, the rate of impairment is not strongly associated with gestational age.[8] As infants got older, minor trends reported in some cohorts often disappear.[9] Many policy statements concerning care of extremely preterm infants use a low Bailey score at 18 months as a definition of cognitive impairment. However, the Bailey score is a screening tool designed to evaluate developmental delay, *not* cognitive impairment. About two-thirds or more of former preterm infants with a Bailey score below 70 at 18 months (in some cohorts more than 80 per cent) do not have cognitive impairments when evaluated at 5–8 years of age.[10] However, many important factors that affect the risk of long-term impairment are usually disregarded in guidelines concerning care of extremely preterm infants[11] (Table 2).

Table 1. Factors influencing survival in ELGANs

What influences survival in ELGANs:
- Official pronouncements of professional societies
- Willingness of Obstetrician to actively intervene
- Birth in tertiary center
- Tertiary center with >100 admissions of ELGANs/year
- Gestational age
- Weight for gestational age
- Singleton (vs multiple birth)
- Female gender
- Exposure to prenatal steroids
- Chorioamnionitis

Table 2. Factors influencing long-term outcomes in surviving ELGANs

What positively influences long-term outcomes in surviving ELGANs:
- Female sex
- Not being SGA
- Socioeconomic factors
  - Higher family income
  - Education of mother
  - Two-parent family
- Absence of perinatal complications: chorioamnionitis, large intracerebral hemorrhage (especially bilateral), extensive cystic periventricular leukomalacia, posthemorrhagic ventricular dilatation, any surgery, postnatal steroids, sepsis/infection, necrotizing enterocolitis, bronchopulmonary dysplasia, and inadequate nutrition
- Breastmilk

---

2. THE DEFINITION OF FUTILITY

If the justification for not offering life-sustaining interventions before 23 weeks gestational age is futility, then definitions of futility must be considered. Futility can be quantitative or qualitative.

Quantitative futility implies that an intervention "does not work."[12] Some suggest that the intervention may have more than a 0 per cent success rate, but "success is … so unlikely that its exact probability is often incalculable."[13] Survival after delivery at 22 weeks of gestational age with intensive care is between 5 per cent and 32 per cent in recent publications.[14] These survival rates do not satisfy the definition of quantitative futility.

Qualitative futility generally means that the intervention is considered to be "not worth it." This subjective consideration of whether the intervention reaches desirable goals may be evaluated by healthcare providers or patients. Schneiderman defines futility as "the unacceptable likelihood of achieving an effect that the patient has the capacity to appreciate as a benefit."[15]

However, when using a qualitative definition of futility, the important question remains: What is "unacceptable"? What is a "benefit"? Who assesses the goals of care? When futility is invoked in ELGANs born at or after 22 weeks of gestational age, is it the qualitative, value-laden futility ("it is not worth it")? It is imperative to determine how and by whom the goals are established as well as to recognize the variations in values that may lead to differing goals.

Whenever the word "futility" is used, it should be explained. In Sam's case, it would have been more honest for physicians in the first hospital to say: "Intervention for a baby with 30% chance of survival, months in the NICU, and a high risk of disability is not worth it, *in our opinion*. We think comfort care represents more appropriate goals of care." This statement is morally superior to statements such as "This is futile and unethical" or "Intervention would be irresponsible."

It is not clear if there have been survivors with confirmed gestational age below 22 weeks; gestational age before 22 weeks could therefore almost certainly be considered to be qualitatively futile at the present time. This would be consistent with other policy statements regarding resuscitation for older patients who have an acute life-threatening even that may lead to altered neurological outcomes, such as a cardiac arrest, a stroke, or a head trauma:[16] *"When is a rate of survival to hospital discharge so low that resuscitation should not be offered to a patient – 5 per cent, 1 per cent, 0.5 per cent? … Resuscitation should be offered to all patients who want it unless there is clear evidence of quantitative futility. Quantitative futility implies that survival is not expected after CPR under given circumstances."*[17]

It has been claimed that life-sustaining interventions for ELGANs are "an uncontrolled experiment."[18] We beg to differ. Neonatologists have been involved in outcome research for a long time,[19] and there are now many thousands of ELGANs less than 25 weeks of gestational age that have been enrolled in comprehensive programs of long-term evaluation with published results. These children have been examined and tested for many years.

3. HOW CAN WE CLASSIFY SAM?

In the first institution, he was categorized as "futile," while in the second, he was considered to be in the "gray zone." In another institution, Sam may have been considered to be in the "beneficial" category. Healthcare professionals define these three zones subjectively.[20] In the policies of industrialized countries, the borders of the gray zone range from 21 to 26 weeks of gestation, depending where the baby is born.[21] In a center that does not provide life-sustaining interventions to babies like Sam, there will be no survivors and therefore no impaired survivors. Another center that might treat *some* babies like Sam will have some survivors, some of which are impaired. However, the center that treats *all babies* like Sam will have more survivors and likely more impaired survivors. However, there will likely be proportionally fewer impaired survivors, since the quality of care for the frailest of neonates is improved by practice.[22]

Practice variations for babies like Sam are driven by explicit philosophic principles. Those who are more interventionist think that life-sustaining interventions for ELGANs are ethically appropriate. Others think that over-intervention is more problematic than under-intervention. Both argue that they are doing what is in the "best interest" of the baby and the family. There is an iterative relationship between policies, guidelines, and facts.[23] If Sam's parents are told that Sam's chances of survival are low, they will be less likely to choose intervention and less children will survive.[24] A high mortality rate will then be used to justify a policy of non-intervention for babies like Sam.

Practice variations raise important questions about informed consent. What, exactly, *should* Sam's parents be told about survival? *In the story above, Sam's mother could be at 22, 23, 24, or 25 weeks of gestation.* Parents are often given a gestational age "formula" that "at 22 weeks intensive care is futile; at 23 weeks it is 'experimental'; at 24 weeks it is ambiguous; and at 25 weeks, it is beneficial."[25] Clinicians may be uncomfortable dealing with complex probabilistic information and life-and-death decisions, and may feel conflicted by their personal values, and thus try to simplify decision-making by using recommendations based solely on the gestational age. This may be easier for the physicians and other healthcare providers, but there is no evidence that the "gestational age mantra" is better for neonates and their families. Shared decision-making is important for many parents. The provision of personalized and comprehensive information will help to establish a trustful relationship with parents and enable them to make the best decisions for their baby, decisions that will give them peace without regrets in the long term.[26]

4. LOOKING FURTHER AT ETHICAL ISSUES RELATED TO THE CARE OF ELGANS (TABLE 3)

4.1. Survival and the Timing of Death

For ELGANs, the personal values of healthcare providers and parents regarding survival without impairment, survival with any degree of impairment, or death should be explored. The average age at death of neonates who die in the NICU has been increasing. The harm of intensive care before death should be accounted for in ethical considerations. Some babies die in the NICU after many months, suffering a greater burden of care. Such a death is very different in terms of harm to the child than a rapid death at 36 hours of age. We have recently reviewed deaths in our NICU.[27] We realized that ELGANs born before 24 weeks of gestational age tend to die quicker than more mature ELGANs. It is possible that this is because they are physiologically more fragile and die despite life-sustaining interventions. It is also possible that it may be psychologically harder for healthcare providers to withdraw life-sustaining interventions for ELGANs born after 24 weeks for whom a better outcome is hoped for and who were initially classified in the "beneficial" zone. Knowing when to withhold life-sustaining interventions in the delivery room for ELGANs is important, but in our opinion, adapting the level of care in the NICU to prevent late deaths, serious morbidity, and significant burden of care is an urgent line of investigation.[28] Every time a fragile neonate in the NICU has a serious adverse event, such as significant NEC, infection, and respiratory failure, continuation of life-sustaining interventions should be questioned; we should be able to calculate survival and long-term outcomes not only at admission, but all along the NICU stay of preterm infants. The debate on whether or not to intervene in the delivery room has taken all the focus and this aspect has been neglected.

Table 3. Ethical considerations that are frequently neglected and require investigation

---

Ethical considerations: Frequently neglected and requiring investigation:

- Not all NICU deaths are equivalent: early vs. late
- The adverse effect of NICU complications on survival and long-term outcomes
- Death and disability should not be conflated
- Parental and HCP [healthcare provider] values regarding the following issues differ:
  - Survival thresholds at which to intervene
  - Whether disability should alter intervention thresholds
  - Definitions of profound, major, and minor disability; what affects functioning of the child and the family
- How families cope and adapt to the death of their child, life with a baby in the NICU and their life after the NICU: resilience
- The moral difference between neonates and older patients: should this be accepted, recognized, or fought against?

---

5. CONFLATING DEATH AND DISABILITY: A CONCEPTUAL ERROR

Guidelines and "calculators" for decision-making tend to conflate survival and disability.[29] Survival and disability do not have the same meaning for families. Healthcare providers tend to judge disability more harshly than parents;[30] they are much more likely to think that being severely disabled is worse than being dead.[31] The majority of parents of very preterm infants judge the quality of life of their infants good, even when they are disabled.[32] Rarely, some families are devastated by these outcomes.[33] Quantifying survival without disability to make a single dichotomous outcome helps the design of research projects, but conflating them in the clinical setting should be avoided, as it sends an ambiguous message. Parents should be informed of the possibility of survival and disabilities separately because they might have disparate values related to disability than that which is typically presumed in "calculators" and policy statements.

6. LIMITATIONS OF THE "DISABILITY CATEGORIZATION"

Almost three decades ago, children with Down syndrome were left to die because of their "unacceptable" outcomes.[34] The approach to life-sustaining interventions for children with Down syndrome has drastically changed. Despite these changes, many parents have reported that prenatal counseling regarding this condition was unbalanced; that only what children could not do was mentioned, not what they could do.[35] If children with Down syndrome were categorized using "neonatologists" categorization of long-term outcomes, they would be classified as having profound impairments: their long-term IQ averages below 50 in adolescence,[36] many will not live independently, and they often die in early adulthood of Alzheimer's disease. Interestingly, life-sustaining interventions are no longer considered optional for children with Down syndrome. By comparison, neonates born before 26 weeks of gestational age had an average IQ in early childhood of 82[37] and the majority of former extremely low-birth-weight infants can live independently.[38] The quality of life of children with Down syndrome is considered to be good, but so is that of ELGANs.[39] The long-term outcomes of ELGANs are in many ways superior (or at least equivalent) to those of Down syndrome children. It is rare for an ELGAN to have cognitive impairments in the long term as marked as those that are common for children with Down syndrome.

For preterm infants, some disabilities that are labeled "minor" in the medical literature, such as behavioral problems, may be much harder for some families to cope with than "severe" disabilities, such as correctable deafness or ambulant cerebral palsy. By categorizing deafness as major and behavioral problems as minor, healthcare providers have made value judgments that may not be shared by families. Parents of preterm infants – disabled or not – should have a voice in how their children are classified in the medical literature.

7. ADAPTATION AND COPING OF FAMILIES

Many authors have stated that the disabilities of ex-preterm infants cause harm to their families. This has been also assumed for many other conditions such as trisomy 21, 13, and 18.[40] However, there is no empirical evidence that having an ex-preterm infant, disabled or not, causes harm to families.[41] An urgent line of investigation in neonatology is to further investigate how families cope with prematurity. Parents should be partners in this research and not only research subjects. The meaning of disability – and not just the risks of disability and their division into categories created by physicians – and the impact on families should be measured. Valuable research done on Down syndrome is a good example of how parents may deal with disability. In a recent study, the majority of parents of children with Down syndrome felt their outlook on life was more positive because of them, that their siblings had positive relationships, and that their children are great sources of love and pride.[42] Parents recommended that parents with a new diagnosis should receive balanced information, including the challenges of disability as well as the positive transformation that many parents experience.[43]

Sam may die or survive. If Sam survives, he/she may or may not have long-term impairment. In each of these scenarios, the parents and the family may or may not adapt to the challenges. Parents may ask healthcare providers questions that are not about survival and disability: "Will Sam have a good quality of life?" "Will Sam be OK?" "Will we be OK?" "How can I be the mother of a dead child?" "How can I be the mother of a disabled child?" These important concerns of parents are often neglected.[44] To be balanced, we should also inform parents of the infants' abilities and not just disabilities; of what their families can do with them, their quality of life, how they cope, adapt, and what factors seem to influence resilience.[45] We could also inform them about how parents of preterm infants cope with their child's death in the NICU.[46]

8. NEONATES AND OLDER PATIENTS COMPARED: MORAL STATUS, PERSONHOOD, AND JUSTICE

The period immediately before and after birth is a time during which a fetus becomes a person. This transition has enormous moral and legal implications. At the moment of birth, a neonate becomes a full-fledged citizen, endowed with rights that should be no different from any other citizen. In the medical context, these rights are identical to those of any other vulnerable patient who lacks decision-making capacity. Specifically, the preterm infant has a right to medical treatment that is in its best interest.

The Neonatal Resuscitation Programme textbook, which is the standard neonatal resuscitation text used in North America and many other countries states: "The ethical principles regarding resuscitation of newborns should be no different from those followed in resuscitating an older child or adult."[47] In practice, however, newborn infants are treated differently.[48]

8.1. Pain Treatment

Analgesia is grossly underused in neonates.[49] Endotracheal intubation, lumbar punctures, and even sometimes chest tubes are performed without adequate analgesia.[50] Trials comparing analgesia to placebo are not rare despite the existence of many studies showing the benefit of analgesia. This indifference or neglect would be inconceivable in older patients. It is ironic that prolonged pain and suffering are often used as reasons for withholding life-sustaining interventions in preterm infants. Intolerable, persistent, and untreatable pain is an ethically appropriate reason for withdrawing life-sustaining interventions. Failure to prevent and treat pain is not.

8.2. Variations of Practice and the Best Interest Principle

Thresholds recommended for non-intervention in preterm infants are not consistent with thresholds set in older individuals with comparable risks of death or disability.[51] For older children, near-certain death or disability is necessary before withholding or withdrawing life-sustaining interventions.[52] This is not the case with preterm infants, who may have life-sustaining interventions withheld despite predicted survival of over 80%.[53] The best interest principle is not actually applied when considering life-sustaining interventions for neonatal patients.[54] Policy statements for preterm infants often state survival and handicap as justification for optional intervention. The fact that such outcome statistics would not be used to justify non-intervention approaches at to older patients suggests that neonates are treated differently to older patients.

8.3. The Moral Difference between Preterm Infants and Older Patients

Newborn infants are considered differently to older children. ELGANs do not yet have a personality of their own, they did not go home, they may live all their lives in the NICU and die there. The attachment parents and healthcare providers feel toward them may be different. Healthcare providers do not react the same way for the death of a baby with potential impairments at 24 weeks of gestational age than for a 7-year-old child with known impairments.[55] Healthcare providers may also feel responsibility when a preterm infant is discharged from NICU disabled; they may feel they created the disabled preterm infant while they "saved" a child with near drowning.[56]

9. CONCLUSION

In conclusion, there is no easy way to make decisions regarding life and death. Labeling infants according to completed 7-day periods of gestational age is not only scientifically flawed, but ethically questionable.[57] What should we do for Sam? It will not be simple, nor will it be quick. Information related to survival and outcomes should be personalized, following an analysis of the risks for this particular infant, taking into account all of the relevant medical characteristics; the joint decision must incorporate and be consistent with the values and desires of the parents and also incorporate the best interest of the child. In this field there are many opinions but little good evidence.[58] The limitations of the evidence should be an incentive to examine each case in a personalized fashion. Establishing individualized goals of care with families while recognizing uncertainty is morally superior to quickly labeling their child in one of three gestational age categories. New horizons for research should seek to understand and rectify the inequities that exist between the care offered to extremely preterm infants and to similar, fragile populations. Individualizing and optimizing care for extremely preterm infants and their families should be the goal.

Difficult Decisions

Since my preemie-parent experience, I have explored the topics covered in the previous chapter more thoroughly and spoken to hundreds of parents – as a neonatologist or a researcher, and even online as a parent myself, to other parents – who have had to make similar decisions. I still find it disconcerting that the main goal of many researchers is to give information to parents for them to make the best rational decision. Many researchers are convinced that this information transfer is what is most important: if parents only knew all the statistics and probabilities and understood the risks, then they would know what to do. Many research projects are constructed this way. First, parents are exposed to information, either in the form of written documentation, decision aids, or other modes of communication. Then, parents are asked whether they are satisfied and what they remember, their recall. When recall is high, researchers conclude that their communication strategy is good. But knowing the numbers does not automatically help parents decide between life and death. Parents do not decide only with their heads; they also decide with their gut and their heart. Parents may only remember 20 per cent of what a doctor has said, but it may be the 20 per cent that is important to them. They may not have listened to the other 80 per cent or do not remember it because it is less important to them. The stressful situation parents are in may also make them less likely to concentrate or remember long conversations.

Traditionally, behaviour scientists believed that, when deciding between different options, we would choose the option that would maximize our "utility" or our gains. In the past decades, decision-making science, also called behavioral economics, has shed a different light on how we decide under conditions of uncertainty. The way we decide is more complex and often biased. Researchers have demonstrated that we decide intuitively. For example, we are more likely to choose an option to avoid loss and regret than to maximize utility, even if the loss is small and the "positive" utility large. Indeed, the negative impact of losing something we have is more important in magnitude than the positive impact we would experience gaining the same thing. This is called "loss aversion." Daniel Kahneman has won a Nobel Prize examining these issues, and his excellent book *Thinking Fast and Slow*[1] summarizes groundbreaking research in this area.

We also know that emotions are critical in the decision-making process. In an article entitled "How Much Emotion Is Enough,"[2] I discuss the legal and ethical concept of informed consent. When parents make life-and-death decisions for their children that doctors don't recommend or understand, it is not rare to hear that parents are "in denial" or "irrational." Clinicians are taught to engage in the informed-consent process: to give information to parents who listen, understand and weigh different options, ask questions, and decide to pursue the optimal course of action. Clinicians often believe that intense emotions negatively influence competence and the informed-consent process. But we decide with both our evolved brain, which is located mostly in our prefrontal cortex, and our primitive brain, which is located deeper in our nervous system. We have survived as a species by making fight-or-flight decisions using our primitive – or reptilian – brain. When we see a big snake in our path, we do not reflect and elaborate a list of pros and cons: "pro, very nice colors and sleek; cons, large and possibly poisonous." Most of us will run away briskly and have a strong autonomic response, a fear-and-flight reaction. Life-and-death decisions that parents take under conditions of uncertainty are probably to some degree motivated both by thoughtful consideration from our "intelligent brain" as well as from our fear-based primitive brain. Several contemporary academics go further and consider emotions to be more than the dimensions of biological processes; they consider them essential components of our bodily and cognitive intelligence.

In an interesting article, "Is Mr Spock Mentally Competent?"[3] Charland, a philosopher, asks if the flight officer from *Star Trek*, who is part Vulcan and therefore unable to experience emotions, could make truly informed decisions. In Charland's view, even if he is a "perfect cognizer," Mr Spock does not represent an ideal of competence because emotions are morally important. In her book *The Upheavals of Thought: The Intelligence of Emotions*,[4] Martha Nussbaum, a contemporary philosopher, considers emotions as central to our cognition and as important to consider as "the rational" thought. Many of these important factors have not yet been integrated in practical decision-making in neonatology and medicine. Many important decisions we take in life are not purely rational: which partner we chose, whom we marry (or not), and whom we love are good examples. We all have experiences in our lives – both medical and personal – where we may not hear unwanted information. When we advise our best friend not to marry an inconsiderate jerk who has cheated on her several times, she may not listen, even if we present the best decision-aids about getting married. She may be intelligent and educated, she may understand the information, but she decides to go ahead nonetheless. Having children is probably the most irrational decision of all: they eat our resources, our sleep, and our sanity. They pollute the planet and overcrowd it. In a rational sense, the con list is probably longer than the pro list, which is motivated to some degree by our biological wiring. It is surprising that when parents are then asked to decide between life and death, the decisional aids and documents that are made available to them often do not take into consideration regret, emotions, and the parental experience.

In all my years of training and as a young investigator, I had unfortunately not been exposed to behavioral economics, to these authors, and this evidence. Decision-making science is rarely part of the medical curriculum. When it is dealt with, it is presented mostly as a "rational theory": to weigh the pros and cons and maximize our "utilities," such as when we buy a new fridge. Since that time, several researchers, including several on our research team, have integrated this knowledge and made it practical for clinicians. We have proposed guidelines to personalize care during prenatal consultations that aims to inform parents and also to manage and explore their emotions so they can best decide with their brains and their hearts.

I now have the habit of asking research-speakers, after their presentations, "So what I get from your study on how to communicate with parents is that you think that two neonatologists, who know all the statistics about adverse outcomes and the NICU, would be the best at making those decisions. That they would know better how and what to decide and choose what is best for their child?" The researcher generally agrees with my sentence and secretly wishes all the parents were neonatologists.

"Well, I am not sure you are right …"

A person is a person, no matter how small.

Dr Seuss

Naming

There's one decision, at least, that was made painlessly: the decision to call my daughter Violette. During my first pregnancy, I was sure I was expecting a girl. It was after I read Michel Tremblay that my fetus, which I had until then called "LB" (for lima bean), became Violette. When I realized I was going to have a boy, we named him Axel, but the name Violette was reserved for our next child.

I adore children, and I adore Michel Tremblay, a great Quebec author. No connection, you think? But there is one. Starting at the age of 10 – very early, I agree – I would write down potential names for my future offspring in my school agendas. One list of girls' names and another of boys' names. I would have liked those lists to be used when it came time to choose a name for my last sister, who was born when I was 11. I applied considerable pressure to get her named Mélissa or Vanessa, but without success. She's called Gaëlle, and the name suits her very well. Vanassaaah, as it's pronounced here in Quebec, doesn't always sound great.

With time, my tastes have changed, and some names have been crossed off the list. Others have been added, usually spontaneously. Sometimes I would discreetly write down a name heard in a movie or a conversation. When I first started dating, the guy would sometimes see me taking notes.

"What are you writing down in your agenda – our next date?"

"No, your sister's name. Coralie, that's really cool!"

"What do you want with Coralie? You don't know her!"

"No, but if I have a daughter one day, I may call her Coralie!"

I've observed that this obsession had quite a contraceptive effect. But it's a test that has good predictive value for a quick PD (potential dad) screening. I've often recommended it to my friends whose biological clocks are ticking.

One name has been on my list for seventeen years: Violette. That name came up when, at the age of 15, I read *The Fat Woman Next Door Is Pregnant* (*La grosse femme d'à côté est enceinte*), by Michel Tremblay. I remember finding the title a little off-putting, but I devoured the book. In it, Violette is an old ghost. But in my head, Violette was a Little Miss Curious with blue eyes and very blond, almost white, hair like in the ads for the Timotei shampoo that my cousins used and that smelled really good, but that we did not have at our house because it wasn't sold at Club Price in a giant economy size.

During my bed rest with Axel, I lived in a blue house on De Bullion Street near Prince Arthur Street. Coincidently, it's the house shown on the cover of the collected Plateau Mont-Royal chronicles by Michel Tremblay! I got the book as a house-warming gift. There wasn't really a house-warming party, or a poetic moment while repainting the house or deciding which shelf in the new fridge should hold the strawberry jam. Instead, I made a Frida Kahlo–style entrance into my new house lying in my bed, carried by the movers. While I lay in bed under the threat of preterm labour, I had decided to read everything, absolutely everything, Michel Tremblay had written, starting by rereading *The Fat Woman* (suggestion for Tremblay's publishers: you should add an appendix with the family tree of the Desrosiers tribe; it would help). That reading confirmed that Violette's name was the winner, not Ariane, Zoé, Coralie, or Mélissa. I was sure I was carrying a girl – I could feel it. I often talked to her. I called my fetus Violette up to 25 weeks, until the day I was told it was a boy. So the fetus changed names. Arnaud doesn't work well in English. As for Ariel, Keith found it suggested both the little mermaid and the prime minister of Israel, a toxic combination. Axel was original, pronounceable in all languages, and above all, easy to write if he had problems in school because of his potential prematurity. Sold! "Patience, Violette, your turn will come," I thought, but she was in too much of a hurry.

In the beginning, lying upside-down in obstetrics, when the nurses asked me if I had chosen a name, I found the idea completely ridiculous. I was struggling perilously with life-and-death decisions for my daughter, while they, to chat, would ask me about her name, as if that made any difference. I would mumble an answer, then sigh. After pouting for a whole day, I began to answer "Violette." The name just came out – my daughter's name. She was no longer an anonymous fetus. Nurses, once again, I love you. You made my daughter a person. When you came to see me to ask me routine questions, it was always personalized: "How are you feeling? Is your slipped disk still hurting? Is Violette moving? All the time?" You gave me hope again. I felt like my daughter and I both counted for you. Thanks to you, I felt that my daughter wasn't "optional," that she was someone important. It wasn't pressure to make me decide on medical intervention if she were born now, but I began to see things differently. Regardless how long her life would be, she was someone.

In some hospitals, mothers who are at risk of giving birth very prematurely (as in my case, at 23 weeks) are told that the situation is hopeless and that it's no use sending them to a hospital with an NICU; or they're offered oxytocin, a drug that stimulates the uterus in order to induce labour. In fact, since intervention and intensive care are optional before 25 weeks, some people believe it is preferable to deliver the baby before then, rather than to wait for it to be born later but still very prematurely, in which case they would have an "obligation" to give intensive care. There are even tertiary care hospitals that don't want to provide intensive care to babies at less than 24 or 25 weeks, and that state this explicitly. Sometimes, they may even offer an abortion when there's a risk of extreme prematurity. At that time, I was so vulnerable that I would have been easy to convince that everything was going badly and that Violette would be better off dead. But I was not in one of those hospitals. I was looked after by sensitive, smiling professionals who were capable of personalizing their care and who knew Violette by name. I knew the statistics were against us. Nevertheless, I didn't want others to be as pessimistic as I was. Maybe if I had been excessively optimistic, the staff would have acted in a more pessimistic fashion. Violette was never treated like a baby with no future, even though her prospects were pretty dim.

Michael Hébert, the father of Domenica, a little girl born at Sainte-Justine Hospital at 22 weeks' gestational age, is one of the authors of an article written by parents, entitled "Our Baby Is Not Just a Gestational Age." He's a calm, smiling man, and is in great physical shape. One day when Domenica was recovering from a bad night and we were talking about the seriousness of her condition, he said to me, "We don't know the winners at the beginning of the race. We don't know who's going to finish. Thank you for giving her a chance despite the risk of a false start, even though we can't yet see the finish line." It was his way of telling me he understood what I was saying to him. The parents who wrote that article were not against comfort care; some of them had lost their babies. They were against life-and-death decisions based only on gestational age, which is uncertain.

My research in recent years has focused on the thoughts that beset me in that room. I look at the questions parents ask themselves when facing the risk of their baby being born sick, when dealing with their fears. The parents are, of course, concerned about the child's development and the likelihood of death. But they also ask themselves all kinds of other questions. How can I be a parent in the NICU? What does the NICU look like? Who will be able to come to see my baby? How can I be a parent to a disabled child? What will happen to my family? What will happen to the other children? What will visits be like? What about nursing the baby? How do we include family and friends? What will my baby look like?

Although the first year – or years – is difficult, families usually recover from that difficult time. Most of them say the impact of a child who is born sick (whether disabled or not) is mostly positive. Adaptation and resilience are important, and they have an enormous effect on the families' quality of life. Adaption is based on many factors. People's outlook on life is a big factor. Some are more optimistic than others. Faced with adversity, I was cynical, ironic, and withdrawn, no doubt a natural defence mechanism arising out of fear of having the door slam shut in my face as soon as I opened it. In such situations, serious isolation, whether economic, emotional, or social, often prevents healthy adjustment. Parents who have the support of friends, family, or their community are the ones who adjust best.

What would I have liked to hear in 2005? That "things will get better," as is often the case, and that this reasonable optimism is based on empirical data and research. I would have liked to learn earlier that we're stronger in adversity than we think. Later I became friends with some researchers who examine quality of life and adaptation. I wish Peter Ubel's book *You're Stronger Than You Think: Tapping into the Secrets of Emotionally Resilient People*[1] would have been available when I was on bed rest, or the wonderful book Saroj Saigal wrote, *Preemie Voices*[2] (a wonderful video was also made based on that book). These books should be recommended reading for medical students and residents.

Parents don't want to know "the risk of cerebral palsy" (approximately 9 per cent before 28 weeks); they want to know how cerebral palsy will affect their child: Will he have friends? Will she be happy? Will he be able to live a rewarding life? How will she integrate in the family with the other children? Will our vacations be the same? Will we have to move? Decisions based on gestational age, with only a list of potential problems, depersonalize care and prevent good communication with parents. They leave too many questions unanswered.

19 May

Violette's gestational age: 24 weeks, 2 days (well … between 23 weeks, 4 days, and 25 weeks)

Dear Computer,

My water has broken. The river has overflowed its banks. I was trying to suppress a sneeze while turning over onto my side, because my back was hurting after hours of immobility. I had just asked Philippe, a wonderful nurse practitioner, to go buy me some French fries with ketchup and mayonnaise on either side of the plate. I was drooling at the thought of them. I was obsessed with a desire for fries while Violette was in mortal danger. That'll teach me. I wasn't careful, and "atchoo," splash, I was drained with a sneeze.

My hopes ran out with my water. Now I have to recalibrate them. Again. That's all I've been doing since I've been here in this bed waiting for nature's verdict. In the beginning, like all parents, I hoped for a baby born full term that I would breastfeed and take home after a few days. Yesterday, my hope was that my baby would get past the 28-week mark, which would be the super-jackpot in a sea of consolation prizes. Since my water broke, the contractions have again become very regular. I'm bleeding and in pain. I don't want an epidural, I'm afraid to sit up, afraid that even more water will run out, that the umbilical cord will drop and I'll crush it, that Violette will suffocate for lack of blood with the cord clamped between my legs. And this means I'm going to give birth. I'll have to readjust my goddamn hopes again. Now that the simple,

28 weeks hope has become completely unrealistic, I'm going crazy. Who would have thought that, one day, I would reach the point where I was hoping with all my heart, with every fibre of my being, for a baby born at 26 weeks! Yet that's what I'm doing now.

Breathe in, 26 weeks; breathe out, 26 weeks; 26 weeks. More time, MORE TIME!!!

Philippe has come back with my fries, and he understood immediately that the situation has changed. I'm not allowed to eat because I could give birth at any moment. I've been forbidden to eat every time the contractions became more frequent – that is, almost every thirty-six hours. But I'm still allowed to have little chunks of ice.

I would like someone to tell me that I'm capable of dealing with what's coming, but that it will take time. That would help me. Not just "everything will be fine" – that's just bullshit. When there's a catastrophe, there has to be a little hope, right? Either that or I'll throw myself out the window. It won't be easy, because the window is screwed to the frame. What's more, the air conditioning is on the blink and I'm baking here, although, when it is working, it's always on full blast and it's freezing. I can't even put on a sweater or turn on a fan. I'm hooked up and I can't put anything on because of the intravenous, aside from the gown that leaves my ass hanging out. In winter in this hospital, you go around in a T-shirt, and in summer you have to wear a wool sweater. It's with our taxes that the hospital is either overheated or refrigerated, but it's also our taxes that pay for me to be here, for my rectum to be emptied, and for me to be taken care of, so I'd better just shut up. Maybe the windows are locked because this room is the one where they put the mothers who, like me, are waiting for a possible death sentence. I wonder if the other windows on the floor are also locked. Maybe some of us get crazy enough to try to open one. But with the intravenous, the catheter, the monitor, and my head down, good luck trying. It would be a bungee party.

Never deprive someone of hope; it might be all they have.

H. Jackson Brown Jr

20 May

Violette's gestational age: 24 weeks, 3 days (give or take 5 days; you're beginning to get the idea, Computer)

Dear PC,

WOW, I have not yet delivered; I've bought myself (and Violette) another day. Maybe I will be lucky and make it to 26 or 27 weeks? Twenty-seven is pushing it, though …

These thoughts make me remember a great family I met, and it really helps. When I was a neonatology fellow, in 2000, I met a couple during the night. She was in the room I am in now. I was called to see them urgently because the mother had just arrived and would deliver soon. She had a fever and her waters had broken too early because of an infection. They had named their son two weeks earlier after the ultrasound informed them they would have a boy. His name was Aaron. He was a very small baby, born at about 23 weeks of gestational age, very quickly. The mother had a severe uterine infection and was preparing to push Aaron out when I started talking to them. I only had minutes to speak to them while the resident was preparing the resuscitation material. With the baby's estimated weight, size, and condition, survival of this little boy seemed unlikely. I told the parents he was unlikely to live, even intensive care and a respirator would probably not help him survive. I told them that many parents in this situation would decide to hold their baby and love him, and explained what we did in the delivery room, what would happen with and without intensive care. I also told them that, if they survive, many babies like Aaron are disabled but that most of their families report they have a good quality of life. I myself was not sure intensive care was the best thing for Aaron – would it prolong his life or his death? They said they wanted to give their Aaron a chance.

When he was born, Aaron was so tiny, so translucent, so fragile. He died several hours later because his lungs were too immature to get oxygen to his body. It was clear shortly after his birth that he would die soon. Little Aaron stayed blue for most of short his life. He was given medication to make sure he was not in any pain. I remember telling the parents that the respirator could not add many minutes to his life, but that they could add love to these minutes. Did they want anybody else to be there, did they want a religious or spiritual ceremony, a special song? The parents had two other children, twin girls, 7 years old, who were at home with their grandmother. They asked if the twins would be terrified to see Aaron. Usually, small kids are not terrified of machines. They see only the small baby. And I knew a family picture could be meaningful in the long term. Coming home without a baby when siblings are waiting for a baby to come is often worse for them than seeing a sick baby.

The grandmother rushed to the hospital with the girls by taxi, at about four in the morning. The two sisters were very blond, one with long hair and curls and the other with a short bob. I remember noticing the different haircuts in the twins, thinking it was unusual. The one with the long hair had a big green-grey teddy in her hands. One could tell this was her "old" security teddy that went everywhere she went. He had signs of teddy surgery around his neck. With one eye missing and his stuffing mostly in his feet and head, the bear draped awkwardly on both sides of her arm. The other little girl was holding a book. My niece had the same book, one with pictures of all sorts of animals inside, with many textures the kids like stroking: a lizard with rough scales, a frog with a sticky tongue, a lion with a furry mane. Their parents told them that Aaron was very sick and would not be with them for long: he was too small, too sick, he came way too soon … The dad took the teddy girl and the grandmother took the other. The mother was sitting next to the incubator. The adults were crying, the two girls were watching their small brother and asking questions about the "red light" (the saturometer indicating how much oxygen is in the blood) and asking why his eyes were always closed. I answered that the light was to know how he was doing; the light told us he was sick. And Aaron's eyes were closed because he was very small, too small to open them. I wondered on and off later in that week if I should have told them they were fused, if I should have explained that, if it might have helped.

Aaron would not live much longer. The sister with the shorter hair said that she had brought the book to read to him: "I bring it because when he moves too much in the belly, we read it. Then he sleeps and mama can sleep," she said. The mother, who was trying to hold back her tears, fell apart. She was sitting on a hospital rocking chair that was squeaking with her shaking. She wore a hockey sweatshirt over her blue hospital gown. She looked like such a loving mother, not knowing what to do with this tragedy her life had become. The animal book doesn't have much of a story, so I do not know what the little girl said. I remember she was holding her tiny brother's hand and making him feel all the textures. The scales, the tongue, the soft mane, the textures on all the pages. The book was much bigger than Aaron and the side of the incubator was up. When they got to the monkey, the girls decided to tickle him with the tail instead. One of the girls said "Shhhh, he is sleeping." It was so touching I was crying at the back of the room. I remember a great nurse who brought a camera at that moment and took pictures of the family. The five of them, all around this small baby, being a family for a short time. Then the grandmother took the little sisters out to another room to draw some animals, and the parents stayed. Aaron was dying on the respirator, so we stopped the machines and tubes to allow him to be in his parents' arms during his last moments, free of machines. We took the best pictures we could for the family.

A year later, I sent a card to the parents, a small note about Aaron and how we were privileged to have been part of his short life. I wrote a short paragraph about the sisters, the teddy bear, and the book and how touching I thought they were. The parents called days later and thanked me. They were each on separate telephone lines and it was unsettling. The mom told me she remembered me offering intensive care, not knowing if it was the best thing for Aaron. She remembered my honesty. The dad thanked me for telling them what I thought was best when they had asked, but respecting their wishes. And they wanted to answer my question: they felt they had prolonged Aaron's life not his death. I spoke about a good death; they thought it was a good life. It was a tiny life, but it was a precious life. I was crying, and I had not closed the door of my office. I had thought this was a phone call from a pharmacy or from a parent asking a medical question. I remember the faces of concerned co-workers who walked in front of the office. I asked the parents what we could have done better to help them, if there were things that doctors should know, or that other parents in their situation should know. Before the mother hung up she said something like "You must know it is not about statistics; it is about life and love, living with yourself, regrets, being a good parent. I think you get it. How can I help you or parents? Me, us? Asking parents if they want to hold their baby for a certain death or want to try and save his possible life is … I do not know how to make it easier. But it is not about numbers. It is about speaking to the parents' guts, not their heads." "Meaning more than numbers." The father said this last sentence. He was a computer programmer. I thought it was an odd comment for him. Aaron's mother continued, "I think of it as the luggage we carry around, our back pack. My parents taught me that all of us have a backpack and we have to carry it around all our life. Sometimes bad stuff happens and puts heavy rocks in your backpack. Death of a loved one is a rock, a short life is a rock, a sick child is a rock, a disease is a rock, divorce is a rock, and marriage can be a rock. Anything you regret will be a rock: this is what my parents used to say. How much can parents lift in their backpack, for how long? What about their kids? How much do the rocks weigh for them, their family? For us, meeting Aaron, loving him during his tiny life, was important for us, even if we lost him. Giving him a chance was important. Knowing we did not have any regrets was important. This was the lightest rock for us. I think for Aaron's tiny backpack, meeting his sisters and his family was probably better too, but we will never know. Also for the twins, I think it was better. I guess it depends what kind of rock weighs less in all the backpacks. I think it could be easier to explain it this way to parents, maybe …"

I keep thinking of these parents. I would like to speak to them but resist, as it would not be acceptable physician practice. It would really be weird to want parents of my ex-patient to help me, a neonatologist in preterm labour. Even so, I feel their words could help me more than all the doctors' words I hear. How much do the rocks in my life weigh?

My dad's death, my mother's prolonged grief, my cancer, my divorce, the craziness at work when I decided to live with Keith. The grief after my first abnormal pregnancy. What would I do if I were Aaron's mother? Previously, if she had asked me for a recommendation, I would have said "hold your son and love him." Now I am not so sure anymore.

But aren't numbers like rocks? Do they have the weight of rocks? Maybe some people can lift more rocks? I always thought I could lift more rocks than anyone, but today I feel crushed. How are we supposed to know how much each rock weighs? Do rocks weigh less each year? I am thinking about this with crusty salty tears in the corners of my eyes, I have to be careful when I cry because I lose precious fluid when I cry hard. So hush, hush. OK I need to try to go to sleep. They gave me a sleeping pill. I did not take it before, afraid of what it might do to Violette. I know it does not do any harm – I am a doctor. I'm just trying to do what a good mother would do. But tonight, I think I will take the sleeping pill. Maybe it will keep me calm and prevent my losing more fluid.

*T*he following article was written by a great stimulating group I have worked with for many years and that has taught me many things. All of us have seen many parents, and our research careers are dedicated to the investigation of parental perspectives and how to support and help families.

Many articles around fragile babies and decision making are theoretical and ethical. While it is relatively easy to say that we recommend decisions to be individualized and not based only on gestational age, practical articles, to help clinicians communicate with families, are rare. The goal of this article is to provide a framework for clinicians who want to engage in personalized counselling with families. Unfortunately, in this field, clinicians often consider that the more information there is, the better. We see more and more decision aids, written information for parents, and so on. But parents are all different: while some may want many details, others just want general information. Recently, John Lantos has written a great article that summarizes the subject well.[†]

The aim of this article is to help physicians adapt to families, to help them do a "controlled improvisation" with each family and give them personalized care.

Personalized Decision Making: Practical Recommendations for Antenatal Counseling for Fragile Neonates

Marlyse F. Haward, MD, Nathalie Gaucher, MD, PhD, Antoine Payot, MD, PhD, Kate Robson, MEd, Annie Janvier, MD, PhD[‡]

Fifty years ago, it was not rare for infants born with congenital anomalies or near-term to die. Neonatology is a recent specialty, emerging in the 1960s as a discipline dedicating itself to the care of sick neonates.[1] Rapid advancements, such as assessments of fetal lung maturity alongside consensus statements on antenatal steroids in the mid-1990s, helped care for premature deliveries. Technological advances in ventilators, exogenous surfactants, and parenteral peripheral nutritional support improved management and survival for these young patients.[2] Neonatology was born and excelled in keeping young fragile infants alive.

DEVELOPMENTS IN NEONATOLOGY AND CLINICAL ETHICS

Coinciding with these medical advances, changes in the bioethical decision-making landscape, rising consumerism, and federal legislation regarding children with disabilities led to increased recognition of the role of parents as decision makers.[3] The climate in the medical arena, previously marked by maternal-infant separation both in terms of parental physical absence and exclusion from decision making,[4] evolved as seminal work championing maternal-infant bonding,[5] and patient-centered care emerged.[6] In North America, the President's Commission for the Study of Ethical Problems in Medicine and Biomedical and Behavioral Research[7] and the Royal College of Physicians and Surgeons of Canada[8] endorsed parents as surrogate decision makers for their infants when best interests were unclear, exploring moral boundaries of sanctity of life and quality of life. A landmark statement by the Institute of Medicine equated autonomous decision making and patient-centered care with "quality" of care so as to deliver "care that is respectful of and responsive to individual patient preferences, needs, and values."[9] In pediatrics, patient-centered care became synonymous with family-centered care, and the concept appeared in several policy statements, including Guidelines for Perinatal Care published jointly by the American Academy of Pediatrics (AAP) and American Congress of Obstetricians and Gynecologists.[10]

Concurrently, in bioethics, new models of decision making challenged physician authority and paternalism, as patients exercised their autonomy and demanded informed choices; physician obligations were defined and interactions between physicians and patients changed toward a more collaborative approach.[11] These partnerships between providers and parents became especially important in the neonatal intensive care unit (NICU) as younger infants were being resuscitated and evidence was mounting about risks of disabilities in survivors. Decision-making frontiers were propelled into areas of uncertainty, unpredictability, and value exploration. Evidence derived from neonatal outcome studies divided fragile neonates into "decision-making zones": (1) beneficial, where intervention was indicated because of good outcomes; (2) futile, where intervention was not recommended because of improbable survival; or (3) "gray zone," where outcomes could justify either life support or withholding of life support.[12]

INFORMING PARENTS AND DECISION MAKING

Shared decision making recommends that physicians and parents work together, requiring at a minimum physician-parent exchanges of medical information and explorations of values resulting in decisions attained through mutual consent.[13] Medical information considered essential to inform parents is based on presumptions of rational and informed decisional processes.[14] Reaffirmed as recently as 2015, this includes information about infant outcomes, with both local and national data, available options, and supplementing verbal communication with other modalities while being sensitive to parental values.[15] As stated by the AAP, the "primary goal of the antenatal consultation is to provide parents with information that will aid their decision making."[16]

However, prioritizing information exchange and suggesting a standardized set of facts is too simplistic. Decision making is multifaceted, and understanding risk information is dependent on relationships, trust, balances between cognitive and affective elements, life experiences, subjective interpretations of decisional outcomes, tolerance of risk/uncertainty, and other personal factors. Furthermore, a multitude of behavioral decisional processes, including biases, impact decision making.[17] In addition, information exchange/transfer represents only the first of 3 phases important in decision making, of which the other 2 include deliberation and defining roles involved in making a decision.[18] Patient preferences can vary in any of the 3 phases; in the amount and type of information desired,[19] preferred processes for deliberation,[20] and defining roles in assuming decisional responsibility.[21]

The goal of the antenatal consultation should not be to prioritize standardization of information nor to give it in a uniform/neutral fashion, but rather to adapt to parental needs and empower them through a personalized decision-making process, acknowledging individuality and diversity. In this article, we will describe why and how to personalize antenatal consultations and empower parents. The goal of this process is for parents to feel like parents and to feel like they are good parents, before birth, at birth, and after, either in the NICU or until the death of their child.

Personalizing the Evaluation of the Situation: Avoiding Decisions Based on Gestational Age

Gestational age (GA), the framework on which these decisions are sometimes approached, is insufficient, inherently flawed, and simplistic as sole predictor of outcomes including neurodevelopmental disability and quality of life for extremely premature infants.[22] First-trimester ultrasound GA estimates incorporate an SD of ±4 to 7 days,[23] meaning for extremely premature infants GA can be miscalculated by a full week. This difference may result in foregoing resuscitation in more mature infants while resuscitating less mature infants. Furthermore, 4 other prognostic indicators, female sex, birthweight increment of 100g, antenatal steroids, and singleton birth, have been shown equivalent to the arbitrary 1-week prognostic milestone.[24] Although fetal estimations of weight before birth are flawed, the other 3 indicators can help refine antenatal counseling regarding the prognosis for the individual infant.

Categorizing care as beneficial, futile, or "gray" by GA alone carries important ethical considerations.[25] Arbitrary rules inevitably lead to self-fulfilling prophecies perpetuating outcomes and beliefs about futility.[26] Although some institutions report 32% survival at 22 weeks,[27] whole country cohorts, such as the French EPIPAGE study, describe 0% and 1% survival in France at 22 and

23 weeks, because of nonintervention.[28] There is tremendous variation in GA thresholds for resuscitation between professional societies.[29] It is comforting to observe that some professional associations, for example, the AAP, no longer have GA as the sole factor for judging whether life support is indicated for a preterm infant.[30] Although relying on GA boundaries in communicating prognostic uncertainty may seem to simplify information for the physician, falsely implying a sense of certainty to the data,[31] there is no evidence that this simplification serves to empower parents, enhance decision making, and lead to better neonatal/parental outcomes. To the contrary, personalizing the situation by considering factors beyond GA is an essential first step in respecting each vulnerable patient as an individual and ensuring that reliable and accurate information serves as the basis for medical decisions.

Communicating with Prospective Parents: More Than a Transfer of Information

In theory, communication of all options, outcomes, risks, and benefits empowers and informs patients by equalizing information asymmetry.[32] According to classic rational choice theories, this thorough transfer of information facilitates probability assessments and decision making.[33] However, the problem is that the facts considered important (outcome data) are chosen by physicians without parental input. For example, families are generally informed of the risk of severe neurodevelopmental impairment: cerebral palsy, visual impairment, hearing impairment, and low scores on a developmental screening test, most commonly more than 2 SDs below a standardized mean score on the Bayley Scales of Infant Development. Physicians should recognize that these classifications have been made using their own values; they have not asked parents of premature infants to categorize their children at 18 months, nor to describe their child's health. Some disabilities that are labeled "minor" in the medical literature, such as behavioral problems or conduct disorders, may be much harder for some families to cope with than "severe" disabilities, such as hearing loss or some forms of cerebral palsy. This leads to biases reflecting interpretation of risk.[34] In addition, those chosen facts are rarely based on an exploration of values or preferences of the individual parent at the time of consultation.[35] Yet unfortunately, in many investigations, assessments of information transfer, such as retention and comprehension of predetermined medical facts, often remain proxies for robust decision making, leading interventions to focus on improving complete transfer and recall of information, rather than personalizing the content of antenatal consultation and decision-making process.[36]

In neonatology, for prospective parents of unborn fragile neonates, transfer of information is often limited. Risk communication becomes increasingly challenging as prognostic uncertainty escalates and values diversify. It is known that risk communication can be influenced by framing effects when preferences are uncertain; for example, using percentages for mortality as opposed to percentages for survival.[37] It is also known that comprehension of statistical information and numeracy are difficult even for highly educated populations; for example, 4 out of 10 can mean something different from 40% for some individuals, depending on the risk it expresses.[38] When making decisions, there exists variability in the utility of risk information at baseline.[39] For some, risk information is dismissed in favor of more intuitive decision-making processes[40] if it does not conform to lived experiences, assumptions, or beliefs.[41] For example, a minimal-risk procedure may seem overwhelming to a family who lost a loved one in the operating room and may lead them to refuse treatment based on assessments other than probability. On the other hand, for others, it is an essential element in more analytical deliberations,[42] and omission can be misinterpreted as an intentional nondisclosure...[43]

THE LIMITATIONS OF DECISION AIDS

Decision aids for antenatal counseling have attempted to overcome some of these challenges by using multiple modalities to improve comprehension of medical information and treatment options.[44] However, as with the professional guidelines, assumptions of rational decision processes prevail and only a few neonatal decision aids have been constructed with parental input.[45] None have been designed primarily, or only, by parents. In current neonatal decision aids, although survival and mortality statistics are generally balanced, depictions of long-term outcomes are not. In some, pictures of wheelchairs or of brain bleeds, as opposed to disabled children with their families, may reinforce fears of disability.[46] Furthermore, data representing parental perspectives, quality of life, and adjustment/resilience literature are missing;[47] these outcomes, rarely included in risk communication, frequently frame patients' decisions and perceptions of risk.[48]

Although decision aids assist comprehension of chosen medical risk information, the question remains whether standardized facts are sufficient and appropriate/optimal for all prospective parents. Given that neonatal decision aids have focused predominately on informational needs, and less on the processes of value exploration or how to be the parent of a sick infant, they may be most effective as a tool used after relationships have been built and specific informational needs determined. It also has been suggested that too much information, not considered central to the parents' deliberative needs, can be overwhelming or harmful.[49] Although some informational elements considered pertinent from parent perspectives[50] have been recently explored, it still remains unknown how information relative to medical risk is operationalized.

Decision Making: More Than a Rational Process

Prenatal consultations with prospective parents, for prematurity and other serious antenatal problems, should move beyond exchanges of medical facts. Narratives have described these processes as complex deliberations between multiple interests, not reliant on medical information alone nor completely rational.[51] Emotions are increasingly recognized in neonatology, bioethics, and decision sciences to be critical for enabling robust decisions.[52] For example, patients often make decision to avoid regret, rather than maximize benefits. Antenatal consultations that exclude discussion of complex emotional and social needs led to decreased parental confidence in decisional outcomes.[53] For decisions of extreme emotional gravity, parents report reliance on intuitive processes[54] and frequently suggest attention to issues other than medical facts, such as the emotional climate and presence of both parents during the consultation.[55]

Decision-science theorists have argued that emotions are beneficial to help decision makers prioritize pertinent issues.[56] Neglecting feelings can inhibit questions, diminishing the ability to gather information and engage in successful patient-physician encounters.[57] Neuroscientific evidence has demonstrated poor decisions when emotions are hampered due to neurologic conditions.[58] Bioethical models of autonomy are calling for physicians to address emotions, thereby assisting patients in considering them when making choices.[59] Personalizing also means acknowledging these affective elements as integral in deliberations.

Certainly for highly complex, intense decisions related to life and death of an infant, disregarding emotions should be avoided. When preterm birth is imminent or inevitable, a multitude of feelings can dominate the parents' minds. Decisions are made as much with the heart as with the brain.[60] It has been suggested that incorporating these emotions, or at least acknowledging them for certain decision makers, leads to increased decisional competence by refining and clarifying moral values and personal priorities.[61] Personalizing information to correspond with a parent's primary concerns and fears, and addressing emotions alongside other nonmedical elements, strengthens relationships, facilitates clarity, and improves the comprehension and application of this information during deliberation.

PARENTAL EXPERIENCE AND CONCERNS

Women at risk of preterm birth report feeling powerless and experience a sense of loss of control.[62] As stated by one: "Uncertainty, it's like vertigo or a precipice. And there is a lot of uncertainty. We don't know when I will deliver. We don't know how I will deliver. We don't know how it will go for the baby. We don't know what awaits the baby after. And we can get surprises, good or bad, for months after that."[63] Furthermore, individual families exist within their own social structure or microcosm, influencing their ability to manage and cope with uncertainty and stress. Although their infant's well-being is generally their primary concern, they bring lived experiences and additional worries related to other children, maternal health, or finances.[64] In addition, each parent may have his or her own separate set of concerns and worries, influencing their personal experience with threatened preterm delivery.

Faced with the possibility of having a premature infant, prospective parents have the task of conceiving a new "parenthood vision."[65] Some may focus on the long-term well-being of their infant, some aspire to become primary decision makers, and/or some want to be caregivers, bathing and singing to their infants. Despite these differences, most parents do not want to assume the role of a bystander.[66] They want to feel like they are "real" parents, invested and present for their infant to the best of their ability.

PERSONALIZING THE AGENDA

In the antenatal consultation, neonatal providers have an opportunity to identify prenatal concerns and offer support. An evolution in consultation approaches has begun favoring a "controlled-improvised" agenda.[67] This contrasts strongly with the traditional physician-driven agenda, focused on conveying standardized medical risk information to all parents, supporting essentially rational decisional processes based on detailed information regarding outcomes. These new models of antenatal consultations favor a parent-driven agenda, and focus on building relationships permitting parental concerns to frame the conversation,[68] helping to diversify, strengthen, and personalize the consultation. Relationships begun in the antenatal consultation have been shown to be important determinants for future adaptation, by decreasing decisional regret and enhancing trust between physicians and parents.[69] Trust in turn improves risk comprehension.[70] Perceptions of risk are not constructed on rational assessments alone; therefore, building relationships and focusing on trust increases the credibility of the informant and the validity of the decision.[71]

RECOMMENDATIONS

Personalizing Conversations with Parents: A Controlled Improvisation Addressing What Matters to Parents

Personalizing conversations is not simple. It requires an assessment of the situation, an understanding of the parent and family, including previous experiences, emotions, and decision-making preferences, and an ability to support parental values and goals of the consultation. Approaching the consultation with an open and flexible mindset is essential; attempts to predict what parents want to discuss before meeting with them could compromise opportunities for a productive exchange. The consultation should not follow a prewritten script or an agenda, such as outcome boxes to tick or percentages to give; however, it can still be structured, for example, by using the SOBPIE[72] framework (Situation, Opinions, Basic politeness, Parents, Information, Emotions). By using the vignette below, the following section will be dedicated to practical recommendations to personalize antenatal consultations for fragile neonates in the gray zone. (Figure 1 summarizes suggestions for guiding the consultation and teaching these skills, incorporating the SOBPIE framework and broadly defining the consultant's role as establishing trust and tailoring information.[73])

Josephine is in premature labor at 23 weeks. She had not planned this pregnancy, but when it happened, she felt it was fate. Her mother had just passed away a year ago, and as her caregiver, she had had a particularly difficult time adjusting. This pregnancy, however, had rejuvenated her spirits. When the contractions had begun she blamed a stomach flu and remained optimistic when

Prenatal Consultation Checklist   Mother's name: _____

___/___/___   ID:_____

Reason for consultation: _____   OB name: _____
☐ Communication with OB team: _____   Joint consultation with OB: ☐ yes ☐ no
Parent told about consultation: ☐ yes ☐ no   Significant person present: _____

Allow enough time / Limit interruptions (phone/pager) / Ensure privacy (# people) / Sit down

Establish trust with parents
☐ Neonatologist introduction / role
☐ NICU team introduction
☐ Ask about the baby
 "Do you have a name?" _____
 "Tell me about your baby"_____
 "Does he/she have siblings?"_____
☐ Ask and Listen to parents' main concerns
 - " What is your greatest fear?"
 - " What is most important to you as a family?"
 - " Is anything worrying you at home or work?"
 - " What do you expect from this consultation?"
 - " What can I do for you?"

Address personalized parental concerns & questions
☐ Ask parents if they prefer statistical data,
  general terms, or both
☐ Discuss potential complications of prematurity
  relevant to them
☐ Explain their role as parents of a premature baby
 - Parental roles: touching, talking, family attachment
 - Baby appearance and behavior
 - Parent as caregiver: feeding/breastfeeding, clothing
 - Parental involvement in future decisions
☐ Explain how the NICU works
 - NICU visit offered ☐yes ☐no date: ___/___/___
 - Allied HCP visit offered ☐yes ☐no

Comments: _____

NICU team members (Name, role):_____

Follow-up
☐ NICU visit done (Date: ___/___/___)
☐ Allied HCPs consulted (Role & date):
 _____

☐ Follow-up visit (ideally) by same neonatologist
 - Date: ___/___/___, GA: _____
☐ Written documents given
  Further comments: _____

Figure 1. Antenatal consultation page 1. HCP, health care professional.

her obstetrician suggested that with a little hydration they might stop. However, her optimism did not last, as her labor has progressed. Instead, she feels alone, anxious, angry, sad, and scared. The obstetrician tells her that she should prepare for the worst: delivering in the next few hours or days. She is alone in the hospital, as the father of the baby is out of the country for his work.

Inarguably, conversations related to life and death of children generally constitute the worst possible moments in a parent's life. No parents want to have this conversation, nor would they ever wish to be in this circumstance. Expectations suddenly and dramatically shift. Although many neonatal providers focus on the management of the unborn infant, prospective parents are also in a process of grieving their pregnancy and their parenthood project.[74] In this situation, they will generally focus on prolonging the pregnancy and stay in the pregnancy phase, as opposed to entering into the "baby phase."[75] Health care providers have to fulfill multiple roles at once; they should display empathy toward the parent and compassion toward the infant within goals of a consultation that may either be known or unknown, and fluctuate between informative and supportive.

All providers, obstetricians, neonatologists, and nurses should take care to deliver the same message after assessing the Situation. We recommend that obstetricians and neonatologists meet to discuss these cases, if only briefly, before the antenatal consultations. This first assessment determines whether a decision needs to be or should be made; for example, if intervention is unlikely or likely to lead to survival. Ideally, the antenatal consultation should include a member of the obstetrics team (staff, resident, or nurse). Conducting consultations in unison promotes trust through continuity and coherence of care. As depicted in figure 1, "establishing trust" is an important element of the antenatal consultation.

Next, Opinions and biases should be recognized by health care providers, taking care to examine the particularities of each consultation (for example, not making decisions based only on GA), with the aim to avoid interpretations of risk and values that would inappropriately frame the conversation or the decision.

Third, providers should practice Basic politeness. To optimize consultations, environmental factors should be considered: making sure to avoid distraction by cell phones and pages, meeting in private locations with a limited number of individuals, staying sensitive to the nature and urgency of the consultation. In some hospitals, distractions are reduced to a minimum because a dedicated team, not responsible for intensive care patients and transport calls, is responsible for these consultations.

Nonmedical people usually do not know what a neonatologist is. Introducing oneself as a "baby doctor/nurse," taking care of babies being born too soon, for example, ensures that Parents understand what neonatologists do.

Some sentences can help to set the stage of a personalized consultation. For example, asking parents:

*Have you been told the baby team would come and speak
to you?*

What were you told?

The answer to these questions can help us understand what
parents have heard from other providers. Josephine may give very
different answers:

*I was sent here from my village. They told me you can do mira-
cles with the smallest babies.*

*The other doctor told me that all babies who are born at
23 weeks either die or are disabled.*

*Are you here to convince me to resuscitate our baby? I don't want
any experiments done on her.*

You are supposed to give me information about small babies.

*I don't want to hear bad things at the moment, I have heard
enough. My baby will survive. She is kicking strong and she
wants to live.*

Asking parents *"Do you have a name?"* enables personalization of the conversation about their child, and understanding the
place of this child in their family. Here too, answers can be drastically different:

Samuel!

She will die; I don't think I want to give her a name.

I don't even know if it is a boy or a girl …

*Me and my husband, we are not sure. We have a James in every
family for generations; we do not know what to do in case he dies.*

*Her name is Amelia; we chose it years ago. We have waited for
Amelia for the past 3 years.*

In our religion, we name children after birth.

Questions such as *"Tell me about Samuel – what do you know about him?"* also help. If there are other children, asking who is taking care of them shows interest in the family unit, providing insights into who the parents are and the context in which they live.

The neonatal provider can also ask parents what their primary concerns are. Questions such as *"What are your concerns?"* may help address misperceptions early on, and help team members understand parental expectations. Certain parents may have already decided on a course of action, so that the goals of the consultation shift from a decision-making deliberation toward one tailored around supporting coping mechanisms, or addressing fears and concerns. Questions such as *"What can I do for you?"* or *"Tell me what you understand"* can help anchor conversations, as do investigations such as *"Do you have any experience with prematurity?"* Answers Josephine will give help us to personalize information and the remainder of the consultation:

> *I don't know what you can do. Can you save my baby? Is my baby going to live? Why is this happening?*

> *My mother died last year. She was very disabled. She had a trach and a G-tube. She was in and out of the hospital constantly. She could not live on her own. Can my baby be this disabled? I don't think I could handle that.*

> *What do parents do in my situation?*

> *I know this is in God's hands. I don't know why this is happening, but I know my mother up there is looking after me; she gave me this gift and I know she will help Lauren survive. She is a fighter and will beat the odds. She is a survivor; do what you have to do to help her.*

> *I don't know. I'm scared. What should I know?*

> *How long will she be in the hospital? Will I be able to see her, hold her, give her my milk, be there?*

Each of these answers would prompt very different responses. Parents generally pay more attention to information addressing their pressing concerns. A question that is often helpful to frame the consultation is *"What are you most scared of?"* Parental answers can be very different:

I don't want her to die.

I am afraid she will be in pain.

What if she survives and is handicapped, and cannot have a normal life? Would this be fair?

Doctor, I want to speak to you just the 2 of us. I just arrived from the airport. I am afraid for Josephine, my wife. We have been going through 6 rounds of IVF. She is not very strong at the moment, physically and emotionally. And she is bleeding more. I am afraid she will die – can she? She wants a transfusion, but should the baby come out? She will choose the baby over her. But I am scared for her. I am not thinking about the baby right now, more about Josephine.

Sometimes one parent is most afraid of death, while the other fears disability the most. Some parents will also have others concerns; some women may face deportation as illegal immigrants; others may be concerned about their potential loss of income, or for the other children at home. Addressing these "extreme" concerns is important. For example, telling a partner that a woman's life is not in danger, or informing parents about how other parents cope with death or disability can help address their strongest fears. Dealing with their strongest fears often helps parents focus on other concerns they may have, or on information the medical team may give them.

Other questions that can also shape consultations include trying to ascertain the level of involvement desired in making decisions and what sorts of information are most useful: *"Some parents want a lot of numbers and information, and others want the big picture; what kind of parent are you?"* Some parents may prefer statistics and numbers, whereas others might not. Some would benefit from decision aids, whereas others may not. Based on qualitative research, most parents want to know about the complications of prematurity for their infant while simultaneously trying to understand how they can contribute as a "NICU parent."[76] You may have to answer questions such as the following:

How can I help my baby?

What can I do for my baby?

Can I touch or hold him?

Can I breastfeed her?

What will she look like? Are the organs all formed?

How will he be fed?

Do I need to bring clothes?

As seen in figure 1, after establishing trust, the antenatal consultation can now focus on tailoring Information toward needs of the parents, individualized for the infant's condition, parental experiences, and goals of consultation. Parents strive for a "scientifically competent and humane medical team":[77] trust is not only engendered by a knowledgeable and expert NICU team, but also by an open and compassionate approach to patient care.[78] Therefore, throughout the consultation, Emotions are important to support. Emotions can help to identify, explore, and construct values but also serve as a vehicle for building relationships. They provide opportunities for empathy, support, and trust between patients and physicians. The following sentence can help address/normalize parental emotions: "*I can see you are angry; many parents feel this way.*" Asking parents if they want the team to leave and come back later is often helpful.

Sometimes, parents do not want to engage in conversations, others do not want to hear about "scary statistics," and others can also cry for a prolonged period. In these cases, it is important for neonatologists to be comfortable with silence and to tolerate it. There is some value in holding space with parents, being there in silence when parents cry, or giving parents time to process their situation or a difficult conversation. It is not rare that, after a period of silence, parents communicate something that is important.

Additionally, it is helpful to inform parents that neonatologists are part of a larger allied health professional team and additional consultation with these professionals can optimize family-centered care. Follow-up visits by neonatologists and allied professionals are strongly encouraged, especially when pregnancies have progressed and the situation has evolved/improved, or when parents and providers are involved in complex decision-making processes.[79]

Lastly, attempts to minimize uncertainty and unexpected events before and after the consultation can help mitigate the stressors caused by threatened preterm birth, such as feelings of powerlessness and the "precipice of uncertainty."[80] Before consultation, parents should be made aware that a neonatology consultation will take place so they can prepare for it. They should know that a neonatal consultation does not mean an imminent delivery. They should also be told when the meeting will occur, so that both parents can be present.[81] Providing parents information about the NICU and how it functions, including written information and prenatal NICU visits, are important steps in preparing parents;[82] they decrease the double shock of meeting their premature baby for the first time while discovering the NICU.[83] Neonatologists should be cognizant of the tone portrayed during the antenatal consultation. Allowing parents to maintain hope for a happy and healthy baby[84] and avoiding overly pessimistic outlooks on prematurity can temper unnecessary worries.[85]

In summary, a personalized approach to antenatal counseling seeks to meet the following objectives: (1) to respond to the stressful experiences of parents at risk for early preterm birth, (2) to address parents' authentic concerns, (3) to avoid creating additional stressors, and (4) to help them make a decision if there is one to be made.

INSTITUTIONAL PRACTICES

Simple institutional practices can encourage personalized antenatal consultations for threatened preterm birth. These include accommodations, such as dedicating one neonatologist to serve

as the antenatal consultant without additional responsibilities
of managing a busy NICU and systematically offering follow-
up NICU visits and consultations with the neonatologist and
allied health professionals including multidisciplinary meetings.
Frequent discussions between obstetricians and neonatologists,
as a team, are also recommended. Parent-centered tools can be
created to teach and support personalized consultations (see
figure 1), and consultation notes should reflect these practices, as
proposed in figure 2.

PERSONALIZED DECISION MAKING

Deciphering preferences in decision making is important. For
many, shared decision making implies that parents want to col-
laborate in decisions with physicians. In theory, clinicians should
learn to discern between parents' informational needs for deliberation and their desires to be involved in making the decision,
broadly defined as "problem solving" and "decision making."[86]
Some parents may want information but not involvement in the
decision, some parents may want both, or some may want neither, relinquishing the entirety of the process and decision to the
medical team.[87] Assumptions about preferred role in decision
making are often misjudged.[88] Evaluations that have surveyed
parents involved in neonatal and pediatric end-of-life decisions
reveal heterogeneity; some prefer sharing the decision with physicians, some prefer making decisions independently, and some
defer to the physician.[89] Decision-making preferences are influenced by age, gender, cultural norms, and specifics related to the
decision.[90] Although those who participate in decision making
for extremely premature infants find psychological short-term
and long-term benefits,[91] excessive information or incorrect
assumptions about decision-making roles may impede decisions
for others.[92]

Problem-solving or deliberation processes not only differ
between decision makers but preferences change with the time
and characteristic of the decision. True risk comprehension inter-
prets objective information with subjective preferences to clarify

Date: __/__/__

Mother's Name: _____
DOB: __/__/__

OB Name: _____
Reason for consultation:
Prematurity   Other

Room nr.: _____
Hosp. ID: _____

BABY
GA: _____ (U/S _____ LMP _____)
Singleton   Twin
EFW: _____ (__/__/__) Gender: _____
ß-methasone __/__/__   __/__/__   __/__/__

MOTHER
Age: _____ G ___ P ___ A ___ Blood Gr: ____
Serol.: _____
Habits: _____

Medications: _____
PMH: _____

OBST. H: _____

CURRENT PREGNANCY
T1 _____
   T1 U/S(__/__/__) _____
T2 _____
   T2 U/S(__/__/__) _____
T3 _____
   T3 U/S(__/__/__) _____

DISCUSSION   Mother   Father
                      OB present: _____
                      Baby's name: _____
Parents' main concerns: _____
Family situation: _____
Information discussed relative to parents' needs:

Other significant: _____
NICU Team: _____

Complications of prematurity   Parental roles
How NICU works

☐ NICU visit offered   Written documentation provided : ☐ yes ☐ no

Follow-up
☐ NICU visit done (Date: __/__/__)
☐ Allied HCPs consulted (Role & date):

Neonatologist Name: _____

☐ Follow-up visit by neonatologist: _____
   Date: __/__/__ , GA: _____

Signature: _____ Date: __/__/__

Figure 2. Antenatal consultation page 2 (parent-centered)

choices leading to decisions consistent with values and beliefs.
It is beyond the scope of this article to explore the multitude of
cognitive biases and behavioral decisional processes that could
potentially impact individual decision making, but it is important

to personalize precisely because each person approaches decisions differently.[93]

A parent's approach to decision making has no relation to her or his ability as a parent. "Good" parents may choose to receive information so as to make decisions, "good" parents may choose to defer decision making to physicians, and "good" parents may choose to receive information alongside medical team recommendations sharing in the decision. And, for other "good" parents, there is no decision to be made; rather, they feel "fate" or God is in control and to suggest a decision may in fact increase their distress. All of these "good" parents make reasonable decision for their infants in a manner consistent with their preferences, frameworks, and beliefs.

SUMMARY

Decisions in the gray zone are complicated. They are reliant on personal viewpoints balancing sanctity of life and quality of life, and reflect preferences for rational and intuitive processes and roles in decision making. Instead of aspiring to achieve mutual consent in shared decision making, physicians should seek to practice personalized decision making. Personalized decision making would take into consideration a parent's preferences for decisional responsibility and deliberation and thereby informational and supportive needs. When relationships are built based on personalization, parents are empowered. For decisions of this magnitude and complexity, any decision made by a parent or physician is one they never hoped to make. Parents and physicians try to make the best decision possible on behalf of fragile neonates under very difficult circumstances. Good clinical practice is contingent on both adequate clinical knowledge and support from compassionate, human interactions between physicians and patients. A good outcome for the antenatal consultation is a successful interaction in which parents frame the consultation and are empowered by support and resources to participate in problem solving or decision making to the extent with which they are comfortable.

part two

THE DELIVERY AND THE FIRST DAYS

The Delivery

Violette was born at 5:21 a.m. in Operating Room 1 at the Royal Victoria Hospital in Montreal. A room that looks like so many operating rooms: too cold, highly impersonal, brightly lit. In some places, they call this an operating theatre, with the OR fluorescent blue light pointing to the main actor and to the precise spot where all the action was focused: my *tsouin-tsouin*. Whether there was to be a caesarean section or not, all the sick babies were delivered in that room, as the resuscitation room was adjacent to it. The "resusc" room was overheated so that babies didn't drop their temperature. Dropping temperature is a big concern when tiny babies come out. Their little bodies are wrapped in a plastic bag or under plastic wrap in order to keep their temperature stable.

I remembered three months back, when I was 12 weeks pregnant, nauseated and on call, that I had been urgently woken up at 3 a.m. because a 25-week baby was about to be born. After driving madly through red lights and arriving on time, I felt sick. The mother who was delivering had fulminant chorioamnionitis (a uterine infection) and the smell in the OR was not pretty. I took the baby to the resusc room. The baby stank, a tiny stink bomb, the whole resusc sauna room stank of old diapers and septic tanks. Her heart rate was not coming up with only the bag and mask. I needed to intubate her (place a tube down her throat into her windpipe). I was gagging while I was intubating this poor little girl, but managed to intubate her quickly. Thankfully I had a mask on. The junior resident asked what he could do, with both his eyebrows raised. I hadn't worked with him before. He was still showing me what the heart rate of the baby was, and his finger was going up and down, but I guess he did not know the protocol for dealing with barfing staff, which list to check, how to assist. When the baby was stable, I asked the resident for some ice. As the main assistant for the resuscitation, he ran out to get some. I am sure he did not know why we needed ice, since we were supposed to keep the baby warm. When he returned, I asked him to place some of the ice in a plastic bag on my head. I felt like I would pass out. This baby did well, though. She was still on the unit weeks later, learning to feed, while I was pushing.

Why was I remembering this baby while I myself was giving birth? I have often tried to understand why over the years. Maybe because I thought my situation was slightly better: I did not stink, plus my physician was not about to puke on my baby. Or maybe because I wanted to vomit with despair. Or maybe because I wanted to remind myself I was not only a failing vessel, a broken belly, the owner of an "incompetent cervix"; I was a strong physician who could intubate a tiny baby in under thirty seconds while puking in her mask. Or maybe because I wanted to think about this pretty little girl who was doing well, in our hospital, with the same care Violette would have, her little preemie-roommate.

Axel had been born by Caesarean section, but Violette used the good old "natural route" at a highly unnatural time. So many people were around, but at that moment there could have been a TV crew, a clown, a deep-sea diver, cows, whatever, and I don't think I would have reacted. I wasn't supposed to be there. Why not another day, week, hour?? Why had I turned around in bed a week before, when my waters broke? That was a huge mistake. This is all a mistake, I wanted to scream. This is not happening. This cannot be my life. This is my husband next to me, with so much love in his eyes, so much despair, and so much hope. I realized it was really happening. When Axel was born, I couldn't successfully push him out of me. I thought this would be easier. How can a 700g baby be tough to push out? Well, it was not easy. I think I pushed hard, but my OB seemed not to think so. The whole team was counting, encouraging, telling me this was serious. Maybe I was not pushing because I did not want her to come out. This was NOT a happy moment; this was one of the worse moments of my life. This was failure. A big maternal blaaaaaaaaaaah in broad florescent light for everybody to see. I felt her coming out, heard a little cry and closed my eyes. I saw Gene right there, our great colleague who was a neonatal fellow at the time. I knew Violette was well taken care of. He took her into the resuscitation room. Keith and I both knew what was happening out there. At least Gene was not vomiting and asking for ice. He intubated her when she was stable, gave her surfactant to open up her lungs and took her to the NICU. She needed only room air to breathe, 21 per cent oxygen, what healthy human beings need. I did not want to see her. I wanted to disappear. I wanted to be alone.

Keith went to collect Axel from my mom's place, and I was taken to the prenatal ward. I was so grateful to go there. I had been in the team recommending that all mothers of very sick babies be admitted there after birth, so they did not have to be exposed to the bright balloons, the damned joy and happiness of the other mothers, the first meconiums, the crying full-term monsters, and the chattering, smiling, noisy relatives. I was with the waiting ones and the sick ones. It was silent. I went to sleep.

May 22nd. This is the day I learned the definition of emptiness. I did not feel pain, sad emotions. I felt nothing – such a big black hole, a void. I was empty; nothing had any meaning. I learned the definition of nothing, of meaninglessness, the meaning of meaninglessness.

A mother who is really a mother is never free.

Honoré de Balzac

22 May 2005

5:40 a.m.: Baby admitted to intensive care. In a plastic bag. Intubated in the delivery room by Gene Dempsey, ventilated by Dr Willis. Surfactant given in the delivery room. Baby pink, endotracheal tube connected to Babylog. R: 60 X 11/4, O^2 50 % then RA in 5 minutes. To = 37.5oC …

Weight in NICU: 730 g.

Father arrived 10 minutes after birth.

6:10 a.m.: Catheters (UVL and UAL) inserted and fixed by Gene Dempsey, blood taken for cultures, CBG, CBC, blood group, gluco. Chest and abdo XRay: position of catheters OK. Gluco 3.5. $TcpCO^2$: 54. Eyes fused: erythromycin not given.

Memories from Gene Dempsey

The call came sometime around 4.30 a.m. This was a call I had been expecting, but was not welcome. It was Keith on the phone, and I am not sure exactly what he said but I knew what was about to happen. I got up, dressed quickly, my wife saying very little other than hoping for the best for all. I felt guilty as I left my 5-week-old newborn girl lying in her crib sleeping soundly.

I walked across the rugby pitch over to the hospital. This was a walk I had made thousands of times before, but this was different. Very different. Much quicker and with a great deal of purpose, reminding myself along the way of how to look after little babies, as if I had been doing it only for the past few weeks. The only problem was that this was not any other little baby; this was the baby of two close friends and colleagues who had looked after my wife and I for the past three years. There is nothing in the Neonatal Resuscitating Program about how to do that. Sure, follow the algorithm, and so on, but this was different. I met Lucie, the obstetrician, at the main door of the hospital; very little was said, other than a nod to each other and a mutual appreciation that neither of us wanted to be here. I went and dressed, and prepared the resuscitation room for all eventualities. I looked in to see where things were and how things were progressing.

It was all a bit surreal, Keith sitting there as the "dad-to-be" of a 24-week baby, and Annie about to deliver a baby at 24 weeks' gestation.

I could hardly believe it. I had been in the same room myself (where Keith sat) almost six weeks earlier, but our baby was seventeen weeks later in gestation (41-plus weeks and refusing to come!), and it was a really joyous affair. This was not. Guilt felt again.

I waited inside the resuscitation room as the contractions went on. Then I heard screams and knew the baby was coming. These were screams that have stayed with me. These screams were followed by a weak little cry, her opening address to this world. Violette was here, and lots of people's lives changed instantly. Significant uncertainty lay ahead. We brought her to the resuscitation room, all 670 grams of her. She was spontaneously breathing, with some recession. She was active, pink; we gave her peep (positive airway pressure) and then electively intubated her. It was all technically very straightforward – a single attempt, right nares, surfactant administered, tube secured. Annie used to joke about how fast she could intubate, but I beat her record that night! Keith waited inside with her.

We brought Violette to the NICU. It was all very strange and extremely quiet in the unit. The nurses were ready for her, but did not know what lay ahead. I set the respirator, and her settings were relatively low in room air. I think I had annoyed the respiratory therapists for the three years I was there, but there was no point in attempting to change now. I went about preparing for her central line insertion, and also preparing myself for Keith and Annie coming over. What does one say? Congratulations? Hardly. Sorry? Hardly.

Keith arrived on his own. He looked in shock. Violette was in the upper section of the ICU, in the second bed on the left. This was the bed in which I first intubated a baby in the unit under Keith's supervision. We stood there often on ward rounds listening to Keith pontificate about the evidence for one intervention over another, and now I stood there about to talk to him about his 24-week baby. I felt extremely sorry for both of them. How would they cope with this irony of all ironies? Keith, head full of up-to-date evidence, short- and long-term outcome data, now has to contend with an n of 1 – his n of 1.

Very little is said, a hug is given, a chair to sit on. A long silence, tears. A hand on the shoulder. "Things will be OK" is what I recall saying. There was no evidence whatsoever to support this statement. "Tell Annie we are thinking about her." "Head on back and we will put the lines in." Keith headed back to Annie, and I went ahead and placed the central lines. The first hour went very well, the baby was female, the weight was OK, and steroids had been given, so perhaps the subconscious "things will be ok" had some evidence to support the sentiment. We spend years training in neonatology to look after newborn infants, and we must remember it is a privilege to look after newborns and their families at difficult times. It was a privilege to care for Violette.

Gene

22 May 2005
10:50 a.m.: Extubated by Dr Sophie N. NIMV: 20 x 15/5. Mom came to visit, saw Violette extubated. TcpCO^2: 53. Bradycardia ad 50, need for stimulation 2+.

23 May

Violette's corrected gestational age: 24 weeks, 6 days

Dear Computer,

Yesterday when I saw Violette, I burst into tears. I was shocked. The same sensation I had when I was 14 and flubbed an acrobatic dive from the five-metre platform and hit the water with my back: the blackout, the hot flash, the acid taste; shaken, broken, dizzy, the wind knocked out of me. This time, there wasn't only the physical pain, there was a violent emotional pain. And I couldn't swim to the side of the pool to catch my breath.

It's hard to see Violette like that, but I have to "woman up" and not fall apart this morning the way I did before. Plus, it's really great – Violette has been extubated! She no longer has a tube in her trachea. Her lungs are working. She only has tubes in her nostrils to help her to inhale and push the air out, but she's breathing on her own, even though she often pauses. These are the apneas of a premature baby. It's normal, but … And all the sharp decreases in her heart rate at the same time, bradycardias. I know that too is normal for a 24-week baby, but she does it a lot.

Things will be okay!

23 May 2005

6:15 p.m.: Neonatologist on duty. BB reintubated because of +++ apneas and bradys. Atropine fentanyl mivacurium per protocol. Intubation right nostril,

1st attempt 15 seconds, no desaturation. Endotracheal tube fixed 7 cm. Pulmonary RX pending.

Sophie N.

24 May

Days of life: 3

Violette's corrected gestational age: 25 weeks

Dammit, Computer, NO!

Holy fucking shit. It didn't work. Violette's lungs are working but she had pauses too often, having too many apneas. With each apea, the oxygen level in her blood drops and her heartbeat slows. It's all very well that Keith is the expert on apnea in premature babies, but I shouldn't have assumed that would help Violette. A ladder, then a goddamn snake. Sophie put the tube back in right away. I love her. Here we go again on the respirator – we'll just have to deal with it.

Finally, Lorraine and Debbie are Violette's primary nurses, the ones assigned to her while she's in the hospital. When either one of them is working, she'll always be caring for Violette. WOW! We met with the head nurse, who told us that a lot of the nurses, about a third of them, have asked not to take care of Violette ... Dr Janvier and Dr Barrington's baby scares them. Maybe not the baby, but the parents. I understand, but I'm not very frightening. I'm not the Annie they've known. Do I even look like a doctor?

Debbie and Lorraine are "matrons" in the NICU, the lionesses of preemies. Nurses who don't shrink from challenges, who've seen it all, and who know their "primary" baby. If they say they're worried about a baby, it means things are going to go badly. They have a sixth sense, a magical intuition. They also know how to stand up to doctors. Residents had better not try to show off with them. Maybe that's why they're Violette's primary nurses. When they say they don't think a baby is ready to be taken off the respirator, you'd better listen. They won't have to fight too hard with me. But they're going to keep away the students and residents who want to examine Violette for no good reason, and they'll make sure no one draws blood just when she's sleeping soundly.

Good news after the reintubation. Sigh of relief!

Half Mother at Home

Violette was born at 24 weeks, 5 days. Twenty-four hours later, I was discharged from the hospital, impatient to go home to be with my little prince again. I felt both relieved and guilty. Empty, too. A part of myself amputated, still in the NICU. I felt like a deserter, like a mother who had abandoned her child. A mother who was torn. I wanted to take Axel in my arms, give him a big hug, and tell him that his *maman* wouldn't leave him again for a very long time. Axel was 2 years old and had reacted to my extended absence.

As a doctor, I knew very well that ten days is not long. A lot of mothers have to stay in the hospital longer. But I felt as if I had been there a lot more than ten days. It seemed like a whole month. The only consolation I had after the birth was seeing my prince again, something that mothers with their first child in the NICU don't have. Who is waiting for them at home? Their bathtub, their shower, their fridge, their bed? I was lucky to have Axel. Going back to my little routines with him revived what was still healthy in my mind. I couldn't stop bringing food to the table and eating with Keith, James, and Axel. Changing diapers, singing him lullabies at bedtime, washing his sheets and our clothes.

Axel couldn't really understand why his mom had been away, or why a baby would want to be born too early. We couldn't either, as a matter of fact. He already had his *Baby Bunny Was Born Too Small*, a little colouring book published by Préma-Québec. It deals with a lot of subjects that help brothers and sisters adjust to new routines, and it's really very good; Daddy and Mommy rabbit frown; Mommy rabbit has to pump her milk; Daddy rabbit has to take the milk to the hospital. To Axel, it was only a book. He didn't understand why his mom wasn't there, and, when I'd leave for the hospital, he would ask when I was going to come back. I didn't know myself when I would return, or in what state of mind. What had happened to Annie the fighter, the bulldozer, the leader, the chief organizer, the camp counsellor? I felt like a drugged mouse, paralysed under the lights of the lab, unable to move, gripped by fear.

I was going back to my 24-week baby in the NICU. During my medical training and my PhD studies, no one had taught me about this devastation. We learned about the shock, but not the fact that, after an ordeal like that, you were never the same, you lost yourself. This reality was broached neither in med school nor during my residency nor during my fellowship nor in any of the complicated books I've read on ethics or neonatology. And yet there are research and articles on all kinds of traumatic experiences, which I discovered years after Violette's birth. One of the researchers working on this subject has become a friend. Peter Ubel studies patients who are in wheelchairs or disabled after an amputation, a transplant, or a colostomy (a surgical procedure that leaves the patient with a bag outside the abdomen that collects the stool). He investigates how people perceive their future quality of life immediately after the accident or intervention, and for years afterwards. At first, they are usually very pessimistic; they don't know that their quality of life may turn out to be very good. They completely underestimate their strength and their capacity to recover and be happy. In 2005, I would really have liked to be reassured. Someone should have told me that it's entirely possible to get back on your feet, to rediscover yourself, to redefine your goals and your vision, to rewrite your unfinished story. That the upheaval was normal. That even though it was impossible to imagine, things were going to get better. That it wouldn't always be like this.

Eighteen years of university and nothing on that, even though I was going to spend the rest of my life with devastated parents. "At least university costs less there than in the United States," my American colleagues tell me after my lectures. "No one gave us any detailed information on that either, and it cost us $40,000 a year not to learn it."

The very fact that you worry about being a good mom means that you already are one.

Jodie Picoult

26 May

Days of life: 5

Violette's corrected gestational age: 25 weeks, 2 days

---

26 May 2005
3 p.m.: PICC line inserted, 28F after topical EMLA + sucrose. Inserted first try right brachiocephalic vein. Measured at 8.5 cm, withdrawn to 7.5 cm after RX.

Dear Computer,

So cool! I've just received a huge bag of gummy bears from Catherine, one of my best friends, directly from Boston, where she is doing her fellowship. There are only red, white, and green bears. She knows that the horrible yellow and orange ones have no business being there; someone should tell them not to make them anymore. She must have performed a gummy-bear-ectomy, an excision of the yellow and orange ones. What did she do with them? Did she give them to some unsuspecting person? Or worse, did she eat them? Eww! I stuffed my face like a real pig.

Violette weighs only 655 grams. I know it's normal to lose weight in the first days of life, but still. She now has a catheter in her arm, and they've taken out the one in the vein in her umbilicus. Plus, I've held her in my arms, and it wasn't as bad as the other times. Holding a baby skin to skin, as I held Violette on my chest, is called "kangaroo care." In the sense of putting Violette in my pouch, not of jumping like a kangaroo. I don't like it much, but that will probably come with time, when her heart stops slowing down so often. Debbie and Lorraine are pushing hard for kangaroo care. The nurses here really believe in it and support parents when they do it. Thirty minutes is the minimum time you can hold a baby on a respirator, like Violette, because it takes a lot of fussing about to organize a fragile baby on the parent, taping the tubes so that everything's held in place and safe. I do my thirty minutes. I force myself; I can't do more now. Keith, my hero, does it two and sometimes even three times. I'm REALLY stressed during kangaroo. With my eyes closed, I count to "sixty Mississippi" thirty times. So that I won't lose count, I focus on each finger in turn for a minute, then one toe, that makes twenty minutes, and then I know that I only have the two hands again and then it's over, YES! My new challenge is not to look at the clock, just to count to sixty, thirty times. I keep being disturbed because Violette is desaturating† and her heart is slowing down, so they stimulate her and check the tube and everything, and I open my eyes so I don't seem rude. I pretend all is OK, but I mustn't look at the clock.

I haven't told anyone this! There are so many moms who seem to love it, and I don't. Today, someone said to me, "Wow, I thought you were sleeping, you were so relaxed, I didn't dare wake you. That makes exactly thirty minutes that you've been calm like that." Oh yeah, thirty minutes? I really need to pee, could we put Violette back in her isolette? I should have gone into acting.

---

† The saturation is the amount of oxygen in the blood. When a baby desaturates, it means she does not have enough oxygen in her blood. When the desaturation is serious, the heart rate of the baby slows down, which is called a bradycardia.

30 May

Days of life: 9

Violette's corrected gestational age: 26 weeks

Computer,

Twenty-six weeks. Violette has regained her birth weight. The second ultrasound of her head is normal. A little party all by myself. Bravo, bravo. Hurrah! All we need now is for her to stop her acting up on the respirator. She tolerates a little milk, but has frequent desaturations, low blood oxygen levels. Then her heart slows down a lot: this is called a bradycardia when it slows down too much. She constantly has apneas, which means she stops breathing, which is normal for preterm infants: they do not have a mature "pacemaker" in their heads to drive breathing. She's the queen of apnea-bradys. She suddenly turns purplish blue and has to be stimulated. Not cool. But I know that's part of the game. I know it with my head. I go nuts when her heart rate slows down. I close my eyes, I hold my breath. MY heart speeds up.

Also, I forgot to tell you, about her name. When I was on bed rest, some nurses came to offer encouragement. Some of them raised questions about Violette's name – not the best one when you're at risk of turning purple all the time. Wouldn't Rose be better? I hadn't thought of that. I said, "Whatever. We'll call her Violette Rose, if that'll help." And they took me at my word! The name written on her incubator is Violette Rose. It sounds like a colour of bubble gum, with sparking unicorns on the package, but I said to myself, that's the way it is. I'm not in the mood to fight. Besides, maybe I'll jinx her if I take off the "Rose," who knows? She has enough blue and violet in her life as it is; more pink would be good for everyone.

31 May 2005

Second course of indomethacin started. Increase ++ of As+Bs. Transfusion 20 ml/kg. Blood culture r/o infection, cefo-genta started.

3 June

Days of life: 13

Violette's corrected gestational age: 26 weeks, 3 days

Computer,

Keith and I have just received the violets we ordered when Violette was a week old. We went to a little basement jewellery store on Saint-Denis Street, and we asked the jeweller to make us two pendants shaped like violets, with mini-amethysts. Maybe they look like violets only to us. We're not going to take them off. They're like a talisman, a good luck charm, a *gris-gris*, even though I know that the violet stones around my neck won't ward anything off. It's nice we're both wearing the same thing. And our Violette is in both our hearts.

We're going to need those talismans. Violette is again on antibiotics for a probable infection, and her ductus arteriosus, an open structure in her heart, doesn't want to close. For the third time, she's on a medication that's supposed to close it. She's still winning the bradycardia competition, although she's intubated.

One thing that's going well is food. She's digesting my milk well. She still needs her intravenous, but not for long anymore.

However, I feel pretty useless at gavage feeding. Here, it's the parents who give the feedings when they're around. Gavage, you're probably thinking, sounds like the force feeding of geese and ducks. Not at all! In gavage feeding, or tube feeding, the milk is administered directly to Violette's stomach using a little tube inserted through her mouth. Or sometimes through her nose. Since she can't eat on her own from a baby bottle or at the breast, it's the only way to give her milk. Anyway, my milk is put into a syringe, and there's not a lot of it: 6 ml now, almost half a tablespoon. You have to give the contents of the syringe over about fifteen minutes.

I have trouble doing it, but the parents around me manage it. Nothing difficult about it. Why am I having a hard time? It seems to me it's not a parent's job. It's a medical thing to me and has nothing to do with my being a parent. But that's my hang-up. And maybe it's by caring for your baby that you gain parenting experience. I told Debbie I'd rather have her do it. She said, "Oh, come on!" but she gave the feeding. That's cool. I just have to make sure I come between feedings, but it's hard – Violette feeds every two hours, and now the nurses wait for me so that I can give the feeding. Maybe I should just come right out and tell them it's not my thing. What will they think? Unless I change my mind.

6 June

Days of life: 16

Violette's corrected gestational age: 26 weeks, 6 days

Dear Computer,

It's so easy to type in this position. What a relief! Although I had become an expert in using a laptop in the Trendelenburg position.

Violette's prematurity, as I said, occurred because of the incompetence of my cervix. Axel's premature birth was caused by an infection and pre-eclampsia. Why the infection, the pre-eclampsia, the cervix that doesn't work? I know very well that, most of the time, prematurity happens just like that, for no apparent reason. Almost every time, it's nature that goes awry, and that's why premature birth occurs. Very rarely, it's because, for example, the mother consumed cocaine. Sometimes, doctors implant more than one embryo during in vitro fertilization, even though they know that 50 per cent of twins are born prematurely. In short, it's nature that screws up, sometimes the doctors, almost never the mothers.

So I mustn't feel guilty, since it's nature's fault. I mustn't feel guilty. I mustn't feel guilty. I mustn't feel guilty. I mustn't feel guilty. I mustn't feel guilty. I mustn't feel guilty. I mustn't feel guilty. I mustn't feel guilty. I mustn't feel guilty. I repeat this mantra to myself, choking on my sobs, tears blurring my glasses. If I keep repeating it, will I eventually believe it?

"Madam, the prematurity was caused by the incompetence of the cervix." It's not me who's incompetent, it's only my body, my cervix, the barrier that was supposed to keep my baby inside. For years I've been telling women it's not their fault. One of my patients blamed her new liquid detergent: "An energizing detergent, that doesn't sound harmless, and I've been doing a lot of dishes lately." Many mothers believe it's because of sexual relations – but I've never heard a man blame sex. I've heard a father suggest that it was because of a decrease in sexual relations: "Her cervix was used to daily exercise; maybe it got soft out of laziness." I've heard everything. "It's because I did thirty minutes a day on the Stairmaster, it was too much!" "It's because I didn't do enough exercise." "It's because of that corn roast that made me go to the toilet so often." "It's because of constipation; when I'm pregnant, I get constipated, and when I go to the toilet, I push too hard." Women generally feel guilty if their pregnancy doesn't go perfectly or if something happens to their child.

When a woman comes to me, or I meet her next to her baby, the first thing I tell her, as a doctor, is "There is nothing you could have done to prevent what happened." Life is like a lottery. Some mothers will have miscarriages, others breast cancer or a car accident. In the baby lottery, we encounter premature births, birth defects, asphyxia, infections, and many other things – a life that begins with an accident of nature, with getting dealt a bad hand. However, you can still win the game. It wasn't the mother who chose the cards; it was nature. Some people believe it's God himself who visits those ordeals on families. Why do people who believe in God think Him capable of doing such things to children? Sometimes nature is a real bitch. God too, maybe. But I can't tell families that.

However, Computer, I'm sure that, for me, there must be a reason. There has to be a reason in my case. It is absolutely necessary that this situation have a meaning, so that I can change it, so I can understand it. To plan better, to be better organized. To finally answer the questions "and if I had …?" "why didn't I …?" and "shouldn't I have …?" I keep replaying the movie of the week before Violette's birth. I see at least twenty things I should have done differently. Would all that, put together, have changed her story?

Did I need all that? Why me? I believed I had already proven to the world, to nature, to the cosmos, to all possible and impossible gods, saints, and angels that my body and my mind were strong. I thought I could get through my pregnancies as I have overcome obstacles, with determination. Since I was little, I've wanted four children; so is that dream now no longer possible? I had already planned four chapters of my book on my four perfect pregnancies, chapters in which I was the hero, an adorable wonder woman in my sexy little maternity dress with boots. After my divorce, I had even considered artificial insemination if I didn't find the man I needed (and who would put up with me). That was Plan B. Artificial insemination, or even natural insemination on "day 14," with the help of a guy who was a virgin so I wouldn't catch any diseases. And if my soulmate came along too late in my life, there was always in vitro fertilization. That was Plan C. But prematurity? Me? What an idiot! I never thought it could happen to me, and it's my job to know that it can happen to anyone. Really pathetic.

I remember saying, when I was doing my residency, that if I had to give birth to a premature baby some day, I would go into the woods to do it. Goddamn imbecile! Other health professionals also say this kind of idiotic thing. Yeah, sure! Nature is now putting me in my place with a nasty laugh: "So you didn't go into the woods after all? You did it in a university hospital near Mount Royal ... Not so far from the woods after all, eh, smarty pants?" How can health professionals say such stupid things? In Quebec 8 per cent of births are premature, and there are no births in the woods, or almost none. Sometimes in taxis or toilets (and the mothers don't do it on purpose), but not in the woods.

But then, Computer, why me? I have to find the answer to this question. I don't believe in a supreme test that's supposed to make me grow. Some people think that's what these things are. I often think about that. I know that not all dreams can be fulfilled, that not everything is possible. I know that positive vibrations and smiles are not necessarily going to save us. I know that sometimes we feel ridiculous and powerless when we roll up our sleeves and put on a Botox smile in the face of an inevitable death. I know that a positive attitude alone cannot heal cancer: surgery, radiation, and toxic drugs take care of the rest. During my dad's long, painful dying, I learned that the impossible is sometimes our lot in life. That even when you really want something, sometimes you just can't have it. That even if you're always optimistic, there are things that are lost, marriages that break up, and cancers that continue to grow. I know that by trying to catch a star, you sometimes don't get anything but sore arms. And the stars stay where they are, inaccessible. That people who've died of cancer don't make the news and don't take part in pink marches. That only the "positive" survivors get a spot on the podium. I already know all that.

But most of all, why does Violette have to go through all this? I'm in the habit of facing adversity head-on, with an unbeatable plan, an appropriate action, a structured, arrogant response, while giving the finger. When Violette was born, my miniature flower, the nurses and the doctor offered me their "congratulations," and that killed me. If the father drops the baby on a tile floor, do they congratulate him too? Congratulations for what? For a screwed-up cervix? I'm obsessed with "what if I had …?" and "what should I have done?"

And more than anything, Computer, I'm afraid to go see Violette. That's pathetic for a neonatologist. Even more for a mother. I'm afraid something will happen. I didn't want to see her immediately after her birth. I wanted to crawl under my bed and wake up twelve months later; I wanted to climb aboard a rocket with my 2-year-old son and my husband and go hide in a cosmic cocoon and come back when the earth stopped shaking under my feet. I was afraid of going to the NICU to face the daughter I had brought into the world much too early. I knew what a "24 weeker" looks like – I see enough of them in my work. And I didn't want to see my 24-week baby, all the time knowing it's not cool to think like that, that she's not a generic baby, she's mine. That can't be my baby – look at her all red and translucent, with jellied raw skin! How could I have done such a thing to her? What would it have been humanly possible to do to prevent all this?

Computer, I know everything mothers can invent to blame themselves for in the case of a premature birth. I know those reasons have no scientific basis. But I know that only in my head. And my head refuses to connect with my heart, with my gut, with every fibre and every cell of my being. That's what I feel. And I keep telling myself there must be a reason for all this. I have to find that reason in order to know what to do now, to move on.

7 June

Days of life: 17

Violette's corrected gestational age: 27 weeks

Computer,

It would have been so cool if I'd been able to give birth today: 27 weeks, wow!

Violette no longer has a PICC line today, a good thing, another little party. A PICC line is peripheral intravenous central catheter, an intravenous catheter that can stay in place for a long time, because it rarely gets blocked. It's a miniature tube, the thickness of vermicelli, that is inserted in a small vein and then advanced up into one of the larger veins of the body. It is not easy to insert. It was Gene who inserted Violette's PICC.

Even with her status of queen of the tummy, Violette is still on the podium for the apnea and bradys – she has the gold medal on the unit. Her heart slows down constantly to punish her dad for doing so much research on the respiratory drive and apneas. It's driving him crazy. At least Keith checks everything, all the lab tests, the X-rays, the feedings, makes sure Violette has her sucrose before they prick her. I love him so much! He says he's only the dad, but he can't help it – he does it on the sly. He's a great doctor, a wonderful dad, and the best lover in the world. He doesn't back down, and he looks like he means business. He's the king, and he keeps his eye on his princess, her X-rays, and the weather.

I'm just pretending. I don't want to know anything. When they try to tell me the number of bradys, desaturations, grams, millilitres, the sodium levels, I feel like covering my ears, closing my eyes, and screaming "aaaaaaaaaaaaaaaaaaaaaaaaaaaahhhhh!" Do what needs to be done, don't tell me any numbers. I'm just here and I'm doing what I can!

10 June

Days of life: 21

Violette's corrected gestational age: 27 weeks, 4 days

---

 22 h 50: Serious deterioration this p.m.: distended abdomen, increase in
O2 needs, ++ desaturations. Good AE bilateral, no murmur. Resp acidosis: pH 7.05 CO2 : 107 … increase in resp parameters? Pneumonia
on CXR vs atelectasis. Plan: NPO, continue ATB, monitor, follow ABG …
Father here, aware of the situation.

We must accept finite disappointment, but never lose infinite hope.

Martin Luther King Jr

11 June

Dear Computer,

Violette stopped eating yesterday. It may be pneumonia. That slows down her intestines. Antibiotics again. The intravenous lines are difficult – they may put back the PICC line, which they took out yesterday. Almost back to square one: she's again today taking tiny quantities of milk, and I'm going to have even more milk to freeze. I'm trying to stay positive. She weighs more than 1,000 g today, finally. That's one good thing. She's growing.

I'm trying to pump my milk and type at the same time. I'm going to explain to you why I'm pumping my milk, so I'll sound a little more like a doctor again and not just a pseudo-nursing mother. A baby like Violette cannot nurse at the breast. Not only because she has a tube down her throat and her trachea (windpipe) to help her breathe, but also because she hasn't developed a baby's reflexes that would permit her to feed at my breast without danger. When you swallow, you don't need to think that you have to stop breathing and you don't have to retract your tongue so you don't spit up your food. It's automatic. But Violette's nervous system isn't developed enough for that. It isn't enough for her to even breathe regularly. That "wiring" develops near the end of pregnancy. There are 34-week babies who can't take the breast either, even if they're in relatively good health. So Violette has to be fed with a naso-gastric tube or oro-gastric tube, which is inserted into one of her nostrils or her mouth and goes down to her stomach, into which the milk is deposited very gently. There are things she can do, such as suck on her soother and digest my milk. And her little belly is functioning well in general, which makes me happy. This is not the case for all babies. Babies like Violette have to be fed through their veins at birth. Milk is introduced in the belly in small quantities, which are gradually increased while decreasing the liquid nutrition the child is given intravenously through the PICC line. The fact that she tolerates my milk is very good news. The faster we can eliminate the intravenous, the better. With the central line there's a high risk of infection, and babies like Violette are not very good at fighting off infections.

I still consider myself lucky in at least one thing. Thanks to my milk, I'm helping her grow. I'm providing her with antibodies, lactoferrin, and all kinds of good things. It seems I still have girl things that work. I can do something for her. Well, less now that she barely eats.

I had intended to give Violette my milk for the first six months from the day she was supposed to be born, to be fair to Axel, whom I nursed for six months. But she was born four months too early. A disaster! I'll have to pump my milk for ten months, or hope that she takes the breast at some point! In medical language, we say "express" the milk, but we mothers speak more often of "pumping" our milk. It's more realistic. It would be a real disaster if I would have to stop pumping my milk tomorrow, because she wouldn't survive, but shit, I don't want to think about that all the time. You have to have hope. When babies die in intensive care, it's usually in the first two weeks of their lives; 70 per cent of deaths occur quite early. But even when the risks are lower, death is always lying in wait. Violette has made it to two weeks. Breathe in, breathe out.

I've given my breast pump a name. Since I have to share my life with that plastic thing, I might as well give it a little humanity. So I christened it Big Bertha, or *Dicke Bertha*, the nickname the Germans gave to a very powerful howitzer during the First World War. Big Bertha was also the name of a cow that held two Guinness records for milk production; she lived for fifty-nine years, which is a very long time for a cow, and bore thirty-nine calves. And she helped raise $75,000 for cancer research and various other causes. She died in 1993. So Big Bertha was both a powerful gun and an incredible cow. When I'm getting ready to pump my milk, I change into either a sadistic German war criminal or a proud farm woman who owns a super-cow. I act like an idiot and say things like "Ich muss jetzt pumpen" (I have to pump now) or "Bertha, Dicke Bertha, mein Schatzi, wo bist du?" (Bertha, big Bertha, my treasure, where are you?) or go "Moo, moo!"

13 June

Days of life: 23

Violette's corrected gestational age: 27 weeks, 6 days

 13 June 2005
3 p.m.: PICC line inserted, 28F after topical EMLA + Sucrose. Inserted
first try right brachiocephalic vein. Measured at 8.5 cm, withdrawn to
7.5 cm after RX.

Gene Dempsey

Computer,

I'm still pumping my milk while typing. I've pretty much had it. Violette
is on her third central line, and her third intubation. Today, she lost her
breathing tube. I don't know how she managed that. To be positive, I told
myself that it might be time to consider what she can do extubated – that
is, without the goddamn tube. Failure.

I'm a control freak, but I really have no control. I absolutely must control the damn milk pump, since I don't have control over much else. I am
the master; the pump is the slave. I can organize at least something for
Violette. I've always been an organizer, a maniac for lists. I devour Post-it
Notes. I made my first list when I was 10. The first item was "Make a list,"
which I crossed out as soon as the list was completed. I thought that was
pretty clever. Before I had Violette, my lists were impressive: organize

the summer vacation, plan the family weekend, write an article, prepare a three-hour class, write a lecture, freeze a whole month's worth of
lunches, schedule a follow-up ultrasound for my neck, plan my mother's
birthday, make an appointment for my Pap test, and so on. Now my lists
are simpler. Yesterday's, for example:

> **Pump** (7 a.m.)
> Wake up (I'm not joking – it was really on my list yesterday.
>   Sometimes, I pump without waking up, believe it or not.)
> Take a shower
> Make coffee
> Make toast
> Wake Axel
> Change Axel's diaper
> Dress Axel
> Take Axel to day care
> **Pump**
> Sit with Violette
> Go to the office (1 p.m.): check email and write articles
> **Pump**
> Be with Violette
> Eat
> Kangaroo with Violette
> **Pump**
> Go see Violette
> Fiddle around in the office for an hour
> Pick up Axel at day care
> Make supper
> Eat
> Take a bath with Axel
> **Pump** while Keith reads to Axel
> Put Axel to bed (with Keith)
> Watch *The Thin Blue Line* with Keith (and drink as little wine
>   as possible)
> Play Rummikub (win)
> **Pump** (while Keith goes to see Violette in the NICU)
> Set the alarm for 4 a.m. to pump

Try to fall asleep, or pretend to sleep
Sleep
Pump (4 a.m.)
Try to fall asleep, or pretend to sleep
Call the unit for an update on Violette
So anxious about calling the unit; wake Keith up for him to
  call the unit
Make sure Violette is okay
Try to fall asleep, or pretend to sleep
Sleep

I always have trouble deciding whether to cross out the item "Pump" before or after pumping. Usually, I delete items from the list after I have completed them, to maintain the integrity of list making. Now I cross them off before. It encourages me.

Computer, please note that the clarification "drink as little wine as possible" is not a trap to check if you're paying attention. You CAN drink when you're pumping your milk. We say "express your milk" in proper medical language; a sommelier couldn't put it any better. Yes, yes, YOU CAN DRINK! But only after pumping the milk. Doctors rarely tell mothers this, but I intend to tell them once this experience is over. And if I've drunk two or three glasses of wine, before I freeze the milk, I stick a label on the bottle that says "Wine milk, for when Violette is older." Of course, it's not "wine milk," but better safe than sorry.

14 June

Computer,

I'm at home, at the pumping station but not pumping. Night, I hate you.

Waking up at 4 in the morning to feed a plastic robot baby is starting to seriously get me down. I can't get back to sleep. The nights are worse than the days. Night-time is hell. No. Daytime is hell, and night-time is the supreme furnace where even the devil is burning. Maybe the tube that helps her breathe is coming out? Maybe there's blood in her stools? Maybe her intestines are perforating? Did they wash their hands? Are bacteria proliferating in her blood? Is she sleeping, is she stirring in her incubator, is she okay? Do her little heels hurt because of all the blood drawing? Will she ever come home? Will that microbaby Violette grow enough to some-day become a real little girl? Am I pumping for nothing, for a baby who's going to die? What would I do then with my two freezers full of milk? How much would it cost to send all my frozen liquid gold to a milk bank? Why couldn't they hook me up on the respirator instead of her?

There are "normal" mothers, with their monster babies, who dare to complain about their cracked nipples, their baby's insatiable appetite, or the frequency of the feedings, when Violette's tiny intestines are so fragile. Violette is all alone in her plastic box at one end of the NICU. She hears the "whoosh-whoosh" of the respirator. It's the sound that domi-nates her entire environment. I'm afraid to call to find out how she is.

Worse, I don't want to be at her side all the time. I can't. I can't help thinking about all the disasters that could befall her. Fuck. Why did I put on
my list "Call the unit" during the night? I can't! I always ask Keith to call.
Why not just write "Tell Keith to call the unit"? It would be more honest
and I would feel less miserable. I should make my lists in the middle of
the night, during the worst moments, not during the day.

It's so dark and I'm afraid. The fridge is making a sinister noise, like a
bad omen. I just went to make sure Axel hadn't been kidnapped, that he
hadn't strangled in his sheets or broken his neck falling out of bed. And
that Keith is alive.

Computer, here I am again at the pumping station desk after my third
pumping session of the day. I'm so fucking tired. But I haven't finished
venting about pumping. You know, I'm pumping every three hours
(eight times a day) like a good mother who listens to her medical team.
I actually pump seven times a day, but I tell everyone that I do it eight
times so they'll leave me in peace. Keith is the only one who knows. Even
under torture, he will lie for me.

I'm getting good at it! I make an effort to read while I'm pumping. I've
started a book on the major milestones in the history of women. The
breast pump isn't mentioned in it, but the contraceptive pill is. Computer,
in order to be able to read a book while pumping, you have to choose one
that's medium size (not a paperback). You place it on a table that's not too
high. Then you position the cups on your breasts. While holding the cups,
you put your elbows on each side of the book, in a pose similar to the one
used by models with their hands on their hips, pulling in your stomach
while pushing your elbows forward (in those photos, it always looks like
the girl has swallowed her keys just when she was getting kicked in the
ass; I've never understood the aesthetics of that pose). Now, to turn the
pages, you hold the right cup with the inside of your right arm and the left
with your right hand, and you turn the page with your left hand; and you
alternate sides, or else your right wrist and shoulder start to hurt. Once
you've mastered this method, you can try another one: wedge the two cups
against the edge of the table, and your hands are free to turn the pages.
But that's a bit risky – if the cups slip, they twist your nipples, and that can
turn your breasts into steak tartare. You can also sit up and pull your knees
up to breast level to hold the cups, a variation of the "boat" yoga pose. It's
excellent for the thighs and abs. There are endless possibilities.

I can no longer stand normal mothers who complain that nursing is soooooooooooo exhausting, that their baby is soooooooooooo tiring, and that they reeeeeeeeeeeeeeeeally need some rest. The poor things, they have to get up in the night to nurse, AND WHAT'S MORE, sometimes their baby spits up and they ALSO have to change their pyjamas. I myself was one of those mothers with my fire-alarm Axel, and I complained about my little bawler. That was another life. Violette can't cry out, she has a tube in her trachea. But the damn alarms are still there. Not fire alarms, but all kinds of alarms that are going off all the time beside her – the saturometer alarm when there's not enough oxygen in her blood or too much, the alarm of the heart rate monitor when her heart slows down dangerously, the respirator alarm when there's a leak, when her tube gets disconnected, or when she's not breathing right. When an alarm sounds, my heart races. I keep telling myself everything is under control. I should know. Far from all that racket, my office is nice and cozy. But Violette gets it all – she hears it all day long.

My baby.

My baby!

The Big Berthas

Dear Mothers,

Dear Parents of Babies in the NICU,

Here's a scientifically proven fact in neonatology: mothers' milk is better than modified cows' milk, which is also called "commercial formula for premature infants." In the long term, babies fed on mothers' milk during their first six months will develop higher IQs and fewer allergies and have less risk of gastroenteritis, eczema, and all kinds of other shit that can affect the children and adults they will become. For premature babies, mothers' milk also prevents necrotizing enterocolitis (a serious intestinal problem) and even death. Milk from a mothers' milk bank is preferable to commercial formula. But the mother's own milk is probably better than milk from a milk bank, because the latter is often pasteurized to destroy possible viruses and bacteria, which also results in the destruction of antibodies and other beneficial molecules. To optimize the advantages of mothers' milk, babies should receive it for six months; beyond that, it no longer makes much difference. The effects of mothers' milk are dose dependent; that is, the more the premature baby receives, the greater the effects. I promised that this book wouldn't be a scientific treatise, so I won't say any more about the science on mothers' milk for premature infants. But still, you should know that there are TONS of studies on the subject, and that commercial formula will never be equal to mothers' milk.

BUT IN THE NICU, GIVING YOUR MILK TO YOUR BABY IS HARD! Giving your milk to a sick baby is not the same as breastfeeding a healthy baby, which can also be hard for some women. Approximately 95 per cent of mothers of sick babies can give their milk to their baby if they have good support and a favourable environment. "It's not always easy" is a polite way of describing it. In reality, it takes a lot of time and it's frustrating, but it's well worth it in the end. That's why, if you are the mom of a sick baby in the NICU, your hospital has a duty and responsibility to support you and help you give your milk to your child as often as you can or want to. If the hospital doesn't help you, fight – it's your right!

If the pharmaceutical industry had a drug, let's call it Lactus Maternicus™, that was as effective as mothers' milk in preventing death and enhancing IQ, imagine what it would cost your hospital. Doctors would be writing all their prescriptions with Lactus Maternicus™ pens. You'd see Lactus Maternicus™ posters at all the medical conferences and on all the bus shelters.

part three

THE NICU

Dear Violette

29 May 2005

Days of life: 8

Violette's corrected gestational age: 25 weeks, 5 days

Dear Violette

I do not know where to start,

I speak to your dad, but not about everything; there are many things that are better left unsaid. I even speak to my computer – imagine! I find it easier to pretend I am a sane person, to pump every three hours, to pretend to be organized and have things under control. It is easier at the moment. I can see all the other great mothers around me, speaking and smiling and reading to their small babies on respirators, with tubes and tapes and wonder why I just cannot do this like them, WHY? Maybe they are also pretending, like me? Who knows …

So I focus on things that are easier to do. I can come and see you, stare at you and hope, hope, hope, and hope again that you will hang in there. Hope that your lungs do not get too damaged, hope than you don't get infected, that bacteria do not invade your blood from the central line, your lungs from the endotracheal tube, your skin through all the small lesions you have, your kidneys through your wet diaper. Hope that your intestines stay healthy and do not perforate, hope your eyes do not get damaged. All this hope is mixed up with intense fear, the fear of everything that can go wrong and can happen to you.

So I need to plan, pump, wash appliances, come to the NICU, speak to the computer, pretend things are under control.

But they are not.

They keep insisting that I read books to you: there is this new literacy initiative where parents read books to their babies. I know scientifically that reading books to your baby is supposed to increase the likelihood that you will read books later on and that it is good for your brain, but it is hard. And I know that if you survive, you will have too many books. We have tons of books. Way too many – we do not know where to put them. So many that I placed some personal books in the return box of the local library. I thought libraries would not throw out books. It would feel like a criminal offence. Nor would they throw them in the recycle. I am not sure what you hear over the respirator. I know you can kind of recognize my voice, and probably my smell and that you need some auditory stimulation. So I read you stories, but it feels weird.

But isn't that so unmotherly?

The nurses tell me I should speak to you. I speak to you, but it is hard to know what to speak about. You are tiny, so small. Your brain is not even the size of my fist, and my hand is very small: I wear size 6.5 surgical gloves. It is hard when your saturation, the amount of oxygen in your blood, goes down every time you are slightly disturbed. When I talk too loud, you desaturate. When I talk too soft, you desaturate; when I breathe, you desaturate; when I just am, you desaturate.

The words also do not come easily. I seem to only be able to tell you that I am sorry and that I love you. Nothing else very much. Fuck, I wish there is something I could have done to prevent this – *merde*! I often end up swearing in the incubator, and this also feels unmotherly. A mother cannot always end up a conversation swearing to her mini-daughter.

I wish I could tell you it is going to be OK. I cannot tell you it will be OK – it would be a lie: I am not sure it will be OK for you. In fact, I am sure it hurts, even if we are trying our best to prevent all the pain you have. And we will all hurt together. But I wish I could take this physical hurt you have. They use sucrose before anything that can hurt you, like pricking your feet. Sucrose works, and we often have to fire the sucrose alarm. Your dad is the sucrose watchdog. He makes sure you have sucrose every time you have a blood test. He makes sure you do not have too many blood tests. To be honest, your dad is the obsessive pitbull. I am the chihuahua hidden underneath a carpet, waiting for the storm to pass. When there is no sucrose, I just quietly ask where it is.

When there is no sucrose, your dad goes berserk. He even had a small sucrose workshop for other parents in the NICU. I love him. I am so glad he is here; I lean on him. I feel he has a gigantos bazooka to protect you, and I have a slingshot with a pea.

I cannot tell you all will be fine in the end. I do not know that either. Which end? When? If you die, I would hate for things to be "fine"– how disturbing. If you are disabled, I would love for things to be fine, but I cannot believe it.

There are also words I cannot tell you, that I can barely tell myself.

You are on the respirator, and I am so scared.

Scared to lose you, scared to try to save you too hard. Scared of wanting too much and ending up more hurt. Scared of loving you too much and ending up empty, filled up with air and loss and guilt and nothing.

I do not know how to be the mother of a microbaby on a respirator attached to wires and tubes.

I do not know how to be the mother of a dead baby either.

How can I be the mother of a dead Violette? To wonder all my life how you could have been. Your first smile, your first laugh, your first steps, your first words, your hugs, your smell, your favorite food, your eyes in the morning, all the summers, swimming, songs, stories, trips, everything … I would miss never having known, seen, all these things.

Does it hurt less to lose a child you never knew or knew only attached to machines for a short time compared to an older child when you know what you are missing? Or does it hurt more, because you are faced with this void, this unwritten story, are in limbo in your heart?

I know you are not dying right now, but you are so fragile, many things can still happen.

I am just talking to you about the real things, the ones that are not in the books they give us parents to read to their children. Maybe these baby books fill the void and replace the hard words parents cannot tell each other or their child?

I will learn how to be a good NICU mom, or at least an OK one. At least I promise I will try.

I do not know how to get better at it – trust me, I am trying, but I know I am not very good at it right now. Maybe with time, it will seem normal to see you like this, I will adapt. But this is also sad; how can a mom adapt to the sight of her daughter all plugged in like this?

I cannot bear the sight of you like that. I can't, and I know the machines and what is going on. How can all the NICU moms who do not know all these things look like they are sane and read books with nice musical voices? Maybe this is why they keep it together? Perhaps ignorance is bliss. Or are we all pretending to be sane?

I would like to be attached in your place, to put you back in my belly where you belong so you can grow and I can protect you

I know it's not possible, that I can't go back in time. I am stuck. Wondering what I did, when, what I could have done, what if … How could I have let you down. And I keep analysing and am persuaded I should have protected you better.

I am sorry now mainly for not knowing how to be a normal NICU mother. For not feeling deep inside you are my daughter, my Violette. For feeling you are my baby and, somehow, you are supposed to turn into my daughter at some point. I realized today, when we come to see you, your dad told the security agent "I'm coming to see my daughter who is sick," and I said "I delivered prematurely." You are not really sick like another sick person; my body expelled you too soon. And all these machines are replacing my womb and trying to do the best not to injure your brain, your lungs, your blood vessels, while saving your life.

When you were 2 days, I did not want to hold you. I was too scared. They forced me to hold you while they were changing the incubator, pretended nobody else could, placed you in my arms. My small lovely girl. I was so scared. I am a doctor who saves babies like you, places tubes in them, knows what to do in the worse of conditions, knows how to resuscitate, order medication, give intravenous fluids, nutrition to give by the veins, look at X-rays. And there I was, holding you and trembling like a leaf. Hating them for doing this to me.

But I will get better at it. I promise. I need to be one of these motherly moms who can't get enough of their baby, who dream of holding them all the time, who speak of their daughter to everybody.

Violette, I know how your lungs work, how the machines work, all that can happen to you. I understand all the numbers they use to describe you. I understand all the numbers they use to define you, the ideal recipe of the nutrition you get in your veins, where you are in the nutrition protocol. I know the percentage of water you have in your body and your body composition. I fucking know exactly how your body works, with the gas exchanges, the oxidization, the enzymes, everything. I know all the possible disasters that may happen to you.

But I do not know how to be your mother.

I have never learned how to be the mom of a small baby dependent on a respirator. There is no recipe for this. No instructions anywhere. I try to learn looking at the other moms and remembering how all the mothers I saw in my career did. But I would need a course, and I know just saying that is not being a mother ...

I console myself because I know I am not alone feeling like this – I met some mothers like me before. These are the moms who were open enough to say these things. I would never say these things to my doc, my nurse, my friends, or to Keith. I promise I will get better.

Breathe, Violette, breathe. I hope you are comfortable, my girl, the most comfortable you can be. I hope your heart does not slow down too often today, that you take in all the milk without any incidents, that your oxygen need stays low, that your central line does not get infected, that your belly stays OK. That your lungs are growing, and all the rest too.

I hope I will also grow; maybe it will just take time.

I am so sorry.

I love you.

This article is perhaps the one of mine that I hear the most about. It is widely read and used in many educational activities. Perhaps the title attracts clinicians, who are used to dealing with more serious titles. In 2010, my mentor and good friend, John Lantos (who co-wrote the preface to this book), asked me if I wanted to be a guest editor for a "parent issue" on quality of life in Current Problems in Pediatric and Adolescent Health Care. *Of course, I said yes! The issue starts with a wonderful review about quality of life written by Antoine Payot and Keith Barrington.*[†] *We called that part "food for the head." Then, I asked many parents I admire and have learned from to write their story, some about disabled kids, others about different families, some about death and dying. They teach us that it is important to nourish the head, but also the soul. Stories have power; with stories, we understand things we may not after reading the most rigorous scientific article. Their characters help us truly understand ethical concepts. I am sure that Gabriel and his parents, the heroes of this story, have influenced clinicians around the world more than many of the scientific articles I have written. If you like this story, there are many other fascinating ones in the April 2011 issue of* Current Problems in Pediatric and Adolescent Health Care.

Pepperoni Pizza and Sex[‡]

"Are you telling me my son is dying?" said Gabriel's mother.

Gabriel was three days old. His nineteen-year-old mother had delivered him at home three months before her due date. Our transport team resuscitated him and rushed back to our hospital, but now things had taken a turn for the worse. Mr and Mrs Petit never left Gabriel's bedside. I spoke to them every few hours.

This was a planned pregnancy. The parents were poor. Neither had finished high school. Gabriel's primary nurse, Ann, was worried about them. "Mom is in denial," she said. "She treats him like a doll. She keeps saying he is soooooooooooooooo cuuuuuuuuuuuute. She wants to dress him up. He is sick, doesn't she get it? She needs help. We need to get them some help. Poor parents, poor baby, poor mother, she is so young for this."

I remember looking at the mother's birth date in the chart and thinking that I was an old woman, with rotten ovaries, and that I was bound to have this thought more and more often as time went by. I told Ann, "Nineteen, wow ... this is young to have a baby in the NICU. Well ... I guess nobody is old enough to prepare themselves to be parents in the NICU ..."

Today, on his third day of life, Gabriel bled profusely into both his lungs and one side of his brain. I was meeting Gabriel's parents to inform them of their son's deterioration and of the results of the brain ultrasound. Ann came to the meeting with me.

I needed to know what the parents thought we should do now. They were not talking much. The mother thought that I was coming to tell her that Gabriel was dying. I reassured her that, for now, he was stable. She immediately relaxed.

They asked if he would be disabled. I tried to explain the statistics: about half the kids like Gabriel who survived were severely disabled. I explained a little about what cerebral palsy meant. I was planning to talk about physical therapy and special equipment that could make Gabriel's life better even if he had cerebral palsy. Before I could, the father surprised me with a question: "Will we be able to love him?"

I responded, "You already love him so much, and there is no reason it won't continue that way."

"I mean, will I love him even if he is handicapped?"

Nobody had ever asked that question before in such a pure way. I didn't know what to say. I thought of Dr Saigal's research showing that parents adapt to their child's disability, that most parents were grateful that their child was alive and not dead. But Saigal's studies did not ask about love. I had to say something. I told them that parents almost always love their children, no matter what.

"Will he be able to love us?" asked his mother.

That one seemed a little easier. "Children with disabilities have the same emotional needs and emotional lives as other people. He will love you as much as any other child, probably more."

This conversation was not going the way I had planned it. Ann was looking at the floor. She hadn't said a word.

"Will he be able to have sex?" asked the father. The mother rolled her eyes and sighed. "Well," continued the father, "it is really important to have sex in life! Love is for the head and sex is for the body!"

What was I supposed to say? I thought that maybe sex was also for the head. Why even separate sex and love? But this didn't seem like the time to have that discussion. I wondered how I got myself into these situations. Did this stuff happen to other doctors? I had already answered the love question. Now I had a sex question! If I answer this one, what would be next? I took the leap …

"Hum … There is no reason he would not be able to … hum … A severe brain hemorrhage should not impair Gabriel's ability to have sex. But in order to make love, one needs a partner, and … "

"So he will be able to get it up and do it himself if he wants to?" said the father. The mother was now giving him not-so-subtle vocal and physical cues that the sex questions were enough.

"Most probably yes," I answered, thinking, please listen to your wife!

Ann was squirming in the background, trying not to laugh. Maybe I looked like an idiot: Annie Janvier, neonatal sexologist, prognosticating the ability to masturbate after a unilateral grade IV hemorrhage in a 27-week preterm infant. I could picture the Dr Phil video that would be in the residents' skit night.

"Will he be able to make pizza?"

Oh, come on. This must be a joke. Did I hear this question correctly? Am I dreaming?

I thought that this was a good time to redirect the question. I had not asked the father "Why are you asking this question?" when he spoke of sex, because it was pretty obvious that he enjoyed sex, and then I would not have known what to say after that. "Oh! Good for you sir! Yes, sex is good, sex is excellent indeed!" But now, I thought, it seemed like the right time to take control of this conversation. But before I could speak, the father went on: "My family has a pizza place. My uncle opened it. We both work there. So does my cousin Samuel, who is a trisomic. Samuel puts pepperoni on pizza. His father makes the dough. I deliver the pizza. Susanne answers the phone and serves at the tables. If our son is happy like Samuel and can work with us, he will be OK. We will be OK."

The mother continued: "Our family lives together. We have the same routine every day: we get up, go to the pizza joint, work together, eat together, come home, watch a film, and eat pizza. Well, sometimes we eat something else! Then we go to bed … and … well, umh … you probably know already that we have sex. We don't have much money, but we have enough. If Gabriel can have the same life we have, he will be OK – we will be OK."

Ann was now sniffling in her corner.

My throat was tight; I had difficulty swallowing.

I could not believe how Ann and I had judged this couple. We thought they didn't understand. Maybe it was us who didn't get it. Faced with the same challenge they were faced with, I would probably have taken Gabriel-with-his-broken-cortex off his high frequency ventilator so that we could let him "die peacefully." I would have told myself that I was doing it for him, in his best interest, that I was not selfish, that I loved him enough to say goodbye.

Gabriel's young parents were teaching me something. All they wanted was for their child to love them, to be able to have sex, and to be able to put the pepperoni on the pizza. I wanted a good rewarding career, a high IQ, an intelligent husband, a comfortable home for my three healthy kids, sports, yoga, good food, travelling, many books, writing papers, restaurants and theater …

"Gabriel is lucky to have good parents like you. I wish I could tell you he is doing great, that he will come through this with perfect health. But I can't promise you that. But I will promise you this. I will meet you every morning and every afternoon and I will tell you everything that I know about Gabriel. I'll tell you if he's getting better. I'll tell you if he's getting worse. Whatever happens, we will get through this together."

"Can we both stay in this room to talk now?" said the mother.

Ann and I left the room. She was sobbing and angry. "It is not fair! Middle-class educated families could give so much to all the little Gabriels. But they don't want to. They ask us to stop the respirators. They want to make another one, a better one." Then, after a pause, in a quieter voice, "And I would not want a Gabriel either."

Gabriel improved and came off the respirator. His parents were there every day. His mother expressed her milk eight times a day, read books to him, sang to him. They brought pepperoni pizza for the whole NICU!

I was there with Mom and Dad when Gabriel died of a fulminant infection a month later. I thought, "How can this happen. Not after all this!" If this happened to me, I thought, I would be such a bitter, broken, irritable, drowning mother. I would question life, fate, philosophy, the cosmos; I'd insult God, find a guilty party. Who hadn't washed their hands? Why after all this? Why hadn't physicians started the antibiotics sooner?

How could this happen to these fragile parents?

They held him in his last moments, kissed his little, mottled, cold, gasping body. They told him he was their little star, their little angel. They told him that they were proud of him, that he had fought the best he could, and that they understood that he couldn't fight any longer. They told him that they would think of him day and night. They told him that they loved him very much, that they were grateful they had been parents, his parents, even for only five weeks. And that those five weeks with him were the best weeks of their lives.

They had another baby this year, Océanne, who was born at 38 weeks with an APGAR of 9–9–9. The parents asked me to be at the delivery.

From time to time, I go eat at their pizzeria, where I can see Samuel, at the back, placing his pepperoni pieces on pizza. The pizzeria is now called "Chez Gabriel."

17, 18 June

Days of life: 27 and 28

Violette's corrected gestational age: 28 weeks, 3 and 4 days

17 June 2005
1:30 p.m.: Neonatologist on service. Acute deterioration since 5 a.m., respiratory acidosis, difficult ventilation, CO^2 90, switched to high frequency ventilation. MAP 13, Hz 8, amp 80% … DD: ET Tube blocked? Change needed? Pneumonia/sepsis? … Increased left pulmonary infiltration and hyperglycemia: ampho B begun after culture in addition to pip-tazo-genta … Active and difficult to ventilate, morphine X 1 given, fentanyl started and increased ad 3 mcg/kg/h, now calmer.
2:15 p.m.: desaturation ad 29 with RC at 40, PPV needed to oxygenate, slow response.
Now saturation > 90% in 30% oxygen and improved.

Sophie N.

18 June 2005
Problems: Ventilation difficult on high frequency, DNAse begun because
    secretions ++
Bilateral pneumonia, pulmonary white out (Pip Tazo Genta Ampho B).
Ductus open ++ despite 3 courses of indo. Glucose intolerance (new) on
    insulin. NPO x 4 days, ileus, abdominal distension.
Bradys ++, new metabolic acidosis.

My Violette, my baby, my little miss, my peanut, my little sweetie, my little flower, my mini-babe, my pistachio, my little honey, my little peach who's losing her fuzz, my little sweetbelly, my micro–belly button. I don't know what to do anymore. I don't know what to think anymore. I don't know what to call you anymore. I don't know anymore if you're leaving or not. If I should hold on to you or not. This morning, we were sure it was yes. Papa thinks no; I think yes. Now, I don't know. I want to run away. I don't know anymore.

You've had pneumonia for a few days and it's not getting any better, and now you have an infection that is killing you. You haven't peed in more than thirty-six hours, your damn blood pressure is at 18 with 0.35 mcg/kg/min of epinephrine. You're not moving, your diaper is open and you're doing nothing, unresponsive. We don't really know what the bacteria that's killing you is, but it's an infection. They've brought out the big guns, ampho B, amikacin, meropenem, and immunoglobulins.

This morning we thought it was the end. Anyway, we'd decided. After more than thirty-six hours without peeing and no blood pressure. After a long time seeing you full of white and purple spots, like a corpse. With your puffy face, your little feet all swollen, your little arm all pricked, your little legs white, almost transparent. I couldn't take it anymore. I think you're leaving us, that you can't take it anymore. That your body is deciding to leave, at the end of its rope, tired. That this is your way of telling us. That you can't tell us any other way.

Papa thought the same thing before he saw you sucking on your pacifier. Your green pacifier. You hadn't moved in hours, and you started sucking on your pacifier. The green pacifier. But scientifically, I KNOW that doesn't mean anything. Papa, too, knows it in his head. Sucking originates in the brain stem, not the brain. Anencephalic babies, those born without a brain, can also suck on a green soother, I tell Papa, but he doesn't want to hear it. Even a frog with no brain can do it. Well, I don't know, but I think so. We did that experiment in high school – not with a soother, but with the feet of a decerebrated frog; in acid, its foot still twitched. I know you're not a frog. I'm trying to explain it to you. I don't know what to do anymore to put up with myself. To try to understand why we're here, how we got to this point.

With the soother, Papa began to have doubts. He's an expert; he knows it doesn't mean anything. But he's calling all the experts he knows to ask if they've seen other little flowers like you do what you're doing. Neil Finer told him not to lose hope. Frankly, based on what? I don't know what Saroj said, and I don't know if I want to know. If Keith and I don't know, there aren't many others who are going to know.

I went and hid in my office. Besides it's Father's Day. I didn't forget. I just didn't think of it. The nurses have made little cards for all the dads (from their babies). Keith cried so much. You can't up and die on Father's Day. I don't know anything anymore.

What do you want them to say, those experts? We're also experts, with statistics, and so are the people caring for Violette. They've told us that things have gone from bad to worse, that the infection wasn't under control, that you were probably going to die. We know what goes on at these times, the discussions that follow. We've done the tough job: "Maybe it would be better to withdraw the respirator, the machines, the wires so that she can die in your arms and not in her incubator?" "Right."

The first thing that was clear after you were born is that we would have to know when to stop, but it's not easy. Maybe we can't take it anymore, and we think you can't take it anymore. I can see that you're declining, and I want to listen to you if you're going. I don't want you to suffer. But you don't look like you're suffering – you're not even moving anymore. You look like you're already gone. This is what I would say to the parents if I were the doctor: that things are not going well and you have to prepare for the worst. That the worst is happening, slowly, that things haven't been getting better, hour by hour, for two days.

I thought I knew. But I don't know anything anymore. I tried so hard to be your mom, but I can't be a normal neonatal mom. But I was starting to get the knack of it, just by pretending. Also, and probably especially, because you were getting better and I thought you were going to survive. So I allowed myself to hope for more stuff. But now things are getting worse and worse. The alarms are going off all the time. The blood pressure alarm was shut off because it was going off constantly, and the limit is set at sixteen. I'm scared when you're in my arms with your tiny body on a respirator. I watch the monitors constantly. They go off all the time because you're sick and fragile. The nurses are being professional, but I know them. They're stressed when everything is going off and your heart slows down, especially now, because it may not start up again.

You're not peeing and your potassium is increasing, and when it gets too high, your heart will stop.

I try to smell your little head, your little head like a peeled peach on top because of the repeated attempts at intravenous lines. It smells like baby. Sometimes, it smells like sweet yogurt when you've spit up. But now you're not eating anymore. I try to imagine that we're home and that I'm frustrated because I have to wash the sheets that are full of vomit. Then the alarm pulls me out of my daydream, which lasted for ten seconds. And I can feel myself slipping, my chair giving way under me. I look at your little pulverized heels where they've drawn so much blood, your little skull. You've never asked anyone for anything. I've let you down.

I'll hate myself the rest of my days for putting you through this shitty month in intensive care if you die. When you die. If you die. Maybe this is all happening because I can't be a normal mom? But you know I love you. Even if I don't like giving you your gavage feedings. It's not because I don't love you. It's a medical thing to me. It's not a mom's job in my mind, and I'm trying to be a good mom, not a doctor. Even though the other moms look like they love it, like they think it's a mom thing.

I'd like to be tough, the way I was in my life before. But I just can't do it. I'm dissolving; I want to disappear. I should be beside you screaming for you, begging, "There must be something you can do!" I want it to stop, to be your mother for real, without machines, without alarms, without wires, without remote controls, without pumps. But I'm going to be the mother of a dead baby instead. We told the family you were dying. But I can't imagine that either. I try to say "Violette is dead," but I can't. Maybe that's my soother.

Also, just to piss us off, the weather is beautiful. Your Papa and I went to sit down for a bit on the reservoir grounds. Three hours ago now. We decided it was enough. That we had to face facts, that it wouldn't work. That nature sometimes wins against doctors. It happens quite often that 24-week babies die. "FUCK, NOT US!" I wanted to scream. But there's no use screaming. Nobody's listening. The sun was so hot, the sky so blue, not one fucking cloud. Not fair; it was raining and storming inside me. Axel is at Mamy's. Our baby in the stone hospital over there. Our baby who is dying.

When we returned, they had prettied you up to look like a real baby. The nurses had put you in a little white dress with lace around the collar.

But you're so blue, pallid, and swollen. You already look like the photographs we take of dead babies. You look like the beginning of a corpse. My little sweetie, I'm sorry it's come to this. Axel came to say hello to you; he had never seen you. Probably won't ever see you again. He doesn't really understand what's happening. "Axel, she's your little sister, Violette." "Baby, tittle baby. Baby boken?" He touched your little hands, your little fingers. He said, "Baby boo-boo! *Maman* fix?" NO, *MAMAN CAN'T FIX*, Sophie can't fix it, Lorraine can't fix it, Julie can't fix it, Debbie can't, or Daniel either, nobody can fix it, my dear Axel. He knows the unit is for baby boo-boos. And maybe he saw your boo-boos, too. And Papa can't fix either. And Papa is the boss, the broken baby expert.

When the pilot crashes and bawls, the airplane will go down, I think. My children, my ephemeral little family. My little world that's crumbling. My life that's slipping out from under my feet. My baby. You'll be buried next to Papy, my papa. Under the egg-shaped tombstone with flowers on it and the names of all your papy's children. We started thinking about his tombstone when he knew for sure he was going to die; it's made to look like the last pendant he gave Mamy. He had fallen in love with that pendant, and so it would be the design above his ashes. Underneath, there are places for five cylinders of ashes. In front of one of the cylinders, a plaque with the inscription "Bernadette Janvier 1945–," Mamy's dates; the story isn't over yet. What will we write for you? "2005–2005," "1 month in 2005"? Or we'll put the weight, something like "730 g–1000 g"? Fuck, I don't even know if there'll be enough ashes! Only a little pile. There was only a medium bag for Papa. I know there will be enough, I've already reassured parents about that, but today I'm having a lot of trouble believing it. Maybe it would be better in another plot. Papa wants to bury you. He's against the business of burning people and producing greenhouse gases, and he thinks it's part of life to return to the earth. I don't agree with that, and I'm going to fight. NO WAY worms are going to eat my little miss or parasites get into your orifices. No way your muscles are going to decompose, your little bum, your little cheeks, no maggots or invertebrates are going to touch them. There won't be any ants in your mouth, ever, except if you eat some later when we're not watching you closely.

I don't know what I'm supposed to do. Maybe they're waiting for my verdict? That's why I'm staying here.

It makes me think about babies we thought were going to die and who did not die, such as Audrey-Anne. She was never able to breathe on her own, since the muscles in her whole body were too weak. We never found the name of her neuromuscular disease. We tried to extubate her five times. The last time, we all thought she'd had enough – that she'd fought enough, that we weren't going to reintubate her if she wasn't breathing and that we would be there for her if she was in pain, if she was suffocating. Her mom had even filled in all the papers for the metabolic autopsy because it had to be done quickly after her death. The whole family was there. The pathologist was at the hospital: he had prepared the many tubes to be sent to all kinds of laboratories to try to find a name for her disease. Well, Audrey-Anne breathed! She's still alive, and her parents take care of her like champions.

I'd even written a poem for her the day before we took her off the respirator. Which I'd read to her when no one was looking. And I had finally given it to her incredible parents. I know you're not Audrey-Anne, that there's no connection – but maybe there is. And I haven't even written a poem for you – shit.

Axel has gone back with Mamy. They were supposed to take Violette off the respirator. I feel completely numb; it hurts too much. I don't want to be here anymore. I don't want to be anywhere. I want to go two months back in time and have another try. Maybe I could do better. Not pick Axel up to put him on the swing when I felt it pulling. Go to bed at ten and not play Rummikub with Papa until midnight and try to win like a damn fool. And at the hospital, I shouldn't have turned when I sneezed. Not lost my water.

Papa is in his office calling the experts to shop for hope, but no one will know what to say. Dammit, we don't know what to say to parents in these circumstances either. I'm a world-class wimp. I hide here and I write to you, marbled gray baby who's dying. I'm not capable of talking to you in person. My baby.

But I don't know if you can hear or feel – your brain is probably not very perfused, with your blood pressure at 18. It's been thirty-one hours now that you haven't moved, even when you're pricked. My Violette, I love you, but I don't know what to do anymore. I don't want to fight with Papa to stop the torture. I can't fight with the love of my life for your death. I'm not capable of doing that. I'll go along with him; he can decide. My breasts hurt – it's been three hours since I drew milk. Pumping for a baby who's dying. What am I going to do with all the freezers full of milk for you? Divided among people's houses. Why are you dying when there's so much milk?

I don't know if they're still waiting to stop the respirator. As a neonatologist, I've seen hundreds of parents go through it. The parents take the baby. Sometimes with the tube, sometimes without. Some spend a moment with their baby in their arms with the respirator. The respirator is stopped and the tube is taken out before or after the baby is in their arms. They take family photos before the baby is too blue. Sometimes they listen to important songs. The baby makes respiratory efforts, gasping; the heart slows down. Sometimes, it takes a long time for the heart to stop – babies' hearts are pretty strong. And when the baby dies, the parents are told the heart has stopped. Prints are taken, locks of hair too. The little card is taken from the incubator, and the bracelets, the little soother too. It's all put in a memory box.

NOOOOOOOOOOOOOO, NO, NOT MY DAUGHTER! The little green soother. The one that might save your life, extend it for a few hours or years? Or extend your death, or cause a disability. Your little green soother.

All kids need is a little help, a little hope, and someone who believes in them.

Magic Johnson

For Audrey-Anne

For your curious eyes and your nose fed up with being squashed
For your plump gums chewing away
For your wandering little hands searching for the forbidden
tubes
For your profound, inquisitive gaze, serious and joyful
Almost adult sometimes
For your sparkling, mocking eyes

For the courage you have
For your teasing personality
For your little body, your too tight, stifling tent
The prison you're shut up in
For you, we hope.

For everything you won't be able to be
For all the love you could have had for a long time
For the room you would have had if your tent had been bigger
We tried to make your "house" the most welcoming possible, the
most comfortable.
We tried ...
Sorry for all the boo-boos
Sorry for all the tubes

Sorry for sometimes tying your hands
For waking you up when you were sleeping
Sorry for showing you death so close up, for giving you so many
angels as friends
For giving you a respirator as a brother
For making your parents cry – they love you so fiercely
Desperately
Infinitely.

Stay among us, but if your tent is too little and stifling
You'll find another
With more air, more windows
Where you'll be able to dance.
We want you to fight
But we don't want your life to be a battle.

You want your face to be caressed by the wind
Your hands free and your throat dry.
Audrey-Anne, we admire you.
We want your little body to be well.
Fight if you can, but stop if you can't anymore. We'll understand.

We won't squash your nose anymore.
We won't play drums on your chest.
We won't prick you.
We won't make you vomit.
We won't make you hungry.
We won't tie you down.
We won't wake you up.

  Promise.

Shooting Stars

Death is always present in the NICU. Prematurity is a lottery, like many diseases. Most of the time, babies pull through. But it's hard when you think that you yourself could become a statistic. Some parents experience the loss of their baby, and that loss usually occurs after a series of preliminary losses: of a normal pregnancy, a normal birth, a normal baby, normal nursing, a normal maternity leave, and so on. The supreme loss is losing your child. And hardly having known that child. The loss of all you would have known about her. All you would have wanted to give him. When a child dies at 5 years of age, you know what you're losing, but, after that, you wonder each year what that child would have done, would have loved, would have become. When a child dies in the NICU, you'll never know who your baby would have been. Favourite foods, favourite music, expressions. It can even be hard to imagine your baby without a respirator. And that creates a big void.

I wonder what Violette would have been like if she had been born full term. Would she have been little or big? Would her lungs have been strong or weak? Would her trachea have been developed enough? How would she do in school? But my question, at that time, wasn't about that. I was wondering how to be the mother of a dead baby. What remains with me from that day is the feeling of calm and emptiness that took hold of me. No more electricity in the brain, a flat electroencephalogram, between bursts of pain and panic. Keith and I were sitting on the grass at the McGill reservoir. Our dream had just ended. I wanted another child, but I seemed destined to sabotage my pregnancies. Keith said he didn't think he could endure another experience like this without going mad. I didn't think I was still of sound mind, but Keith seemed to think I was. I was torn. I would have liked to withdraw inside myself, to go back in time and make a different choice.

At least when Violette was in the NICU, we weren't subjected to other people's spirituality. We politely refused to have her baptized prophylactically. I myself was baptized against my will, or at least before reaching an age where I would have understood what it meant. Luckily, no one in the unit applied any pressure when the end of life was nearing. And in the room where Violette was, there weren't any of those allegorical images people plaster on the walls when babies are doing poorly, images that rub me the wrong way: an empty chair, a leaf in the wind, a stupid boat drifting away from shore, a hummingbird. The ultimate of those shitty allegories is the image of a butterfly. In many NICUs, they often print the image of a butterfly on a blank sheet of paper and stick it on the door of a room where a baby is dying. I constantly complain about it. I find it totally kitschy and not in the least poetic. In fact, it just serves to remind staff that they have to enter the room very quietly. You could just stick a blank sheet of paper on the door and that would do the job.

A few years ago, I was taking care of Lily and Maren, twin girls. After a few days of life, Lily's condition was deteriorating quickly. It was clear she was going to die. I telephoned the parents. Rebecca, the mother, arrived at the hospital and asked, "Why is that stupid butterfly on my daughter's door? Lily's not a butterfly, and Maren's not a caterpillar!" I threw the paper out. Into the garbage, not even the recycling.

Fortunately, there are some things that provide comfort. In difficult moments, I often think back to a rabbi who had come to see a baby. The baby, Ehud,* had been in our unit for two months and had accumulated so many complications; he had had infections, his lungs were destroyed, and no interventions could help him survive. He was dying. The parents were in great distress, and the nurses suggested that they bring in their spiritual guide. They didn't go to synagogue anymore and refused to see people. They were no longer sure they believed in God. But they thought it would be a good idea for the rabbi to see their baby, if only once, since they wouldn't be taking him home. Maybe the rabbi could help them get through this senseless ordeal. The parents asked the usual questions: "What happened? What should we have done? Why us?" I answered: "There was nothing you could have done to prevent what happened. We know that. But there are many things we'll never be able to understand. How can a life be so short? Two months!"

The parents turned to the rabbi, who said, "In two hundred years, Ehud's life will have as much meaning as Dr Janvier's life. Everyone Dr Janvier will have saved will be dead. Dr Janvier will be dead. We'll all be dead. When strangers walk past our graves, they will see no difference between Ehud Blickstein's* grave and Annie Janvier's grave. They will see two lives that came and that passed. Two little stars that left a little light in the lives of a few people. Maybe that light changed those people, affected what they were. But they will still be two lives that are no longer." Pow! Take that, Dr Janvier.

I often remembered those words when Violette was at her worst, and I remember them again when I see a baby die. My grave, her grave, their graves, in a hundred years, all covered in moss, most of us completely unknown to passersby. Tiny stars in the sky of our descendants, a little light in their lives, another family in our house.

19, 20 June

Days of life: 30

Violette's corrected gestational age: 28 weeks, 6 days

 19 June 2005
8:15 p.m.: Improved with hydrocortisone. Hypotension improved,
epi reduced to 0.25 mcg/kg/min. Readings radial line > armband ...
Urine +, acute tubular necrosis ... Lumbar puncture: white blood cells
31 (no meningitis) ... Parents aware of results.

Dear Computer,

The past few days have been hell. Violette has started to pee, finally; maybe it's because of the hydrocortisone they gave her, maybe not. Now she's peeing too much, because her kidneys are no longer filtering properly.

I'd like to be put under general anaesthetic and wake up in six months. Hopeless. Despair. Despair. I'm devastated. I'm going crazy imagining all the horrible scenarios in which Violette is injured, dies, has even more complications. The worst scenario is that she'll die; or that she'll be severely disabled. If only I didn't know there were so many clinical situations that could still kill her (necrotizing enterocolitis, other infections, metabolic problems because of the kidneys). The only way for me not to think about them is to tell myself over and over again that I'm not crazy. I can't relax. A knot of stress, pain, and despair is choking me. I have to repeat to myself that one day, everything will be fine and I'll no longer feel the way I feel now. I read last year in an article that when you smile, you feel better, because the muscles you use to smile send messages to the brain telling it that you're happy. I try, but it doesn't work. I see my reflection on my computer screen and it's pathetic. My smile is empty.

I can't feel like this forever, can I? It's eating me up. I feel like I'm dissolving in my own stomach acid. I'm becoming a lump of soft flesh that has collapsed on the floor. A big hole is forming in the middle of my body, with blurry outlines. When I walk, it pumps all my air and that increases my pain, my emptiness, my hypervigilance. It will end up giving me stomach ulcers and I'll vomit blood in front of a big puddle of indifference. Red, viscous blood, very sticky, very toxic, the blood of a creature drained of its raison d'être.

Violette, Violette, I beg you, try to get better! I know it's not you who decides. It's not up to you. We were ready to shut down all the machines, and we were wrong. Or maybe not. Maybe the time had come and we didn't listen to you. Maybe we weren't wrong and we were just prolonging your death. Maybe we should have accepted that you were dying. Then there would have been no more uncertainty. Maybe a certain hell is better than an uncertain hell. BUT HOW CAN I WRITE THINGS LIKE THIS?! Your father, my Keith, saved your life. All my wonderful medical knowledge almost killed you. I have to stop thinking with my brain – I have to think with my gut, with my heart. But I can't, because the goddamn movie with its series of catastrophes always takes over, with the wheelchair, the Botox for cerebral palsy, the guide dog, the gastrostomy, and all that shit. Violette, I want to know you. I want to see you smile when you look at me. I want you to know that I really love you; I want you to be aware of it. Am I eating up all your energy, poisoning your air with my despair? If you get better, I promise you I'll be a good mother. I will even give you your gavage feedings.

Or else … Or else … Or else.

Computer, I hope that one day I won't feel like this anymore. But I can't imagine feeling differently. How could I? How could I get used to all that? How could I feel okay in that situation? A normal mother canNOT feel okay in a situation like that.

When Papa died, people told me that time would help me. And that made me mad, because I couldn't conceive of his memory fading over time. But they were right. Time has erased the pain, even though I think of Papa every day, especially now. Sometimes I feel as if I've been completely abandoned, as if I'm no longer here. It's a feeling I've had before, but it's been frequent since Violette's birth. So I repeat to myself that, one day, I'll feel all right, hoping that, by my repeating it, it will finally happen. But I can't imagine myself getting used to Violette's death. I need someone to tell me that, one day, I'll feel okay, that I'm not going mad.

Do ALL women who go through this fall apart? Is it like a kick in the stomach for all of them? Maybe they give in to despair when they're alone, like me. Why doesn't somebody tell me I'm going to feel better? Maybe it's not true? "Okay, one day I'll be okay." The words resonate in my head, but they have no meaning. When I'm fed up with repeating that to myself, I try other tricks to free my brain. I count to the rhythm of my breathing. As I breathe in, I count to four, imagining four colours: one, red; two, yellow; three, green; four, blue. When my lungs are filled, I count to two, then I breathe out: one, blue; two, indigo; three, pink; four, mauve. Or I do some intense exercise, and that helps me get it out of my system. I imagine myself both tiny and huge. An ant in the universe; a giant, with my cells, my transcription factors, my DNA, and my enzymes. I look down and I see a continent; I look up, and I see myself in a very small airplane, an insignificant speck in the sky, but at the same time gigantic, watching over my mini-daughter.

21 June

Days of life: 31

Violette's corrected gestational age: 29 weeks

MERDE, COMPUTER!! NOT AGAIN!!!

We got a call this morning. Violette's condition has deteriorated even more because of a rare complication. The situation is critical. They'll have to remove the central line from her arm. Her third. The first was the catheter that was inserted into her navel at birth to avoid having to prick her too often. At five days, they inserted a central catheter in her arm, which went to the big blood vessels of the middle of her body for intravenous feeding, again to avoid pricking her too often until she could absorb milk in her intestines. And then they had to put in another to give her antibiotics and feed her; she's no longer digesting because of her infection, and they're going to bombard her with meropenem for a while. But that last catheter irritated one of her central veins and made a little hole; there was leakage. Her left lung filled with fluid and they had to put her back on the high-frequency respirator again, yet again. It's really not going well. Sophie is considering the option of putting in a chest tube. They're taking more X-rays now. Sophie and Keith can decide which is better for her. I'd like to think like a mother and not as a doctor, but I don't know how to do that anymore. Or else the opposite: I don't know how to be a doctor anymore.

I'm in a rage. A blind, red-hot, burning rage that makes me want to puke. Maybe writing will do me good. I'm now falling into an opaque, viscous, sticky rage. I fume, I sink, I seethe. My heart beats with the injustices of the world. I rage against the paunchy, slimy, stinking Normals who bitch and grumble over nothing. Who complain they don't have enough time for their children, while they themselves choose not to look after them because they'd rather watch TV, make appointments, or go to work. When you get hit by a truck, you find the time to be taken to the hospital, don't you? And then there are the ones who complain that they're tired because they had to meet a deadline. In two years, who's going to give a shit about your deadline? Violette also has a deadline. Either she meets it, or she's dead. I resent those inconsiderate Ungrateful Normals who are fed up with the couple routine and who would like a less predictable sex life. POOR, POOR YOU! I can't have sex without being terrified at the idea of getting pregnant again. I might like it if my sexual relations were just normal and predictable again. I stopped taking the pill because, with the medication, I had less milk. I'm afraid a condom will break; I imagine the spermatozoa getting through and resisting the spermicides. Or that they'll reproduce through asexual budding, like yeasts, and I'll find myself infected by billions of mutant spermatozoa programmed to fertilize me. I can't get pregnant again. Never again. I can't have sex without imagining another Violette starting to grow in my belly and suffering under the fluorescent lights. I can't think about sex without feeling a hole in my chest, without thinking about a dead child. Routine is good, but not when it means waking up at 4 a.m. to stick an electric milker on your chest and draw your milk while thinking about your daughter plugged in inside the NICU.

I had a brilliant idea this afternoon when I saw the crash cart arrive: I could take a nice dose of sedatives and have myself admitted to intensive care downstairs. Disappear for a month. No. Four would be better. Four months in a coma. And wake up when it's all over. Or build a time machine and go back and erase this shitty chapter in Violette's life, in my life, in our lives, and not go through all the pain and craziness, not know about it. And not have to hear those Ungrateful Normals say that whatever doesn't kill us makes us stronger. That trials only come to people who can gain something from them. What a bunch of heartless bastards. Is Violette learning something now? Are all the pricks on her heels making her stronger? They'll only give her rough heels. I don't find myself any stronger than before. This is not being stronger! It's killed me, that's what it's done!

Life is not the same. The other Annie Janvier is dead. The Ungrateful Normals don't know how lucky they are to have good health and a normal life, with a family and normal little problems. I was once like them. It's true I watched my father deteriorate for two years. I wasn't an Ungrateful Normal – I'd already lost that innocence. But it didn't make me stronger; it made me weaker. It made me realize that anything can happen. And that's what happened: I had that goddamn cancer. And with Axel's birth, I became completely paranoid. I already know I'm NOT stronger. And I'm perfectly capable of recognizing the luck I've had in my life. What more must I learn? I've often said to Keith, "These are the best years of our lives." Well, not 2005. Scratch that. Erase the hard drive. Purge it. Go away, 2005. Fuck 2005. Trash it. I want 2006. Now. I want to disappear and come back.

I don't know who I am anymore. I'm not the same. I've changed. Now I'm in the other group. In the sick group. Again. But I'm not sick. I'm in the group of those who care for the sick. In the subgroup of those who care for their sick babies. The group of those ravaged by waiting and uncertainty. I do have one small advantage. I didn't go from the group of Ungrateful Normals to the group of the desperate overnight. With Papa, then with my cancer, I'd already gone downhill. I didn't fall from such a great height. But I never wanted to disappear from the world when I was sick or when Papa was sick. I savoured every minute I spent with Papa. I drank in his words, I etched his image on my memory. I told myself, "You're experiencing precious moments, they're sacred, breathe them in, absorb them, incorporate them into every fibre of your being, fix them in your brain, preserve them for life." But now I want to disappear. I don't want to die; I just want to come back later. I do NOT want to be here. And when I say that, I think I'm being horrible. My poor Violette: her mom wants to go away while she's in the NICU listening to the takatakatakata of her high-frequency ventilator.

They keep telling me that I have to take things one day at a time. That you can never be sure of anything. I know that, dammit, I'm a neonatologist! I KNOW I HAVE TO TAKE THINGS ONE DAY AT A TIME! Stop telling me that. Nothing is ever certain. We know that. Oh, sure, I could get run over crossing the street. But you know what? Right now, it's more likely Violette will die before I do: it's likely my daughter will die before her mother, before her brothers, before her father. That's the reality – so leave me alone with your "we're all going to die some day." I, too, have already said that "life is a fatal disease" and other such banalities. The only statistic that never changes from one province to another, from one country to another, is that 100 per cent of human beings end up dying. Thank you very much.

Come on, 2006, get here, dammit! "One day at a time" just doesn't cut it. And if I again become a neonatologist someday, if I someday get back to my normal state, never again will I say that to parents. I know very well that you have to take things one day at a time. One day Violette is extubated; the next day she's reintubated. One day they're supposed to stop the respirator, and then she starts peeing and moving and she doesn't die. One day she's better and stable; the next day she has a pleural effusion and they have to start the high-frequency ventilator again. One day at a time! The nurses are very nice. They try to protect us by warning that a fall is coming, that there's going to be a sharp drop and, after that, a slow climb back up. Like on a roller coaster. Okay, we get it. For almost five weeks now, we've been knocked around like Shake 'n Bake. Anything can happen. I've decided to adopt an original alternative, to no longer take things as they come, but focus on a point on the horizon. I project us to six months from now. I visualize Violette in her car seat. I see her in Axel's crib, which would become hers. I imagine being woken up by her crying, and no longer by the alarm clock telling me it's time to pump. I imagine James holding his little sister in his arms. But, shit, in six months, Violette may not even be here anymore.

Life Trajectories

"Your baby is stable." You hear that often in neonatology. A nice empty phrase. Health professionals, stop saying that to parents. Stop saying it to each other. Talk about real stuff. A stable baby can be in the arms of her mom being nursed, or hooked up to a respirator, ventilated full-blast with 100 per cent oxygen for a few days. For one baby, it's super-positive; for the other, it's a catastrophe.

Parents of a child in the NICU usually need information on their child's life trajectory. Is their child's situation as it should be – is it "normal for a 26-week baby," for example? Is it normal that the child needs an intravenous line or a central line? (Yes, they all have them.) Is it a good thing that the child no longer needs an intravenous line at 12 days of life? (Yes; usually it takes more time for babies to tolerate their milk; so the child's belly is working well. That baby is a tummy champion.) Is it normal that the child still needs a ventilator at three months of life? (No; it means the child's lungs are extremely sick.)

Many professionals help parents understand their baby's life trajectory. And this is how they proceed:

- They know the baby's name and clinical history.
- They ask the parents how they find their baby.
- They listen to the parents.
- They listen to the parents.

- They listen to the parents.
- They ask the parents what they want: do they prefer to receive detailed information or general information on their baby's condition?
- They ask the parents how they can help them and whether they have questions or concerns.
- And they listen some more.
- They tell the parents that Baby is lucky to have parents like them, who are there and who ask questions. That Baby is lucky to have a mom who brings her milk, that this increases the baby's chances of doing well.

What usually helps parents of babies in the NICU is knowing the following:

- What generally happens to babies like theirs, what the average is. For example, that a 26-week baby always needs help to breathe. That the fact that the baby does not need to be intubated is a good thing. That the tube in the trachea may be necessary for a few days and sometimes even a few weeks, but rarely more than four weeks. That, at a month, most of the babies no longer need an intravenous line. That most of the babies have retinopathy (changes to the back of the eye, the retina), although it is usually minor.
- What we hope to see happen: progress with regard to lungs and feeding, a decrease in technological assistance (respiratory and nutritional). "If Baby does what the average 26-week does, this is what should happen: …"
- Is Baby different from the average at birth? Is Baby a "big" 26 weeks, was he or she born with an infection, are there any malformations? What sets Baby apart from the average? Do we anticipate more problems in a specific area, and why?
- What is normal for babies like theirs: apneas and bradycardias, weight variations, regurgitations. X-rays of the belly or lungs when there are concerns, blood cultures and antibiotics when an infection is suspected, etc. These are the kinds of interventions we do regularly for very preterm babies.
- What is monitored at each stage of Baby's life, what progress we hope to see, and what would worry us. What is the next step, if all goes according to plan?

- That we see a lot of babies like theirs, that we're used to taking care of them, and we know what to do with the problems that can occur. The parents should know if their baby is seriously ill or not, according to our definitions. It's difficult for parents to determine that, even if they're doctors or nurses by profession. When your baby is on a respirator, the baby is sick and you are often sick.
- The words "your baby is stable" are sometimes used to avoid talking about the worst. To avoid talking about death. It is not rare for a parent to ask, "Is my baby dying?" "Is she at risk of dying?" "Do you fear for his life?" or "Is there still a risk of death?" Some parents ask those questions when their baby is not very sick; just seeing the baby hooked up to a monitor, with an intravenous line, with alarms going off, can be frightening for parents. With other babies, there is really a significant risk of death. Answering these questions appropriately is important.

The following are the kind of answers to avoid:

"All babies here are at risk – we're in the NICU. But your baby isn't dying now; she's stable."

"Sir, your baby's on a respirator, he's fragile. But he's stable for the time being. One day at a time. Things can change very quickly."

"We can't answer that question very well. Everyone is at risk of dying, even you. But for now your baby is stable."

"We are worried, but, for the time being, she's stable."

"He's stable. He's now at 90 per cent oxygen and may start peeing again. That's really great!"

"Come now, look at her, she's got nothing but a little PEEP!" (Then the dad looks at the doctor as if to say, "WTF is a peep?")

"He's doing fine; look, it's just a CPAP!" (Then the mother wonders, "Is that like a Pap smear?")

Worse still, some caregivers may not even answer, because they don't hear the question. An evasive clinician who's hiding in his office to avoid difficult situations doesn't manage these situations well. Definition of a bad clinician: one who doesn't step up to the plate, who won't get their hands dirty, and who follows the action from a distance. But there are also parents who don't dare talk about these things or ask questions. That doesn't mean they're not scared. Often, they need a little help. They need to be told about the life trajectories of babies, where they started from, what we expect. They need to be told whether we're worried. There are plenty of areas of medicine where doctors and nurses don't have to deal with death. In neonatology, they do. Those who don't want to face the music and talk about these things shouldn't work in the NICU. There are tons of jobs elsewhere in the health care system.

Fortunately, there are many caregivers who are exceptional.

If parents ask, "Do you fear for his life?" on the first day of their baby's life when he is not intubated and is on a little oxygen, we can tell them certain things. First of all, we can ask them how they find Baby. And listen to them. And listen to them. And listen to them some more. We can ask them why they're worried, what worries them most, what scares them most. We can tell them that most babies born at 26 weeks of gestation survive. That when a baby like theirs dies, it is usually in the first weeks of life. That babies like theirs die because of various things: lungs that don't work, infections, and bleeding in the head, mainly. If parents want more information, we can give it.

Some babies die because their lungs don't work. Baby's lungs are working well, he's breathing well with air being pushed through a mask, and we're satisfied. He doesn't need oxygen. But we're going to monitor how much pressure he needs in the mask to support his breathing, and how much oxygen. Most babies like him need a little oxygen – we can expect that in the coming days, so you mustn't be worried if Baby starts to need oxygen. We are reassured with regard to his lungs now, and we are monitoring them closely.

Some babies die from an infection, because they don't defend themselves well against bacteria and viruses. Their skin is fragile. There are bacteria on them, as with everyone, but the risk is greater that the bacteria will get into Baby's bloodstream now because there's a central line piercing her skin and going to the middle of her body. When there's no more central line, we will be far less concerned about blood infections. Another kind of infection concerns us: enterocolitis, a kind of belly infection. Usually that occurs during the first five weeks of life, and after that we are less concerned. Mom's milk or the milk from the bank and the probiotics we are giving her help to prevent enterocolitis. We constantly monitor the risk of infection in the NICU, and we are obsessive about handwashing.

Some babies die because of bleeding in the head. But that doesn't happen often. Also, Baby had a good transition at birth and has adjusted very well. Usually babies like her do not have significant bleeding. After ten days of life, babies no longer bleed in their heads, because the blood vessels are more stable. Then we'll no longer be worried about that possibility.

There are parents who don't want that much information, others who want more. Still others need this information, but spread out over days, or weeks. Parents are all different.

If, in two weeks, Baby contracts a major infection and needs a respirator, it's possible to adjust the story. It will no longer be the story of what happens to babies like him, but the story of what happens to babies like him who have bacteria in the blood. What is the impact of this infection on him? What usually happens to babies who have this kind of infection? What would be worrying, what would be reassuring, what is being monitored?

Also, sometimes, as my friend and colleague Michel Duval, a doctor in paediatric oncology and palliative care, puts it so well, there is nothing to be said. Sometimes, when things are going badly, the parents know the answer to their questions. When a father asks if his child with a relapse of leukemia is at risk of dying, often the best thing to do is to communicate without words. To look him in the eye, sometimes take his hand and give him a hug while he cries. It's the same in the NICU. When a baby is getting worse and worse, often the best thing to do is to take a mom or a dad in your arms and deal with the parent-quake.

If a baby has a head ultrasound, it's an important day for the parents, and the pressure will often subside only after they have the results. Don't wait till the next day to look at it, listen to the report, or ask someone to interpret it. When a baby has a test that is important for the parents (X-rays, ultrasound, blood gas results, eye examination, etc.), give them the results the same day. "I don't have time" is not an excuse; take the time. It's crucial for the parents to feel that their baby has value for the caregivers and that they know her. There's nothing more difficult for a parent than to be told than "I'm only here for the night, I don't really know the result of her cranial ultrasound" or "I'm just replacing her nurse, who will be coming back in forty-five minutes. I don't know your daughter well."

It's okay not to know, but parents should feel that someone is in control of the situation. As parents, we'd rather hear "I've just seen Baby's X-ray. As a resident, I can tell you the things I'm sure about: the breathing tube is in the right place and there's no pneumonia. That's what we wanted to see. But I will look at all the X-rays with the fellow or the chief, as a team; there will also be other things to look at, such as the general condition of her lungs for a baby at 5 weeks of life. We'll look at all the X-rays, and I'll give you Baby's detailed results and keep you informed later today." And no, don't say the X-ray is stable: stable doesn't mean anything, and that means everything.

23 June

Days of life: 33

Violette's corrected gestational age: 29 weeks, 2 days

Dear Computer,

They have to insert a fourth central line, another PICC line, because she has no more veins in her head, or anywhere else. Several people, including the stars, have tried unsuccessfully to put one in. She'll have to go to the Children's, another hospital, for them to put in a femoral line, but I don't want to have her transported over there. Gene is coming back tonight; he's the champ of PICC lines. The superstars here have put back a little mini-butterfly, and we're waiting, holding our breath, for Gene to arrive.

I'm mad as hell! In medical school, I read about the "anger stage" and the "stages of grief." Shrinks get on my nerves with their labels and their systematization. They talk as if everyone follows one recipe and one typical pattern. That's not the way things happen. Not all parents experience these difficulties in the same way.

It comes in waves. I always try to be reasonable. I try to put things in perspective. I love my routine with Axel, and I tell myself, "I'm lucky I have my routine with my boy. That's something half the NICU parents don't have." And there's also James, our teenager, who's trying to deal with the situation as best he can. But I also tell myself that most of the parents around me are lucky to have a baby born well after 24 weeks of gestation. So, to console myself, I think about Keith, my soulmate, my love, who loves me and supports me, while some mothers here are all alone. And then I become obsessed with those who are not as lucky as I am. It's my "coping mechanism," as the shrinks would say.

Yesterday, during my nighttime fears, I told myself that everyone was trying to help my daughter. No one has ever tried to kill her, neither I nor my neighbours nor the Quebec nation nor my culture nor my traditions. I trust those who are taking care of her – that's important. But still, there's a nurse who drives me nuts, who's always fiddling with the incubator: checking the diaper, the pee, the feet, the intravenous line, and then immediately starting again. Leave her alone! The doctors say she's like a nuclear technician who's constantly working in the fume hood and never takes her hands out. When she's there, I don't have the courage to visit the NICU. I'd rather stay home; otherwise I have tachycardia and feel awful. And I'm not capable of saying anything either.

But, apart from that one nurse, I have absolute confidence. I feel like I'm falling, but in a safe world. Then I think of mothers in Gaza or in certain countries in Africa or elsewhere, countries at war where women and children are systematically raped, where children are murdered to hurt the parents. There are still places in the world where a mother has to choose which of her children will die of hunger. And I tell myself that those women are falling in a terrifying world. There's nothing to comfort them. They can't tell themselves, as I tell myself, that everyone is trying to help them. They're doomed to suffer.

It comforts me for a moment to think about my good fortune, but then I start to cry because I pity them for not being born in a rich country, and I start feeling guilty again for having such a crummy uterus. And then I start to imagine Axel raped or killed in front of my eyes, and I panic and feel nauseous. My coping mechanisms are turning against me. When I think about the two-thirds of babies in the world who don't have access to neonatal care, I feel like a fat, selfish bourgeois. Any mom in the world who's seen her baby die because of a simple infection or lack of food must be saying to herself, "Well, the fat, selfish bourgeois has just woken up. About time." So, in order not to go completely crazy, I think about the real Ungrateful Normals, who are also fat, selfish bourgeois but who complain for no reason. It makes me feel less guilty for an instant, then it pisses me off again. Could someone get the *Parents* magazine that is in the hospital lobby out of my sight? Could someone get the Ungrateful Normals who come to give birth to shut the fuck up about their hemorrhoids?

---

 23 June 2005

5 p.m.: 18F PICC inserted in the right hand, brachiocephalic vein up 16 cm, withdraw to 14.5 cm position confirmed with RX. Premed: EMLA, sucrose x 2, morphine.

Gene Dempsey

Red Underwear

At times, I was angry even at objects, inanimate things. When jars would not open quickly enough and offered too much resistance, I would throw them into the garbage. The idiots deserved it – they would die untouched! If my shoelaces tried to put up a fight, I would cut them: they were asking for it. When my computer took too long to open the internet link I wanted, I unplugged the whole thing from the wall. "I'm unplugging you, you comatose shit. Wake up!" If my book would not stay open when I tried to read while pumping, I would forcefully crack it open. "You'll get a page ripped out next time," I would warn him (a book is masculine in French). I was not like this all day. I had spikes of anger through my apathy, and sadness. I generally indulged when I was alone, unnoticed. Like a person with an uncontrollable tic disorder, I felt the tension build unbearably if I didn't explode.

I remember my worst crisis, how scary I once became. I decided one morning to wear sexy underwear, knowing that this kind of thing had always made me feel better in an incognito way. But I could not wear a sexy bra, since it would get all milky and gross. I was wearing the ones with the garage doors in the front, with the pads underneath, so it was no use imagining sexiness there. My boobs had lost any kind of sex-symbol status. They were now important utilities that provided liquid gold to Violette. One day, after I squished empty cartons of milk to place them in the recycle bin, Axel started playing with them. He was familiar with Bertha, the electric breast pump, and put the cartons next to it and said "lait [milk]?" He held these stupid milk cartons all day, and slept with them during his nap. That afternoon, we drew a mama on the sidewalk with chalk, and he placed the empty cartons of milk where the breasts should be. What a clever boy, I thought!

So I had to re-locate what was left of my imaginary sexiness lower down. I had this lacy fire-engine red underwear. I even had remembered a funny incident about that *culotte*. During my NICU fellowship, I moonlighted in the emergency room most Friday evenings to make money. But also to stay capable of communicating with "normal children" who actually spoke, a skill I needed for my paediatric exams later that year. After my shift, around midnight, I would go salsa dancing. So I had a change of clothes for salsa in my backpack. Earlier in the day, I biked around in looser outfits and wore scrubs during my NICU day and my ER shift. Scrubs are really comfortable top you pull over your head, and a bottom you pull up and tighten with a string ... like pajamas. After my shower, right before my ER shift, I changed into my "salsa underwear," the red lacy *culotte*. It can be described as somewhere between a bona fide thong and a full-cover bikini. It exposed half the backside, as my husband refers to it, so they were perfect for energetic salsa dancing: no VPL (visible panty lines) problems or too much jiggle action.

So one evening, I had this sexy red lacy thing underneath my scrubs, and was examining the ears of a kid who was about 2 years old. The parents were young, stressed. The kid had a fever. He was lying down on the exam table. I had his mother hold him so I could look inside his ears. While I was hunched over him, bending down, trying to negotiate a look into his right ear, he pulled the knot on my scrub pants. My pants fell down with a clunk, weighed down by all the stuff attached to them or in their pockets – personal pager, "code blue" pager, calculator – and left me bare assed, butt up, with the kid's father sitting behind me. I could not just let go of the thrashing kid I had pinned on the examining table to examine his ears. If I let go of him, he might end up on the floor, or with a perforated eardrum. I asked the mom to hold him, reached down and pulled up my pants with the most dignity I could muster, attached them with four secure knots, and continued examining his ear. I thought this would have been hilarious in a movie – except that it was happening to me. I hoped the parents would still take me seriously, even with my frivolous underwear. "Your son has a bad otitis," I told them, my face as red as my underwear. I went to write the prescription. I heard them crack up laughing when I left the room. I returned as fast as I could, explained the doses, the time, how to have him take the medicine if he did not like the taste, all as quickly as I could. The father thanked me and told me he thought his son had good taste. I wanted to disappear.

So that morning in July, I thought that I would feel better if I wore the "red otitis undies." They had a funky history. I did not at all have the bum I had BC (before children), though. It felt kind of stretched, wobbly, and elephantesque. But whatever, I thought. It will have to do – there are worse things in life. A new period of my life is starting. So I sported this lacy thing, underneath the only pants that fit me (with an elastic band stretched to bursting). During the day, the red undies became more and more uncomfortable. I felt like a ridiculous mom with my red underwear eating at my lady bits. What was I trying to prove? What was my problem? I was now a Fruit of the Loom lady. I no longer belonged to the world of those girls who dance salsa with Victoria's Secret underwear. At some point that day, I could not focus on anything except my damned cheeky underwear. I am really an Insensitive Rich Bitch, I thought: I couldn't think of anything but my stupid red *culotte*. I have a sick daughter – she is on a respirator. I am supposed to be here to focus on her. Wow, great mother. Violette, I am sorry; your mom has serious underwear trouble. I was holding Violette on me, in what we call "kangaroo," painfully, shifting from one side to the other, trying not to trouble my small baby too much. I could not just reach down my pants and pull the damned thing that kept crawling sideways.

A few minutes later, in one of the breastfeeding/pumping rooms, small rooms where you could pump in private and could talk to yourself without people judging, I pulled the undies back to the middle, with relief, and started pumping. While I was pumping, though, they started crawling sideways again. It was so uncomfortable, I actually started hissing at the cheeky undies: "You red bitch (underwear is feminine in French). You can't stay rigorously in the middle like a thong; you can't even be a solid supportive bikini. You half-assed thing, you half-baked slut. You gotta decide: in or out, not just in between sideways. This is my last warning! I've had it with you. This is the last time I am placing you in the middle. In or out – you decide. Not sideways." It was the most ridiculous blind rage I'd ever felt – this is why I describe it now in so much detail. Blind anger was eating me up and oozing out. I'm really not a frivolous weirdo in real life. But this is what can happen when a Fruit of the Loom tries to be a Victoria's Secret.

I remember pumping, realizing the underwear was starting to slip sideways again. I thought, no way, the defiant slut! "You are really asking for it – you are testing the limits." I stopped pumping (the bra garage doors open, T-shirt up), took my pants off, threw them against the wall, and pulled my lacy underwear off, on a raging mission to tear the enemy to shreds. "You're gonna pay. I'm gonna beat you to some sorry red pulp! I warned you!" I declared out loud. The damned things were resistant though. They were putting up a real fight: they would not rip. Please let me be stronger than a lace *culotte*! I am stronger than her! Above the sinks in the breastfeeding room was a metal box that held rolls of brown paper towels, with a saw-toothed edge for tearing off the sheets. HAHA, I thought, with a crazed feeling and a dried metallic taste in my mouth. Holding the red demon firmly in my two hands and quickly sawing back and forth on the teeth of the metal edge, I tried to cut through my enemy. It took a while, but I succeeded in shredding my underwear into four pieces, won the war, and threw them in the trash. I continued pumping with an empowered feeling. Finally, I was a winner. I was a dominatrix. I had won against the red evil, and her corpse lay in the trash.

But after five minutes, I realized how much rage I had directed at an inanimate object. I realized I was sitting bare-assed on the sofa, pumping breast milk for my critical baby. I had to destroy my underwear to feel empowered. I felt so empty, so lost, so distant, not-there, invisible, so absent from the world, from myself. A non-person was pumping – I could see her from above. Somehow, it was supposed to be me. "I am pumping, I am pumping, I am pumping, I am pumping," I kept repeating out loud, talking to myself in a neutral tone, to stay focused and not lose it again. Describing what I was doing out loud worked very well in scary moments like these, kept me in the moment, kept my wandering brain from scattering completely. I wasn't comparing myself with either the Inconsiderate Normals or the worse off in the world. I just continued talking slowly: "I am me," "I am breathing," "I am unplugging my attachments," "I am washing my attachments," "The water is too hot," "I turn the cold-water tap," "I am screwing the plastic top on," "The milk is lukewarm," "The milk has lots of IgA antibodies," "I am washing my hands," "I am standing up … "

I'd much rather be a woman than a man. Women can cry, they can wear cute clothes, and they are the first to be rescued off of sinking ships.

Gilda Radner

My Love

My dear Keith,

I love you so much. I tell you so constantly; we tell each other constantly. I'm so lucky you're there. There are things I don't dare say to you, or even to myself. I say them only to PC. No, not my lover, my personal computer. I don't know if you'll read this message one day. You'll read it if I die or go mad and someone searches on my computer. There are things already written in our wills, but just in case … and we'll have to talk about the wills again. Maybe I'd be happy in a wheelchair, after all. Maybe don't unplug me in that case. I don't know if you'll read this letter that isn't a love letter. But I can't say it out loud – you'll think I'm suicidal, and that isn't true. I don't want to worry you.

I can see that sometimes you act strong, and so I act strong so that you too can let yourself go and get the bad stuff out. But I'm nothing without you. My bedrock. My beacon. My Ironman of the NICU, who knows all the science, and who knows our daughter as well as Lorraine and Debbie do. My lover, my soulmate. I love the way you take care of her, the way you make sure everything is up to date, her lab tests, her X-rays. And I love the way you say, hypocritically, "I'm only the father," when you go into your office to look at her X-rays in secret (but I won't tell anyone). I love the way you always make sure she has her dose of sucrose before the procedures. I love it that you're the bulldog of handwashing. I love how you hold her close during the kangaroo sessions, the ones that last a long time. She's so at home in your arms. The two of you are so beautiful. The dad-baby unit. She's so secure like that. I love when you tell her you're an international expert on apnea in newborns and that she should take your classes.

If something happens to me, if I really go mad and I don't understand what's happening, I beg you, look after our children: you know exactly what they need. Keep doing what you do with Violette, have confidence in her, have confidence in yourself. If I go insane, please make sure the drugs don't make me grow a beard or hair on my chest. And if there are any hairs, pull them out, zap them with a laser or whatever, but I don't want to have a beard. Even if I look like I don't give a damn. I give a damn if I have a beard, and it's my dignity that will be at stake. It won't matter if I go bald, no need for a wig or a scarf. Please take me outside a little bit every day. Please wash me every day. Please make sure I don't pee in the bed without a diaper, and buy diapers that don't leak. Please feed me things I like. And when I ask stupid questions, no need to always answer the same thing. To keep yourself entertained, you can tell me I was once married to the king of England. If I end up not recognizing you at all anymore, no need to come and see me (except to pluck out my chin hairs). And if I sink that low, find somebody else.

But from now on, you're the one who decides for Violette, for the children. I will always follow you. Always.

24 June

Days of life: 34

Violette's corrected gestational age: 29 weeks, 3 days

Violette,

I am with you. I love you. It's hard seeing you like this. I try to explain to myself what's happening and why it's happening, but the words don't come. You're doing better than last week. But that's not very hard. I'm the one who should be taking the hits, not you. My little flower, who is blooming slowly, who has been a little bud on the surface of the earth for a long time. A very tiny sprout, magical and precious. I'm waiting for you to grow. One day you will bloom, I hope. The more the days pass, the more hope I have, and I need to believe in that in order to help you heal.

But I look at my little sprout every day and I don't see the flower growing – I see the little Violette bud and I HOPE. The snow could cover it, a dog could piss on it, the letter carrier could crush it without noticing; it could be eaten by a squirrel, pulled out by a little rascal, hit by a hailstone. I know you're growing a little every day, but it doesn't show and it's driving me crazy. You're not getting better. You've already had four intubations, too many central catheters, and I don't know how many procedures. It will end up destroying you. How much more can you take? I don't see any improvement from one day to the next. I don't see the little flower developing.

Sophie sat down with me today and gave me a good talking-to. She showed me a progress note from 19 June, then the one from today. It's true, you're doing better. Yes, there are risks but, still, you're improving. We have to look at what's going well: no bleeding in the head, no meningitis with your sepsis, you're no longer on high-frequency, you're completely fed by mouth, although you still have your damn PICC line bombarding you with meropenem, and you don't (yet?) have enterocolitis. It's true, you're no longer a bud, but I'd like you to be less fragile.

I'm not used to so much uncertainty, so much waiting. I want to take charge of things! I just want it to be next year. In 2006, things will have to be better. I don't want to visit you in the cemetery with a pot of violets. You'd have a little white marble tombstone with green or mauve veins, with the design of a little violet carved in the centre. Fuck. Why am I writing this? Come on, HOPE! I'm able to start having it again. We'll have to organize "hope boot camps" in the unit. I'd have a lot of push-ups to do.

26 June

Days of life: 36

Violette's corrected gestational age: 29 weeks, 5 days

Dear Computer,

Things are going better every day. And I'm starting to get seriously impatient! I want to be with Violette at home, I want to watch her sleeping with Axel, I want her to be discharged from the hospital. RIGHT AWAY! The two of us will take care of her, Axel and I.

What will she look like in a year? What colour will her eyes be? For now, she looks pretty much like any premature baby, but with more collapsed veins and not much hair left; she's had so many intravenous lines in her head, it's been almost completely shaved. All she has left is a little tuft like Tintin. But her mouth is different. She already has an adorable little mouth, heart-shaped like a doll's. Kind of a little cherry mouth, with slightly parted lips that will barely show her perfect teeth. I hope her tooth buds haven't been damaged by the intubations. No, it was Gene and Sophie who intubated her. They're excellent. Her tooth buds are okay. Shit, is this the time to think about that? I'm really shallow. She's still on the respirator, she's just had a serious complication with her catheter, and I'm thinking about her tooth buds. What would I have said about a mother like me before I'd had Violette, when I was pseudonormal? "She's thinking about her teeth! Are you kidding?"

Of course, I'd love Violette even if her teeth never came in. Then I'd tell her that when her papy was young, they used to pull out everyone's teeth and give them dentures. And everyone loved Papy! There's more to life than tooth buds. There's more to life than teeth!

Violette could come home. But my throat tightens just thinking about it: the year 2006 is my goal – 2006, 2006, 2006. I have to visualize 2006. I've just spent fifteen minutes writing this. That makes fifteen minutes less until 2006.

27 June

Days of life: 37

Violette's corrected gestational age: 29 weeks, 6 days

Computer,

TODAY IS A BIG DAY: VIOLETTE HAS BEEN EXTUBATED! She's still having apneas-bradys, but they're much less serious than before. I adore hydrocortisone: it saved her life. It helped them extubate her. But, in large quantities, it's not very good for the brain. I think it is not over and we should buy some at Costco.

If anyone dares to tell me again to take things one day at a time, I'll kick their ass. It's funny, they always tell you to take it one day at a time when things are going well. When Violette has a good day. YES, WE KNOW she could die the next day. A good day … I've become a real NICU mother. A good day is when all the gas levels are okay, when there aren't too many desaturations on the respirator, and when we can hope that some day she'll manage without a tube between her vocal cords. A good day is also when I can take her in my arms and she doesn't have too many bradys, and I don't turn pale and get agitated. You'd better believe it, that's a good day for the family. That gives you an idea of how we're feeling. And when one of those blessed days happens, with nice results and fresh, sweet hope, couldn't they just leave us in peace and let us enjoy it? There's no need to remind us that anything can happen. WE KNOW THAT. We know that her ductus arteriosus is open, that there's still slight kidney failure, that she has a little fluid in the lungs.

But dammit, they just extubated her, and she was dying not so long ago! So, what do you want me to say? We also know she could die of necrotizing enterocolitis. I'm not an imbecile, I'm a neonatologist! We should put a note on the incubator: "Things we know and that you don't need to remind us of: the thirty complications that could kill her or leave her disabled for life. Let's hope that those thirty complications won't occur. Let's hope really hard. Just say it's a good day. That's all."

Other People

29 June 2005

Days of life: 39

Violette's corrected gestational age: 30 weeks and 1 day

Dear Computer,

I can't take it anymore. I can't take other people. I'm discovering the true faces of people I thought I knew. There are some I found distant who have opened their arms to me. There are others who had always been close to me who have run away. Since I'm a doctor here, a lot of people know me and try to be nice to me. But I don't feel much like seeing people. Usually I just want to be with Keith, Axel, and James in our little bubble, to hide in our little world, eat my peanut butter toast, pump my milk, and wear sweatpants. I can stand only a small number of people at a time. Is the problem them or me? I don't know.

Computer, I'm going to start by talking about the things that are going well – it will be like therapy. We have great support. People are taking care of us, they really help us, they say nice things, they send us beautiful letters. There are flowers at our house. The flowers are encouraging, and they smell good. Sometimes, the most comfort comes from people you didn't expect it from. Strangers, practically. Often, former NICU parents give us their support, parents I'd stayed in touch with and who had heard that "Dr Annie" was dealing with the same shit they'd had. The connection with those parents is incredible. What's even weirder in my case as a doctor-mom is being comforted by parents whose babies are in the NICU now. Only a few weeks ago, before my twentieth week of pregnancy, I was still looking after their sick babies. All that is so far away now, it feels like another life to me. But they're still here; their babies are doing better, they're in intermediate care now, and these parents know exactly how to listen, what to say and what not to say. They know that the most important thing is to be there, to listen, and to tolerate silence.

Olivia's mother is a good example. I took care of her little girl, who almost died of respiratory failure. One night she was so unstable that we were sure we were losing her, and I took her mother's hand. There was nothing else I could do. Olivia survived. Today it's her mother who tells me that it's okay to want to run away, that she was also on automatic pilot when Olivia was very sick, and she also left when things were going really badly. NICU parents, you have no idea how much you've done for me, and I thank you for it. I've heard you talk about your family crises, your fears, your dark secrets. And I'm lucky to be a neonatologist – right now, my great medical knowledge isn't doing me much good, but my position has allowed me to get to know you, to share a little of the parents' experience. Since Violette's birth, when she seems to be dying, then does better, then starts again and comes back to life again, I remember the stories of those families, and I know I'm not completely crazy. I have no idea how I could have gotten through it, how I could have remained standing, if I hadn't known them.

My own family and friends are also giving me a lot of comfort. People say all kinds of nice things, as in these conversations:

"How are you doing?"

"…"

"I wish things were going better for you and Violette. I hope they'll continue to go well/they'll go better soon."

Or:

"How's Violette doing?"

"…"

"I wish things were going better/I hope things will keep getting better. Is there something I can do for you? Would it help to have company? Do you want me to bring you a movie?" (Not war movies, or movies about cancer or illness.)

Or:

"I made an apple pie. Would you like me to bring it to you? I could come and play with Axel after supper – that way you could go to the unit with Keith."

Those who are really helpful know that when the answer is no, it's no. They don't try to get invited; they just leave the apple pie at the door. They don't try to make us laugh; they're just there for us. When we have nothing to say, they're able to listen to the silence. They listen to our complaints when we have them. They tell us to hang on. They ask us what they can do. And when we reply, "But what do you think you can do? You can't do ANYTHING," they don't get offended, they just give us a hug. If we tell them we want to be alone, they go away without saying that the company would do us good.

My friend Ginette, a former police officer who founded Préma-Québec, the association for premature children, had two premature babies. She told me that when her babies were in the NICU, she didn't want to see anyone except her husband and children. She describes herself as a Doberman that had been hit by a car. The only thing she wanted to do was hide under the veranda and lick her wounds. I love that image. I often feel that way. When the parents in the NICU tell their friends they want to be alone, it's because that's what they really want. Now I understand. I used to think they said that because they wanted attention, because they were depressed, or because they needed company but didn't want to upset people. I was completely out to lunch. I know it now.

I just want to be alone. With my love, in my house, with Axel and James. That's all. Since Violette has been in the hospital, I notice the "snakes and ladders" coming from people around me: the kind words, the low blows. I wrote on the days when I was disgusted with the Others, and the days when I was touched by having people who are so important in my life. Those writings aren't very coherent. I've just put everything together, making a list of the beautiful things, and a list of the poisonous things. I copy-pasted the transcriptions of a few toxic conversations, and I even divided them into categories. It's like a little spontaneous qualitative narrative research project, without having to go through the ethics committee. I must be fed up with navel gazing and now I'm starting to breathe, since Violette is really, truly doing better.

The cool things: sometimes friends, family members, or colleagues surprise me by sending a poem, a letter, a photo of me as a little girl missing her front teeth, body lotion, or flowers. What gave me a lot of pleasure when I was in the delivery room, in addition to the food everyone brought, was a package mailed to me by my great friend Catherine, who's living in Boston during her fellowship. It contained a big bag of the artificial jelly candies I adore, with some kinds I didn't know – and I'm an expert on gummies – with big fluorescent-coloured octopuses dusted with sugar and a horrible pink pen with a cow-head top that flashes, and a SpongeBob notepad in which to write down my toxic thoughts. Another friend, Annabelle, invited us to her house and made us a very simple meal while Axel played with her kids. I remember an evening spent at her house, folding clothes, eating corn on the cob, looking at the sky, and playing Settlers of Catan and Carcassonne. We didn't talk a lot, but it was reassuring being with "normal" people and doing normal things. I remember when Keith showed his friend Pierre a photo of Violette and they fell into each other's arms weeping. Sometimes you don't need words.

Mamy is always there. She often takes care of Axel. She tells me that Violette is my baby. She finds her beautiful. "Look at her, look at her little feet, her little hands, she's perfectly formed, she's so beautiful!" And I'm sure she really thinks that, because my mother isn't the kind of person who goes overboard about beauty. And she's able to see Violette's beauty through the wires, the tubes, and the machines.

And then, Computer, there are the Others, the ones who don't listen, the ones who can't simply be there and are incapable of shutting up for one second, the ones who drag you down when you're soaring, the ones who won't let you sit quietly in peace, the ones who are simply not there because looking at a baby hooked up to a respirator, hoping against hope, smiling when they know you might be about to take a hard blow, is too much for them. Because they can't stand the uncertainty and waiting. Most of those Others don't mean us any harm. But they're often unhelpful and toxic. There are little things that do us a lot of good, but there are also little things that can destroy us. An inappropriate word. A stupid comment. An insensitive remark. For instance, I had this conversation today. I wrote it down to get it out of my system as quickly as possible. Now that I've listed the pleasant things, I can go back and pop the pimples and get the pus out:

"How are you?" one of the Others asks me.

"So far, it's been a good day. Her heart hasn't slowed down too often, she's growing, she's tolerating her milk, she's been extubated! She's breathing, and they haven't put the tube back in! I've been waiting for that for weeks. The next stage: they take out the fourth catheter before another infection occurs or something gets perforated!"

"Don't exaggerate; don't be so negative."

"I'm not being negative, I'm just saying how things are. It's good, I'm positive, she's getting better, she's no longer intubated! Today I feel like we're going to get through this!"

"Be careful. You told us yourself that things are never completely certain. It's hard when you build your hopes up and they're dashed. It hurts even more when you fall from a height. For example, when I was pregnant, I didn't tell anyone before I had passed 12 weeks, in case I had a miscarriage."

"Thank you for calling, it's very kind. I have to leave you; I need to pump my milk."

"Don't hesitate; I'm thinking of you, call whenever you want."

When I feel wounded, insulted, or shocked, when I feel I'm going to explode from hearing all these stupidities, when I have to end the conversation stat (a medical term, from the Latin *statim*, which means "Now! Immediately! Yesterday!" as in "Epinephrin, STAT!"), I use this quick solution: I say that I have had a milk let-down, that my T-shirt is all wet and I have to go and pump. Or that the hospital is calling on the other line.

After a few conversations like this, I understood that it was no use discussing the good or bad side of the situation, or comparing being pregnant with being Violette's mother. It annoys me and offends me to always have to explain why my daughter could live or die. When I'm positive, it seems that the Others automatically try to undermine my mood. They tell me she could have lifelong effects, and it annoys me to have to explain to them that children with cerebral palsy can still have a good quality of life. Parents of babies in the NICU shouldn't be obliged to educate their friends or colleagues about prematurity. It's not up to me to comfort them – fuck! So I cut things short.

The opposite is also true. At worst, they say everything will be okay, and that makes me look like a crazy pessimist. There are people who simply don't understand. Then I go back to my pump while doing "rewind-delete," and I try to let it slide off me like water off a duck's back and not get to me. As soon as I realize I'm in a "rewind-delete" type of conversation, I look for a way out.

As a neonatologist, I've often seen parents being visited by these insensitive people. There have been times when I should have intervened but didn't. You have to be in the situation of those parents to understand them, and I didn't always realize what they were going through. Maybe I also thought it wasn't my role as a doctor to intercede with the families. But if the jerks are doctors or nurses, then I don't hold back.

Computer, I've decided that if I ever become a neonatologist again, if I can still function in that environment of life and death, with the constant alarms, the uncertainties, and the little babies, I promise to try to help parents protect themselves from the Others. I also promise to try to help the Others to behave better with the parents, to become a source of comfort and not a nuisance. Ultimately, what they want to do is help, not harm.

Computer, you're getting all my ideas in a jumble. I've written down the comments that have wounded me and the ones that have helped me. My brain is such mush that I don't know how to classify them so that it makes some kind of sense. When I get out of this hole, I promise you I'll write a kind of guide for parents, friends, and families. A kind of survival guide.

4 July

Days of life: 44

Violette's corrected gestational age: 30 weeks, 6 days

 Resp: stable on nIMV 11/5 X 15, in 23–25%, A/Bs frequent, caffeine +
Fluids-Nutrition: 160ml/kg/d, TPN + EBM24 (120 PO). Lasix stopped
today, less edema. Weight 1350 g, +10 g.
CVS: PDA murmur unchanged, pulse.
ID: Still on antibiotics, CBC, WBC and differential still abnormal.
Imp/Plan: clinically stable, status resp. improving.
Following A/B closely, if we are able: gradually going to wean her off the
CPAP.
CBC: recent infection, to be followed.
Feeding progressing, when FPO X 24h: remove PICC.

Resident

Just Being There

Today, I took you in my arms and fled to another world
I was holding onto you for dear life
On an island of love
On an island of stillness
Holding on my moon
Holding on my *ancre*, by buoy
In a bubble of oxygen and CO_2, generated by the two of us, our bubble
In a suspended life, a security net below us
With roots underneath my chair and organic connections between our bodies
With leaves above us, dew on our lips and warmth

This magical world cannot be reached on demand
I just landed there and we stayed suspended for a while
My treasure on my chest, all my life in my hands
Our bodies connected
The halo of our warmth and our love
A world without "day by day" mantras and roller-coaster analogies
The passport to this world is placing all desires aside
A world of right now, JUST right now

A world with no anxieties regarding the future, no guilt,
A raw world with no promises

A world with no thoughts, no fears
Fear of losing you
Fear of losing all the dreams that I had imagined
Fear of holding you and loving you too much and not being able
to recover from your loss
Fear of falling

Just being there
Not hoping for anything in return

I spent liberated moments levitating with you
Imagining all my organs, the blood circulating
And all your mirror organs, growing slowly
Thinking of my breasts engorged with milk to feed you
Of all the small milk ducts, of the immunoglobulins
Of the curdled milk being digested in your small stomach and
intestines
Of your mini kidneys making urine
Concentrating on my heart beat, on my breath
On your heart beat and your breath
Until you forgot to breathe, your heart slowed down and this
fragile card castle world disintegrated into a spiral of alarms and
you were taken from me
And I felt empty, cold and alone again

20 July

Days of life: 60

Violette's corrected gestational age: 33 weeks, 1 day

Computer,

It's Papa's birthday. He would have been 60 today. I'm sure he would have made us laugh. He would have injected his humour into all this. We're supposed to meet at the cemetery at four this afternoon to sing songs. My heart's not really in it, but I'll go anyway. Maybe it will boost my morale to see the whole family again, the nieces and nephews – who knows?

I tried to breastfeed Violette. Not great. When I just bring her close to a nipple, she starts to have apnea, she forgets to breathe. But with the bottle, she's quite capable of sucking. So we'll have to alternate the breast with bottles. It's hard to provide the ideal conditions for breastfeeding, even though I have all the help I need. But she loses weight every time she tries to feed at the breast. Weight = brain matter = neurons. So I get stressed. Fortunately the nurses are here. Doctors are generally not much help when it comes to breasts.

24 July 2005

Weight: 1885 g (<25 g)

Problems: Apneas + bradys: on caffeine. Neonatal pneumopathy.

Resp: 2 bradys die requiring stimulation, several desaturations.

CVS: breathing stable.

GI: FPO gavage LME q 3h, several suctions non nutritional.

Heme: sp. Infectio: SP. Neuro: ROP + TF ultrasound to follow.

PDA: still open + breath.

FPO: EBM24, growing.

Anemia: on iron.

Possible hypocorticism: to be followed.

ROP stage1 in both eyes: to be followed.

Exam: stable.

Imp: stable.

Plan: idem, transfer to bed.

18 August 2005

2:25 a.m.

Preemie of more than 37 weeks, with pneumopathy of prematurity and A+B.

Post examination of eyes for ROP stage 3 bilateral.

Today, bright blood in stools, abundant, mixed with stools X 2 Clinically stable,

RR = 50–60, indrawing 1–2+

BP normal, urine+;

FPO bottles EBM, abdo normal; Good muscle tone, no evidence of fissures.

BB stable, normal physical examination, active reactive.

Imp: r/o NEC, infection not very likely, no fissure.

Plan: abdo X ray, NPO, labs, intravenous ATB to be followed according to X ray and CBC.

part four

PROGRESS AND SETBACKS

20 August

Days of life: 91

Violette's corrected gestational age: 37 weeks, 4 days

Computer,

Sorry for the relative lack of communication lately. Violette was doing quite well, so I didn't feel much need to write. No major problems, no fits of absolute despair. But a big pile of shit has just landed on us. In fact, two piles. Bloody. There's blood in her stools, and not just a little. I saw Debbie changing her diaper after I went to pump my milk. It was all red. She looked at me; we understood each other. She said Violette looked so well, that it was nothing. I'd like to believe her. I even think she didn't want to go get the resident. Poor resident, what can he do? An X-ray. I asked her to wait for the antibiotics – the first time I've asked for something! Dammit, I'm so fed up.

On the X-ray, no pneumatosis, therefore no enterocolitis, which we were so afraid of. But the plan is still to stop feeding for two days and put in an intravenous, which was so difficult to install. Poor Violette. She lost her intravenous today, and Debbie convinced Daniel, the doctor, to begin giving her milk again. And now it's started all over. There's a tiny bit of blood in her stools, so they're monitoring. Is this ever going to end?

22 August

Days of life: 93

Violette's corrected gestational age: 37 weeks, 6 days

Computer,

Another goddamn pile of shit falls on us, not bloody this time – much worse!

Violette is now 38 weeks old. Everything was going fine, but Keith had to go to England for six days. His sister Janice has been diagnosed with an aggressive breast cancer and has to have an operation. Really, what a rotten year. The whole family is getting hit.

Keith wanted to see his sister before her surgery. His brother Richard has also just lost an eye because of a blood clot. I encouraged him to go. Since Violette was quite stable, I was too. But I miss him. And now I've received this horrible news. I don't know what to do. I feel so alone, really alone. Keith, my love, where are you? I don't know what to do anymore.

I try to tell myself things are going to be okay, that I'm not crazy. I shut myself up in my office to say it out loud and hear it, but it's not enough. If I write it, that might help a little, but I know that it won't work, because you're not here and, no, things are not going well. Things are going badly, in fact. Violette's eyes are not good, the retinopathy has progressed and they have to do something to reduce the risk that she'll lose her sight. I'm so desperate, I'm nauseous. I'm afraid of losing control. I'm an adult, a mother, an educated woman. I can control myself.

I shouldn't have agreed to have my mom take Axel today. With him, at least, I have certainties. He keeps me grounded. With Violette, there's nothing but uncertainty, and I don't know what to do. There's always more bad luck. As soon as I calm down and stop hiding my face in my hands, as soon as I start to relax and I don't have my shoulders up around my ears, as soon as I manage to sleep, I get another baseball bat in the teeth or in the stomach.

Keith, I can't reach you. I press "redial" every five minutes. I call all over. No answer anywhere. You're probably with Janice at the hospital, with your phone turned off. I said it was okay for you to go see Janice, but now, there's a problem with Violette's eyes. She has stage 3 retinopathy in zone 1. They say they would operate on her if you were here, that she needs laser surgery. On top of that there's the unbearable doctor who's substituting (because two neonatologists aren't here – guess who?). He doesn't talk, he yells. When he does rounds with students, he complicates everything. He talks to the parents as if they were 3 years old, while many of the parents know more than the students. I can't stand him. Sophie and Gene are on vacation, and I'm making great efforts not to pester them. They've done more than their share for Violette. The loudmouth came and drew a picture for me, and he'd forgotten Violette's name and mixed up the right eye and the left.

I have no one to talk to who would really understand. What's more, Olivia has been discharged, and her mother was my unofficial "mentor mom." Olivia is at home now, and I don't want to disturb her. Heck, I'm a neonatologist. I know exactly what everyone's going to tell me, and I don't want to hear it. In any case, people don't know what to say anymore. What's left to say?

When Dr Oh gave me the news, I was dumbstruck for three minutes, as if someone had stuck a sock down my throat. I was physically unable to speak, as if I were encased in ice. Freeze frame. Because of your absence, they're going to do another examination in three days, and then they'll make a decision. I'm in no condition to give consent now. I don't know what to say. I tell them I need my husband, it's an important decision, it's an operation with another intubation. And that idiot,

Dr Loudmouth, tells me it's the ophthalmologist who's going to do the operation, not me, Annie Janvier, no reason to be afraid. Oh yeah? Gee, I thought it would be the anaesthesia technician, or maybe my brother – he's an engineer, after all. Dammit, Keith, I'm an expert on informed consent, and I teach the importance of autonomy. But I don't at all feel like making a "free and informed" decision. I haven't been autonomous since I had children, and especially since I've been in the NICU with Violette. And an informed decision for my daughter, who's at risk of becoming blind – dammit, that's ironic. I don't want to have a voice! I just want Dr Oh to give me a hug and tell me what she's going to do with Violette and that everything will be okay. They know their job, why ask me for my opinion? Fuck empowerment! How could I feel strong enough to make the right decision? Poor Violette, we have a big decision to make, one I can't make on my own.

Keith, do I sign? For her to go back on the respirator, with her little lungs that are so fragile? But where are you? The last time I had to make a major decision for Violette, I screwed up completely; luckily, she sucked on her soother, and you were there to decide. So I'll wait three days and the examination will be repeated on your return. I know there's still a risk, but not too much. Do you agree? She can't go back on the respirator, can she? Never again, unless she's in danger of dying, right? We agree, don't we?

Axel is at Mamy's house. She took him so I can devote myself to Violette 24/7 and prepare for her, maybe, one day, to finally come home. It's true I can be here more. I've planned a "weekend getaway" with Violette, although I often feel sorry for Axel. It sure hasn't been an ideal summer for him. Yesterday, he tried to pump while we were waiting for Mamy to come and get him. He even understood how the two buttons work: one speed, one strength. He demonstrated both. So cute.

So I'm here at the office, freaking out. I really wish you were here. You're my man, my soulmate, my rock, my love, my confidant. You're Violette's papa. You saved her life. You always know what needs to be done. You're reassuring. Violette is so beautiful in her little bassinet. She finishes almost all her bottles with my milk in them. She's getting stronger. She has an acid-sweet smell. A taste of yogurt with honey when I kiss her. She squeezes my finger when I put it in her hand. I know it's a reflex, but I like to think it isn't. I like to imagine she's telling me she needs me.

That she likes her milk. That she knows I have milk in my breasts that nourishes her. That she likes it when I hold her in my arms, when I sing her a song. That she knows I would go to the ends of the earth for her. That I'd be willing to spend the rest of my days in a wheelchair for her, to have my legs cut off for her if only it could help her. I am her planet; she is my moon. My pure little moon. If I could, I would give her my eyes.

No! No operation! She can't take it. I can't take it! I need to talk to you, Keith, and I can't get through. So I'm writing to you to try to calm myself. I don't want her to go back on the respirator. I love her. I would sign immediately to take ten years off my life – no, twenty! – if that could bring her home to us and guarantee me that this ordeal would be over. I can't live with this uncertainty anymore. Violette blind? That makes me sad. That stresses me out. But no surgery, not now. Blind, that would be terrible. But the respirator, out of the question!

Dear World

Please, world, be tolerant.
Society, be tolerant of little flowers that are trying to grow …
Do not squish them because they grow too slowly …
Do not dig them out because they look sickly and grow weird leaves …
Do not stop watering them even if they are tiny and grow to be much smaller than the other bigger flowers …
Nurture them, find something beautiful in them even if they have lost some petals and may grow sideways.

And protect my flower, my little Violette.
Protect her when she will go up the stairs, when she will cross the street, when she will play with others, when she will walk with those bigger than her, when she will play sports, when she will try to bike and when she really will succeed, when she will take the bus at night and walk alone in the streets, when someday she will walk with a guy late at night.
Protect her when she ends up at the wrong place, with the wrong person, at the wrong time.
Protect her when she will take her bath, when she will swim in paddle pools, when she will swim in lakes, when she will be in boats, on bridges, in planes, and in cars that go too fast.

Protect her when she eats so she does not choke, especially uncooked carrots, grapes, round candy, and anything that may obstruct her small trachea.

Protect her from all nasty infections, or at least protect her from Intensive Care if she gets hospitalized.

Protect her from pain, at least until she is an adult; she has had enough …

May she be strong, but also vulnerable. May she always walk in life like she did as a microflower.

Hands open, oxygen pumping in her lungs, heartbeat slowing but not completely. May she have the conviction to stand up after she is crushed, the will to continue, the strength to walk with lights in her eyes in the darkest nights, the hope and desire to continue until light comes, until it makes sense.

Guide her to hang around those who will not crush her, who will find her beautiful inside, who will not take advantage of her weaknesses, who will not use her, who will not abuse her.

Guide her away from bullies who will want to steal her pink erasers, but also from girlies who only like Barbies, rainbows, and ponies …

May she realize her dreams. May she have time to smell flowers, taste lemon pies, watch ants, be amazed by nature, children, and the strength of humans …

May she be quick enough for the world we live in, but not too quick to notice the beauty of life that is going on all the time …

Make her always continue to move.

Immobility kills us.

Because if she continues moving, she will go somewhere.

If she moves, it means she is alive.

A few hours of mountain climbing turn a villain and a saint into two rather equal creatures. Exhaustion is the shortest way to equality and fraternity, and liberty is added eventually by sleep.

Friedrich Nietzsche

Learning to Fall

That night, after the news about Violette's eyes, I went home at seven. I gave her a bottle with my milk, gave her a bath, and, when I left her, she was asleep in her little bed. I had spent the whole afternoon with her in the NICU, worried sick and repeating to myself, "No one's going to die. She's not going to die. I'm not going to die. Everything will be okay." I was fighting to keep from crying, to keep from collapsing. I kept telling myself that I had to be strong for her, to nourish her. I had to stop being a bundle of nerves every time I went near her, because that really didn't help her. I also had to remind myself that there was no point hanging onto her like an anchor, wanting to hide her in my T-shirt and run away, far from this senseless world. I just had to be with her and focus on the bottle, the milk, the bath, the diapers. To stay focused on Violette, and stop thinking about "maybe this," "if that," "time will tell," or "one day at a time." Just now. Now was more than enough.

But when I walked into my empty house, I felt lost: no Keith, no Axel, no one. James was also on vacation. I called Axel at *Maman*'s house, but he was already sleeping, because he hadn't had a nap during the day. *Maman* has always been a bit of an anarchist about sleep schedules. We kids had no set bedtime and no mandatory naps. I didn't want her to know how upset I was, so I hung up and decided to go for a run. I was quite plump at the time, but I could still get moving. I'm not the world's greatest jogger, but I needed the fresh evening air. I needed to run or else I would explode. I took my music and my heart monitor. Why the heart monitor? Maybe to get back to my old athlete's habits and try to feel normal again.

Montreal is a beautiful city, and Mount Royal, the mountain that dominates it, with its beautiful trails and magnificent belvedere with a fabulous view of the city, is five minutes from our house. My usual running route takes me up 260 stairs to the belvedere, and I normally go up and down the stairs three times. I left the house as the sun was setting. For the first fifteen minutes, everything was fine. But, suddenly, the song "Mistral gagnant" by Renaud was playing in my earphones. I often used to listen to that song when I was between 15 and 20 years old, and my father also liked it. It talks about memory, about time that passes and never comes back, about the love between a parent and a child, and about the passing years that carry away the laughter of childhood. And this time, it really hit me. My throat tightened, I picked up my pace, I got goose bumps and shivers, and tears began to run down my cheeks. I couldn't see anything or anyone around me. I was in my own world, cut off from everything. Shut up in my bubble of sadness and emptiness. When I got to the bottom of the stairs, I went all out, and I don't think I've ever climbed as quickly, until I was completely out of breath, with a heart rate of 190 all the way. I pushed on for a few more metres, to the base of a tree, where I dropped to my knees. I was crying so hard I could no longer hear the music. I was broken, drained, and I wanted my father. I wanted my old self back, my health, my mind, my spirit, my optimism, my composure. I was weeping, screaming, nauseous with despair. I was suffocating. I curled up in a ball, my head on my knees, with a huge need for all the things I would never have again, enraged at not being able to go back to the person I am.

A little girl, who couldn't have been more than three years old, put her hand on my shoulder. Her other hand was holding her mother's hand. At first I didn't move. Then I took off my headphones. The child had two thin little pigtails, a Holiday Inn T-shirt, and a cap worn backward. Her nose was really grubby. A little late to be outside at that age, but it was summer. She asked, "Do you have a boo-boo? Did you fall down?" I was a bit embarrassed, but at least I stopped bawling. And then I realized that there were beginning to be quite a few people around me who were concerned for me, who thought maybe I had just had some sort of attack. And in fact, I had, in a way.

The girl's mom asked if I needed anything. I remember answering, "I need my life back." She must have been wondering, was I suicidal? Should she call an ambulance? I don't know who she was, or where she is today. I don't know if she even remembers that woman collapsed under a tree one summer evening on Mount Royal, that woman she had wanted to rescue. But for fifteen minutes, I poured it all out to that stranger: my Violette, her lungs, her eyes, her sepsis, my divorce, my cancer, my father's death when I was young, Renaud's song, the reasons for living, the "one day at a time," the tides that repeatedly flung my life out to sea and back onto the shore. "I want to be able to walk on the sand again, I'm scared!" She asked if my baby was going to live. "I think so," I answered. Then she said, "In two summers, you'll come here with your daughter. You'll climb the highest staircase in the world to buy yourselves fluorescent yellow banana popsicles before bedtime. Just like the ones our parents used to buy for us, with the two sticks, the ones we could never finish without getting them all over, especially at the end. Then you'll go rinse your sticky fingers in the fountain and you'll splash each other and laugh. That's what you should think about."

I don't know if she remembers that messed-up stranger who wanted to get her life back. But I wish that, wherever she is, she knew that I have my life back. Every time we climb up to the cross on Mount Royal with the kids, I buy them a popsicle in her honour. Not a banana one, though, because Violette prefers the red-white-and-blue rocket-shaped ones. Just like the ones Papa used to buy me.

A woman is like a tea bag – you never know how strong she is until she gets in hot water.

Eleanor Roosevelt

24 August

Days of life: 95

Violette's corrected gestational age: 38 weeks, 1 day

Keith,

I know you're coming back tomorrow, but I wanted to write you again, just so you know I'm better. I had a realization today: I'm sure now that everything will be fine. I spent the night crying and trembling. I couldn't take it any more. I fell asleep as the sun was coming up. And when I woke up, I thought, "Yes, we can live with a blind child. We just have to buy a dog and move somewhere close to a school for the blind. We'll help her. I'll work less. I like taking care of sick babies. I'll just have to take care of my own, whatever happens. We'll learn braille. She'll learn music – yes, the family will get into music again!"

Despite that, another part of me answered back, "What do you want with me now, you shitty life? Are you kidding? What did I do to deserve this? Or is it something I didn't do? I'll never manage with a blind child. No more bike trips, ski days, and what else? And what about Axel in all this? And my relationship? And my job? And my dreams? I'll have to do something to deal with it all. There has to be a solution!"

But there's no solution. There's nothing I can do. I have to let go a little. Accept whatever happens. I have to control what I can; and I can't control Violette's apneas, her retinas, the weather. I have to swim with the current, not against it. Even though it's really, really scary. Otherwise, I'll become exhausted and end up drowning. Go with the current, focus on the shore in the distance, and convince myself that I'll make it there, calm. And believe that I have the strength to make it. Turn over on my back and float when I have to.

Before, I tried to convince myself in my head. I understood the whole thing about quality of life, resilience. I knew that you can adapt to almost anything that's thrown at you. I understood that, but only in scientific terms. Remember when we talked about Down syndrome? I told you I'd rather get an abortion, but that if my baby were born with Down syndrome, I would love it anyway. We often discussed it. You said, "Since we can adapt, we shouldn't take death lightly, whatever happens." And I answered, "Just because we can adapt doesn't mean we have to choose to adapt." We could also choose to say we don't want that, no need to make our lives even more difficult. But that wasn't where I was at. Now, I really think in my heart and my gut that we'll manage, we'll be okay. When we talked about laser surgery, I was more afraid of intubation than of blindness. I couldn't stand to see Violette on a respirator again, even if she has to be operated on. But I have no choice. We don't need to know everything, and since we don't control very much, the doctors should probably just say, "We're need to operate, we're going in two days." Period.

I also know that I'll love her just as much if she's blind. You can be happy, even with a blind child. We'll deal with it. If we can't go skiing anymore, well, we'll go skating, that's all. We'll hold hands and we'll laugh. She'll have a curious expression as blind people often do; she'll open her adorable little mouth to catch snowflakes. And if she ends up with severe cerebral palsy, well, we'll push her wheelchair on the ice and she'll laugh happily while she catches the snowflakes.

Why this sudden realization? If someone had told me on May 12th that my baby was going to be born at 24 weeks and have prolonged septic shock with almost zero blood pressure, a pleural effusion, four intubations, many central catheters, extended time on the respirator, and end up at the threshold of stage 3 retinopathy, I would have said, "Thanks, but no thanks." Because I would have thought, "She can't take all that. I can't – I don't want to take all that. No one wants to be subjected to that. I don't need it, she doesn't need it." Deep down, I didn't believe (or didn't want to believe) that things always work out in the end, that families manage. No one wants to cope with illness. Yet we have to fight to stay alive (like me) or else we die, and sometimes we die anyway (like Papa).

Keith, do you remember, forty-eight hours after my admission to the hospital, when Violette was still inside me, what was going on in my head? You wanted them to intervene, and I didn't. You were right. I was wondering what would become of our family, of me, of you, of Axel, of our jobs, our future, our dreams, our love, everything. I didn't think I could endure all that. I wanted to change the course of history, but I couldn't. I was in a train racing toward an unknown destination. And I wanted to change all the jerks who criticized me for being pessimistic, and the ones who said everything would be fine. I was resolutely optimistic with those who said that premature babies are left handicapped and that the families didn't recover. I wanted to convince them that the opposite was true. And I wanted to change society because of all the nonsense people write and say about premature children when they talk about miracles or catastrophes. I wanted to change the way the media operate. In Quebec, the media are often biased and they show only the catastrophes; in the United States, only the miracles. An average "ordinary" former premature baby eating her peanut butter toast doesn't make the news. Boring.

I'm no longer the same. I don't know anymore who I am, but I know at least that I no longer have my fists clenched in front of my face and my shoulders up around my ears. I'm starting to breathe again.

I love Violette. I love her as my daughter, not as a-premature-baby-who-will-one-day-be-my-daughter. I love her even more than on that May 12th, when she was still in my belly and I was trying to keep her there as long as possible. Now I have a feeling that everything will be okay, whatever happens. Maybe that's because I don't have an ounce of energy left to keep fighting. I've been burned, but the skin will grow back one day.

Maybe the reason I had that realization was because I was on the verge of really going crazy. But that's not what I feel. I have the impression everything will be fine. That's the way it is. Keith, this abandonment, this new art of letting go, of making peace with my life, is refreshing. It's like catching your breath after intense exercise. Like running, when your heartbeats are synchronized with your stride. Like doing yoga in nature, with your nostrils full of fresh air and chlorophyll, when your body opens up to life and you can visualize the air in your lungs, in your mouth, in your sinuses, in your ears, and you feel yourself levitating. But that's not a new sensation. When I think about it, that's the way I've felt almost my whole life. It's my normal state. Of course, I'm still concerned, but I'm no longer plagued by all the possible and imaginable scenarios. Before, I'd tell myself that everything would be okay, but without being able to believe it. Now I don't need to keep saying it – I finally feel it. I've stopped being fixated on numbers and statistics. If numbers dare to come buzzing back in my head, I shut off the valve and I stow them away somewhere. Instead, I'll play myself some pretty little elevator music. My new muted reality. Violette isn't going to die. It's no longer a question of her dying.

Right now, I feel like going to buy a seeing-eye dog, but I realize that's being alarmist. Do you have to buy one or would they give it to us? You'll have to help me look into that. How to find the best possible dog. I don't know if there are any meta-analyses on that.

I've never felt so calm. Keith, it'll be okay. We'll love her. We'll love each other. She'll love us, she'll love Axel and James. And we'll be the perfect family, even if we're not normal. Violette will have problems, but she'll be absolutely perfect. My Violette. My baby.[†]

---

† Finally, Violette came through without going blind, although she has glasses, like her father, her mother, and her brothers Axel and James.

31 August

Days of life: 102

Violette's corrected gestational age: 39 weeks, 1 day

Computer,

Soon Violette will be 40 weeks old, corrected gestational age! It's strange to think that she was supposed to be born a few days from now. Do you realize? I'm excited: she'll be coming home soon! If we're lucky, that will make five to seven days that she won't have had an episode of apnea or bradycardia, and hopefully she won't hit us with one on the eve of her discharge. I can't stand being here anymore – I want to go home.

Today we talked about Violette's discharge and follow-up. They asked us if we wanted a magnetic resonance imaging (MRI) of her brain, "to make sure everything is okay."

But what would we do if everything wasn't okay?

"Let's stay positive. If everything is normal, we'll be happy. If not, there's a 50 per cent risk of problems, and we'll follow her closely to make sure she'll develop to her full potential."

"But aren't you already supposed to follow her closely? We'll certainly have to come back to the neonatal clinic, and we'll be seeing our paediatrician, won't we? That test has no significant predictive value if it shows that things aren't normal. After all, 50 per cent is not much – it's what you told me in the delivery room."

"But it could also be normal. It would be good to know, wouldn't it?"

"Good for who? For the medical team?"

"No, for you."

How to answer that? We refused the MRI. Enough is enough! I wanted to yell at them, "Leave Violette alone! Stop measuring her! I just can't take any more numbers and information. You tell me to focus on my baby, not the monitor. I don't want more images if we won't do anything special with the results."

Computer, I'll try to be clear. A normal MRI is encouraging. But living with abnormal results is no fun. Another whole bunch of uncertainties.[†] I know that, in some NICUs, only babies with abnormal MRI results get neonatal follow-up. It shouldn't be that way. That's not the way it is in Quebec, and it never should be.

Some doctors always want more details on the condition of their patients; as long as there are tests, they'll ask for them. I know that normal MRI results for Violette would be reassuring for her doctors. The more they know, the better they feel. Who wouldn't want to know everything? We've become hooked on precision medicine. I know it's useful to collect all possible data on premature babies in intensive care. It helps us predict their development in the long term, measure the effectiveness of our actions, and adjust them if necessary. But do we really need all these data, these ever-more-precise images, simply because we have the ability to obtain them? Can we talk about my daughter other than with medical jargon and numbers? For anybody, I am not sure it is beneficial to have an abnormal brain MRI in your chart for your future. Is that labelling useful, especially if the test doesn't change the clinical management? Besides, an MRI costs a lot, and you sometimes have to wait months to get one. There are children who really need them, children for whom the results will change their treatment. I'm overdosing on scientific information and measurements. It's enough.

---

† In 2019, a normal MRI means there's a 90 per cent chance the baby will present no disabilities later (out of ten babies with a normal MRI, nine will be "normal"). When the MRI of a full-term baby is abnormal, there's a 30 to 60 per cent risk of a disability, most often related to cerebral palsy (if ten babies have an abnormal MRI, approximately four of them will have long-term problems, most often mobility problems, especially with their legs).

It's time to go home and start the next chapter in Violette's life – with words, not with numbers! We want to take this story back from the doctors' books and from the chart, to write it ourselves. We certainly needed clinicians and hospital providers to write the first chapters, because, without them, she wouldn't be here. I know we wrote many chapters with them. But now it's our turn. We no longer want others to spend their time predicting what she'll be or what she'll do. Violette is going to live, so leave us in peace. Let me learn to be a mom without cutting-edge technology, just a mom who gives her daughter a bottle of her milk. A mom at home on maternity leave. I have to get used to that idea. This is where I am – I'm preparing mentally to return home, and I keep being bombarded with information. I don't want an MRI now that Violette has reached full term. I don't want to become a paranoid mom who can think only of one catastrophe after another. The stay in the NICU reminds me of what Robert Louis Stevenson said: "Life is not a matter of holding good cards, but of playing a bad hand well." I'm beginning to understand how to be a good mom of a premature baby in the NICU – I have the situation in hand now and I know what needs to be done (I know, it's about time!). Of course, I have to let go; I have to cultivate patience; I have to keep my hopes up; I have to accept that I can't control everything; I have to ignore the "one day at a time" and let myself be carried by the current; and I have to see what card Violette will pick up now, hoping it will be a good one.

But I'm going crazy with the data, the numbers, and the deluge of information. In neonatology, we're driven by data. Before Violette's birth, we received information on the possible outcomes. Since she was born, the flood of numbers hasn't dried up: grams and temperature; blood pressure; apneas and bradycardias (in that regard, Violette was the gold medalist in the Quebec summer games); CO_2 and oxygen levels; ventilator settings; electrolyte, glucose, and hemoglobin values; millilitres absorbed, regurgitated, excreted, transfused; and on and on. Our lives have revolved around those numbers for months. We've become dependent on them.

Computer, go have a look on PubMed or any search engine on prematurity, and you'll see that the field of neonatology is the kingdom of numbers and statistics. A kingdom where the dominant philosophy is pessimistic. We neonatologists are obsessed with measuring everything in premature babies as they grow. Instead of thinking positively about what these babies and their families can do, we're interested only in the ones who are dying or "doing badly" (the ones doctors consider "abnormal"). It's deplorable that there are so many studies of the long-term problems of premature babies and so few on ways to improve their prognosis or on the parents' capacity to adapt. Year after year, new research and technologies are added to our precision arsenal: epigenetics, magnetic fields, MRI results, genome sequencing, questionnaires on autism. These technologies and methods usually describe to what extent children born prematurely are abnormal, abnormally programmed – in short, not quite perfect. Sometimes, premature babies even do exactly what they are supposed to, but in an abnormal way. It is very rare for studies to describe what premature babies are actually capable of doing. And all this money pumped into research and given to researchers to measure children, and not much money invested in research to optimize knowledge of the best ways to help children and their families.

To hell with the damn numbers! You can't call the NICU without getting told "how much," knowing there's always an answer ready, because, without fail, someone is measuring her weight, her hemoglobin, her stools, her breathing, or her heartbeat. At the beginning, when they announced an improvement in her sodium levels (from 122 to 135), it made us crazy with joy – we had something positive to celebrate – while, as doctors, we know very well that it doesn't mean anything. A reintubation plunged us into distress. A normal transfontanellar ultrasound made us ecstatic, and we could fall asleep at night without fear of waking up as the parents of a dead or disabled baby. She lost 10 grams and it was a disaster: it meant 10 grams less of Violette, of her brain matter in particular. We lived in fear of unfavourable numbers, which necessitated new tests to rule out the worst hypotheses. The uncertainty was destroying us, and the "good numbers" were becoming ridiculous band-aids.

I sometimes feel like screaming, "Too much information! Enough numbers, enough data! She's Violette, just Violette. She's healing. Stop measuring her!" But I can't. I listen to the grams, and it does me good to know she's gaining weight every day. It's a vicious circle, and I can't take it anymore. Fortunately, Violette will soon leave the NICU and come home.

Computer, I hadn't realized before how much suffering some tests cause for parents and families. Keith and I feel that we shouldn't do an

MRI at 40 weeks gestational age on a baby born prematurely without telling the parents what that test can reveal. If the result is normal, there's a 90 per cent chance that the baby will have no long-term problems. If it's abnormal, the chances fall to between 40 and 60 per cent. In all cases, the result will not change the care the child will receive. That doesn't mean we have to stop research aimed at perfecting those technologies. One day, MRIs may help us develop specific early intervention programs. But that is not yet the case.

Computer, today I declare that I've had enough, and that there will be no more tests that will have no impact on her care. Violette has overcome so many obstacles, with her intubations, too many central catheters, fulminant septic shock, pneumonia acquired on the ventilator, major pleural effusion caused by one of the central catheters, severe retinopathy, not to mention blood in her stools, episodes of NPO, r./o sepsis X 3, transfusions, NPO r./o NEC, etc. She's exhausted, and so are we. All we want is to go home and get to know our daughter without checking monitors or constantly taking her numbers. A challenge for numbers addicts like us, whose dependence was made worse by Violette's condition. But the thing that interests us least is the pseudo-conclusive and super-precise imaging of her brain. As if we needed proof that it wasn't exactly like the brain of a baby born full-term! Does that surprise us? NO! We don't want to hear the words *abnormal* and *normal* anymore. It's enough. Violette is not normal – she's exceptional. She's our daughter!

*T*he next two articles examine how we measure and predict outcomes of fragile babies.

Seven years after I had written the preceding diary entry as a mother, MRIs were being done in many neonatal units after imperfect communication with parents. I was reminded of this when parents who were in our unit pointed it out. I recommended that they express their opinion in the scientific literature. Sometimes, parents say it best – as in the first article.

The second article examines not only how we measure outcomes, but also how we communicate with parents. Clinicians and researchers are the ones who have decided which outcomes are measured, when they are measured, and what they mean (or how severe they are). But things are changing. Many teams are debating this approach and investigating parental perspectives. Recently, with wonderful colleagues all around Canada, we have been examining what counts for parents and families – PIOs (parent important outcomes) and FIOs (family important outcomes). For the past year, many parents in Canada have been asked to tell us about their children's strengths and challenges. In our unit, we ask all parents what we could do (and could have done) better, how we can improve our care, and what prematurity has taught them, so we can learn from them. Our team (in alphabetical order), Claude Julie Bourque, Paige Church, Magdalena Jaworski, Thuy Mai Luu, Rebecca Pearce, Kate Robson, and Anne Synnes as well as great students (Laurie Anne Duquette, Aurélie Fortin, Émilie Thivierge, and Thuy-An Mai-Vo), is stimulating and our investigations are rewarding. With Camille Girard-Bock, a PhD student (and a 26-week preemie) whose mentor is Anne Monique Nuyt (my boss and one of the reasons I became a neonatologist), we are also asking preterm infants who are now adults about their life and how we can better help them take care of their health.

I am sure that, with parents and patients, we will change the way we measure and communicate outcomes in neonatology in the future. This is an exciting time – stay tuned!

Term MRI for Small Preterm Babies: Do Parents Really Want to Know, and Why Has Nobody Asked Them?

Rebecca Pearce, Jason Baardsnes[†]

The year 2009 was going to be fantastic. Jason and I had great families, jobs and friends, and I was pregnant with our first children, twin girls. Abruptly, proving true the Yiddish proverb "man plans, God laughs," life went off the rails. My mother was diagnosed with Stage IV pancreatic cancer and given months to live. Then, on the evening of September 19, I started to bleed at 25 weeks. We rushed to the hospital where I was admitted in labour and 3 cm dilated.

Maren and Lily were born on September 21, at 25 weeks 5 days of gestation, weighing 760 and 840g, respectively. The girls were whisked away to the NICU, where they were intubated. Our NICU education would be shockingly quick. My parents drove up to see the babies the next weekend; by this point, my mother was very sick, but she was adamant about seeing her granddaughters. That Sunday, September 27, we went out for breakfast before one last visit to the NICU. I missed the many messages that were being left by increasingly frantic doctors. Jason went to his laboratory to do some work and missed the message left at home.

When I walked into the girls' room alone, I immediately knew something was wrong. Lily's incubator was surrounded by people. Dr Janvier came up to me and told me that Lily had suffered a very sudden, very severe infection. She had perforated her gut and had a severe brain bleed. She was dying. Dr Janvier said how sorry she was. Then she hugged me, and I remember she had tears in her eyes. It was literally like being punched in the gut. Jason came from work, crying, and my stunned parents came in. We held Lily while her tubes and IVs were removed, and she died quietly in our arms with her sister sleeping in her incubator nearby. It was the only time that my mother would hold a grandchild; she died just over two months after Maren and Lily were born. Lily and my mother are buried together in a quiet rural cemetery.

The NICU experience is like living through a nightmare that you just cannot wake up from, and the next 2 months were utterly terrifying. Dr Janvier treated Maren as if she was also infected with the same bacteria that had killed Lily. Despite that, Maren developed septic shock but survived. She had a large PDA that required ligation and had a rough postoperative period. She required numerous blood transfusions. Her CO_2 was very high. She developed a fungal infection from her PIC line and needed antifungal drugs and several subsequent platelet transfusions. She required nitrous oxide and a high-frequency ventilator for a long time, which means we had very little chance to hold her. She developed severe BPD. The doctors and nurses told us many times that we had a very sick baby. We were well aware. The NICU is full of numbers: As and Bs, grams per day, ounces of milk, q3 hours, % of oxygen, level of sodium, etc. We constantly read research papers and abstracts, trying to digest the information. Our lives revolved around the numbers, percentages and statistics regarding cognitive impairment, behaviour abnormalities and motor disabilities; the outcomes for 25-week preemies with severe BPD were not particularly great. But percentages are statistics. We did not have a hundred babies. We had two but 50% had died. One was left. What did that mean for Maren?

About 2 months into her hospital stay, Maren turned a corner. She was gaining weight, her CPAP levels were slowly being reduced, no more infections. After 3 months in the NICU, she was officially a "feeder and grower." We started to breathe, but not for long.

At Ste. Justine, all preemies below 26 weeks are given an MRI before discharge from the hospital. This was not presented to us as a choice, and there was no discussion of the pros and cons or even why it was done. Maren was a 25-week 5-day preemie and got an MRI; her roommate, born just 4 days later than Maren, did not. We did not even question the reasoning behind this procedure; to us, it was just another test, medically necessary to her care. It seemed like it made sense, and I think we actually appreciated the thoroughness of the hospital. We were not aware that there is actually a tenuous link at best between MRI results and preemie outcomes. A few weeks before Maren was discharged, she was lightly sedated and wheeled down for her MRI.

I was feeding Maren one afternoon soon after the MRI when a neonatologist came to give me the results. It had identified moderate cerebellar damage from an unrecognized bleed, a bleed that could have happened soon after birth or after one of her infections. At that point, it did not really matter. Our daughter had brain damage. Two of the most horrific words a parent can ever hear. The doctor was compassionate but vague about the possible motor, cognitive and behavioural problems that Maren could face. He also said that it was hard to predict outcomes from MRIs, and it was not certain at all Maren would be disabled. In fact, many children with abnormal MRIs are not disabled. When he left, I thought "okay, maybe this isn't so bad after all." I called Jason with the news, and he soon arrived from work. As soon as Jason got to the hospital and I went home, I looked on PubMed for abstracts about cerebellar damage in preterm infants. One of the few articles that I found (Limperopoulos et al. 2007) was totally devastating. The study reported that babies with cerebellar damage had a much greater chance of expressive and receptive language delays, severe motor disabilities, cognitive disabilities and autism symptoms. This could be our child. We thought that we finally saw the light at the end of the tunnel, and then we were handed this earth-shattering, crushing information.

Maren was discharged after 4 months and 1 week in the hospital. For the first year, we were petrified and hypervigilant, the MRI always in our minds. Was she making eye contact? Reaching for things? Showing any signs of ataxia? Babbling appropriately? Drooling too much? Acting "strange"? She was our first child, so we did not really know what "strange" was, but were watching for it! I would imagine Maren in a wheelchair or with leg braces, in a group home or with severe autism. I started seeing a psychologist on a regular basis. Slowly, as Maren started meeting her milestones, our utter panic settled into something less acute.

In our case, Maren's MRI gave us no information about what she is like today; it served only to completely terrify us. Maren is now two and a half, with no disabilities. She is a gentle, mischievous, adventurous, beautiful little girl, beloved at her daycare for being a sweet, happy child. She speaks French as well as English, and her favourite thing to say "c'est quoi ca?" – "what's that?" – reflects her curiosity with the world around her. Sometimes, we look at her with complete and utter wonder, trying to reconcile this miraculous creature with the tiny, red, ventilator-dependent micropreemie she once was, or the damaged child we thought she could be. It is very possible that a trained psychologist could identify subtle behavioural or cognitive differences between Maren and a term baby, but, for all intents and purposes, she is a normal toddler and we would love her no matter what. We are also well aware that many learning issues in former preemies do not become apparent until they start school, but no MRI could ever give us this information, any more than numbers and statistics could define the person our child was becoming.

Looking back on our experience, parents should be given an informed choice as to whether they want an MRI done on their baby. If doctors really feel that an MRI is absolutely necessary or that the information is invaluable to them (and is this really the case?), then parents should have the choice as to whether they want the results or not. Some parents would prefer to remain "blissfully ignorant," especially if there is nothing medically tangible that they can do. The decision, however, should be theirs. We are not angry at the hospital, but, knowing what we know now, we never would have consented to an MRI, because it served no purpose other than to traumatize a family that had already been through so much and affect our ability to enjoy bonding with our child. Maren still received the same follow-up care; in fact, most of the professionals we had appointments with (physiotherapy, audiology, ophthalmology, speech-language pathology, etc.) said that they never use MRIs in their assessments or diagnoses, because they have such little prognostic value. Instead, they observe and let the children tell the story. Thankfully, in Maren's case, while the story may not be a fairy tale, it has a happy ending.

Measuring and Communicating Meaningful Outcomes in Neonatology: A Family Perspective

Annie Janvier, Barbara Farlow, Jason Baardsnes, Rebecca Pearce, and Keith J. Barrington[†]

INTRODUCTION

Neonatology is a fairly new specialty. In 1965, the first neonatal intensive care unit (NICU) was opened, and in 1975, the subspecialty of neonatology was formally established. Initially, many treatments were administered without rigorous research. Neonatology was once said to be a huge experiment[1] but this is no longer the case; the short- and long-term outcomes of NICU-hospitalized infants have been described and investigated more than any other critically ill patients. In the past 50 years, there have been enormous advances in the survival of sick neonates. Many infants will survive the NICU without disability or major long-term impacts. However, some children will survive with impairments, which may be physical, behavioral, or intellectual.

Many investigators examine the long-term outcomes of groups of high-risk neonates, which serves a number of purposes: (1) quality control within units, (2) comparisons of outcomes between NICUs, (3) investigating whether an intervention improves outcomes in the context of a clinical trial, (4) end-of-life decision-making, (5) to better understand the effects of neonatal conditions and/or interventions on organs and/or long-term health, and finally (6) to prepare parents for the future.

It is vitally important to investigate short- and long-term outcomes to improve NICUs. However, the outcomes that are being measured and examined, those that have been judged as being important, have been chosen by researchers, physicians, and other health care providers. They have become fixed into practice by repetition and have never been evaluated by parents or families in terms of whether they are the most important outcomes for them. Furthermore, stakeholders with different perspectives – for example, neonatologists, nurses, policy makers, fundamental researchers, school administrators, physiotherapists, hospital mangers, and parents – may weigh the importance and the reasons for investigating and describing neonatal outcomes very differently. Sometimes, parents and providers may disagree on the purpose and benefit of measuring outcome predictors.[2] In this article, we will describe parental perspectives with regard to outcome research in neonatology. First, we will describe how researchers measure and report neonatal outcomes. Second, we will examine how potential future outcomes are communicated to parents and families. We will finish by giving recommendations to optimize communication with parents of sick neonates.[3]

DICHOTOMOUS AND CONTINUOUS OUTCOMES IN NEONATAL RESEARCH

Many publications detailing neonatal outcomes, either descriptive or after a clinical trial, report dichotomous outcomes ("yes" or "no"). Certain outcomes are truly dichotomous, such as survival or death, or having surgery for necrotizing enterocolitis. Other important outcomes are continuous variables, such as lung injury, retinal injury, and developmental delay: these three outcomes are usually reported as dichotomous, after being artificially divided into two arbitrary categories, according to whether they have a finding above or below a particular chosen threshold. Lung injury, for example, is in reality a continuum, but creating a diagnosis of bronchopulmonary dysplasia (BPD) and dividing into "BPD" or "no BPD" based on whether the child still requires oxygen at 36 weeks post-menstrual age is an artificial distinction which has questionable implications for families.

Furthermore, such dichotomous outcomes are often included in composite dichotomous outcomes such as "death or BPD,"[4] "death or severe retinopathy of prematurity (ROP),"[5] or "death or neurodevelopmental impairment (NDI)."[6] Dichotomous outcomes are useful for planning sample sizes, simplifying analyses, and accounting for potentially conflicting results (an infant who is dead cannot develop an impairment). Although it may be statistically appealing to combine these competing outcomes together, we should consider how such reporting can affect clinical care and the information parents receive.

Research design specialists have recommended that in order to be included in a composite outcome, components of the composite should (1) reliably change in the same direction, and (2) be of similar importance.[7] For many of the composite outcomes used in neonatal research, this is not the case.

Neurologic and Developmental Complications of Prematurity

The most commonly promoted primary outcome variable for large clinical trials in recent years has been "survival without NDI." This outcome conflates several adverse events into an omnibus composite outcome that has become almost a default when addressing study design or recommendations for antenatal counseling.[8] The components of the outcome (when expressed as negatives) are death, cerebral palsy, visual impairment, hearing impairment, and low scores on a developmental screening test, most commonly more than two standard deviations below a standardised mean score on the Bayley Scales of Infant Development (BSID). The elements of this composite outcome do not reliably change in the same direction, nor may they be of similar importance to families.[9] Even more problematic is the inclusion of low scores on developmental screening tests and defining this as an impairment.

Although this classification may be useful to evaluate how neonatal interventions affect specific long-term outcomes, it may be of little value for parents. Physicians should recognize that these classifications have been made using their own values; they have not asked parents to categorize their children at 18 months to describe their child's health. Some disabilities that are labeled "minor" in the medical literature, such as behavioral problems or conduct disorders, may be much harder for some families to cope with than "severe" disabilities, such as deafness or some forms of cerebral palsy.[10] Researchers could simply report these outcomes in a separate fashion, the way the outcomes of cancer are reported, or the secondary effects of chemotherapy. For example, oncologists/urologists inform patients of various potential outcomes without classifying them as being severe, moderate, or mild: for some men with prostate cancer, impotence will be a severe outcome and for others a moderate or mild one, depending on their life circumstances.

Visual Complications of Prematurity

In a similar way to neurologic and developmental outcomes, "severe ROP," which is not uncommon in the extremely preterm infant, has often been conflated with death in neonatal research. The definition of "severe ROP" has also changed over the years, as have the interventions and long-term outcomes after severe ROP. It is now rare for NICU survivors to be blind.[11] The Surfactant, Positive Pressure, and Pulse Oximetry Trial (SUPPORT)[12] had death or severe ROP as one of its primary outcomes. The trial showed that death and severe ROP differed in opposite directions between the two oximetry target groups; the patients randomized to the low saturation goals had a higher mortality, but a lower incidence of severe ROP. The trial therefore had a negative, non-significant result. We question whether many families would consider the two parts of the composite outcome to be equivalent; particularly as longer-term follow-up has not shown a difference in serious visual impairment between the groups.[13]

Pulmonary Complications of Prematurity

The combined outcome of "death or BPD" is also commonly used in neonatal research. The most frequently used definition of BDP currently is the requirement for supplemental oxygen at 36 weeks post-menstrual age. Is discontinuing oxygen at 35 weeks as opposed to just after 36 weeks truly a good indicator of the impact of lung disease on a child? Furthermore, still requiring oxygen at 36 weeks but then being weaned to room air before discharge has a very different impact on the family compared to going home on oxygen or requiring ventilation at 6 months corrected age. Research with a primary outcome of "death or BPD" may also lead to results that are difficult to interpret. Consider an outcome of a trial in which the intervention decreased mortality but increased the number of survivors who need oxygen at 36 weeks. This in fact happened in many of the trials of surfactant therapy.[14] Is that a good outcome? A bad outcome? Is it really, as the result of the statistical analysis suggests, a null outcome? Families need to know if a treatment increases the chance of a child surviving, and, if they survive, what will be the impact of respiratory outcomes on their life. Many pulmonary outcomes having a negative impact on neonates and their families, such as rehospitalisation, needing oxygen therapy at home, and visits to the emergency department, are not systematically reported. A description of the impacts of the lung injury beyond a dichotomous BPD outcome would be much more useful, both to parents and to the health care professionals who care for them.[15]

Perinatal Counseling

Because so much research has depended upon these dichotomous outcomes, they influence the way the literature is written and analyzed. The reliance on dichotomous outcomes in neonatal research has an impact on what providers describe as "good" and "bad" outcomes, and on how different outcomes are valued. This may influence clinical care and communication with parents. Dichotomous outcomes have been integrated into perinatal counseling for individual patients.[16] Professional societies also use these outcomes to make life and death recommendations for preterm infants.[17] One such example is the use of the NICHD [National Institute of Child Health and Development] extremely preterm birth outcome calculator for antenatal consultation.[18] Many physicians use this tool to speak to parents before a preterm birth – after entering the gestational age and other relevant data, the calculator predicts expected outcomes. One can find the risk of survival and death, but the other outcomes reported are composite outcomes, such as "survival without profound neurodevelopmental impairment" or "death or moderate-to-severe neurodevelopmental impairment." For a parent, the outcomes of death and survival with serious impairment may be very different. For many parents, it would be more useful to hear about the chances of survival and then about what happens to survivors. There are remarkably limited data concerning the outcomes that parents think are important for decisions about withholding or withdrawing life-sustaining interventions. One study in which parents of extremely low birth weight infants in an Icelandic NICU were questioned[19] found that the outcomes which parents felt to be appropriate for consideration were a certainty of death and/or certainty that the child would be unable to communicate. Further research of parental views regarding this issue is vitally important.

When patients with colon cancer are counseled prior to surgery, we doubt that they hear about the percentage chance of "survival without a colostomy" or "death or incontinence." When two outcomes have potentially very different values to patients, they should be discussed separately.[20]

PREDICTING THE FUTURE

Neonatal Tests to Identify High-Risk Patients

There are a number of reasonable indications for performing investigations in the NICU, which are designed to predict future neurological or developmental outcomes of preterm babies, but these investigations can lead to potential problems.

Confusing Screening Tests with Disabilities

A low Bayley Scales of Infant Development score is not an impairment. A generalized problem is the use of BSID scores at 18–24 months of age as a way of defining infants as having "cognitive impairment." However, in extremely low birth weight infants (ELBW) and extremely preterm children, BSID-II scores have been shown to poorly predict cognitive scores at school age.[21] Hack et al.[22] showed that the positive predictive value (PPV) of K-ABC Mental Processing Composite of 70 at 8 years given a BSID-II MDI score 70 at 20 months was only 37% for an ELBW cohort overall, and just 20% for the neuro-sensory intact subgroup. In the Caffeine Therapy for Apnea of Prematurity (CAP) trial cohort, only 18% of the former preterm infants who had BSID-II MDI scores <70 at 18–20 months actually had an IQ <70 when re-examined at 5 years.[23] Not only are the BSID scores of limited predictive value for cognitive function[24] but they also have no significant correlation with quality-of-life scores, or with measures of family function. Prospective investigations of extremely preterm children using the more recent BSID edition, the BSID-III, have demonstrated that delay on cognitive and language scores at 24 months is not strongly predictive of 4-year cognitive impairment, although BSID-III scores are associated with later Differential Ability Scale scores.[25] We suggest that BSID testing at 18–24 months should be recognized as a tool of potential value for identifying infants who need further evaluation and for possible intervention, but does not reliably classify infants as having future significant cognitive impairment.[26]

Autism screening tests. A few years ago, an article reporting the high frequency with which former extremely preterm infants failed an autism screening test made a great impact,[27] with articles in the lay press, and statements about the enormously high frequency of "autism" in former preterm infants. On closer inspection, however, the autism screening test (the M-CHAT) was just a screening test designed to have a high sensitivity but low positive predictive value, intended to detect infants who may need further evaluation, and not designed at all for a population of infants who frequently have speech delays. It is now clear[28] that the majority of former preterm infants who screen "positive" for autistic traits have developmental speech delay which usually improves with time.[29] The true prevalence of autistic spectrum disorder is indeed somewhat increased among former extremely preterm infants than the general population,[30] but is far lower than that suggested by inappropriately interpreted screening tests.

NEW TECHNOLOGIES TO PREDICT LONG-TERM OUTCOMES

Cerebral MRI

In recent years, many groups have investigated the long-term outcomes associated with abnormal cerebral MRI results.[31] For neonatal asphyxia and congenital anomalies associated with severe lesions – such as lissencephaly – conventional or structural MRI may be useful for evaluating the clinical situation and for decision-making. On the other hand, for preterm infants, most investigations have been aimed at determining whether there is a significant statistical correlation between cerebral MRI findings performed at term equivalent age and "NDI" in early childhood. As yet, there is no intervention that demonstrated differential effects according to MRI findings.

For a preterm infant, a normal term equivalent age conventional MRI has a high negative predictive value (NPV) for cerebral palsy, but a much lower NPV for developmental delay;[32] an abnormal MRI is much more troublesome. Although there may be a statistically significant association with adverse outcomes, the PPV of moderate-to-severe white matter abnormalities for either cerebral palsy or developmental delay is below 50%.[33] With such a low PPV, does it really help to know the results of a term MRI for a specific baby when no interventions are available?[34] Does changing the probabilities with the MRI really help parents prepare for the future? Percentages may be useful for some parents, but they also want to know what will happen to *their* child, not just to a previous hundred similar children. Today, if we type "MRI preterm brain" on PubMed, 1131 articles can be

found, reflecting enormous research funds. None of these studies demonstrate that this technology helps parents and families
of preterm infants. Parents have described the negative impacts
of an abnormal MRI on their family: "For the first year, we were
petrified and hypervigilant, the MRI always in our minds. Was
she making eye contact? Reaching for things? Showing any signs
of ataxia? Babbling appropriately? Drooling too much? Acting
'strange'? … In our case, Maren's MRI gave us absolutely no information about what she is like today; it served only to completely
terrify us."[35]

Genetic Testing in Neonatology-Perinatology: An Ongoing Research Project

Infants with congenital anomalies often undergo genetic testing
in order to confirm a clinical diagnosis or, at times, to suggest a
diagnosis when one is not clear. In the neonatal unit, in the past
decade, microarray testing – which has in many places largely
replaced karyotyping – can detect the presence of much smaller
chromosomal aberrations. In a few institutions, whole exome
or genome sequencing is also performed regularly.[36] These new
techniques are far more likely to produce abnormal results, which
are often of unknown significance (at the present time). While
for some neonates, the genetic anomaly is clearly related to their
condition, for many, the penetrance may be variable and lead to
uncertain clinical importance.

Genetic investigations and technologies have developed at
an astonishing pace, but do more detailed genetic tests in neonatology improve the outcomes of children? Do physicians
and parents share common goals and are these goals eventually
achieved? Precise genetic tests may positively affect the treatment
of children on some occasions. The development of personalized
pharmacogenomics in oncology is an example. But at the present
time, in neonatal patients, the results of such tests rarely alter a
child's clinical care. All the specialists agree on one aspect: they
recommend that providers adequately inform parents about the
potential benefits and risks of these tests and obtain adequate

informed consent. However, even for the most common and best-understood chromosomal anomalies in children – trisomy 21, 13, and 18 – counseling has been reported to be pessimistic, devoid of parental experiential outcomes and unbalanced by families who lived with these children.[37] Without adequate research about the impacts of these investigations on children and families, optimal informed consent cannot happen.

The Blurry Border between Clinical Care and Research

A recent publication has identified, as part of a "choosing wisely" approach in neonatology, that routine term equivalent age MRI for extremely preterm infants was one of five tests that should be avoided[38] because there is insufficient evidence that it can be used to improve long-term outcome. Although MRI and detailed genetic screening tools are of limited clinical utility at the present time in neonatology, continued investigations into the utility of these technologies for neonatal outcomes are important nevertheless. They help us better understand the underlying mechanisms of neonatal disease and aid researchers in finding beneficial interventions. These investigations are likely to have a positive impact for *future children*, which implies that they are for research and not for standard clinical care.

Informing Parents

Research in these areas is being done in "the best interests of children," according to the opinions of professional experts. However, the subjective nature of "the best interests of the child," leaves parents out of these discussions even though they are key stakeholders. These discussions are *about* parents, children, and families, when they should be *with* the families.[39] When screening tests or other research interventions are offered to parents, they should know that they are unlikely to alter the care for *their* child, but that they may help future children. For example, some parents may consent to a term MRI for their preterm infant, in the context of research, because it may appear to be of minimal risk to the family. In this case, some parents report that they would not want the results disclosed.[40]

OUTCOMES OF IMPORTANCE FOR FAMILIES: GOING FORWARD

What Standard Should We Use?

To be useful for families, an outcome variable should reflect the functioning of their child, and/or the functioning of the family, and/or the integration of their child into the family/society. Other important outcomes are the happiness of the child and how this child enriches the family/society. Cerebral palsy, by any definition, is something we would all like to avoid. But physicians should be able to inform parents not only about the risks of cerebral palsy as a diagnosis, but what that means – in a practical sense – for their child, her quality of life, and their family. There has been remarkably little empirical research about what outcomes matter most to families, which outcomes have the most impact on family functioning, on other children, on parental well-being, or indeed even what outcomes have the most impact on the daily life of a former extremely preterm infant. There is also a paucity of research that relates to the value and importance of disabled children to families and society as well as a description of quality of life of the child living with disability.

Feeding Problems

Feeding problems are one example of a significant but under-evaluated issue. Many former extremely preterm infants have difficulty with normal oral feeds,[41] many require tube-feedings at discharge, and may have serious oral aversion. Such problems can last for many years and have major impacts every day on the life of a family.[42] A small preterm infant may be considered without impairment, but if they are losing weight, cannot feed orally, or have oral aversion, they can seriously disturb the functioning of a family. What proportion of extremely preterm infants has such an outcome? Currently, the question is difficult to answer as this outcome is rarely examined in neonatal research using "traditional" outcome measures. Parents of preterm infants are often not informed that difficulties in feeding are common in preterm infants. Many parents are inadequately prepared and discover this after discharge, when feeding problems become more apparent and inadequate growth occurs.

Coping Mechanisms

In general terms, human beings are resilient. When faced with difficulties, especially if those difficulties are likely to be permanent,[43] individuals generally find ways to cope with adverse conditions. They most often adapt their lives and find ways to adjust.[44] This is not to say that problems faced by ex-NICU patients are unimportant. Some families will be faced with considerable challenges. But on the other hand, a family with a child who has severe cerebral palsy, for example, will find meaning and hope in the life of their infant, even if they wish it was otherwise.[45] The same can be said about families of children who have home ventilation,[46] Down syndrome,[47] trisomy 13 or 18.[48] Adaptation and coping have been measured in older patients,[49] but neonatal research is lagging behind. Several studies have noted that the adverse impact of a child with neurological or developmental difficulties decreases markedly over the years.[50] A recent study of families with children who have intellectual disabilities[51] was almost universally positive about the impacts of having such a child on themselves and their family. Interventions aimed at families with poor resilience predictors could improve neonatal and parental outcomes. How can we improve a parent's sense of control, of "being a good parent," give more power to them, and enable a positive adjustment?

COMMUNICATING WITH FAMILIES ABOUT THE FUTURE

When there is clinical information that has potential impacts on the future of a baby, how and when should that information be communicated with the family?

1. *Provider knowledge is critical*: The caregiver should themselves be informed regarding the condition, the risks, and the potential impacts of the condition for children. A recent publication about how to share a diagnosis that increased an infant's probability of developing cerebral palsy demonstrated how poorly informed the caregivers were regarding the population prevalence of CP, overestimating the true incidence by 10–100 fold.[52]

2. *Avoid conflating neonatal outcomes*: Remember that, for a parent, death is not the same as disability. When indicated, clinicians should speak about the risk of death, and then of disability in survivors; they should also avoid speaking to families about dichotomous outcomes when there is a clinical spectrum.

3. *Children are more than a diagnosis*: Parents should not only be informed of potential adverse conditions or diagnoses. *They should know what these diagnoses mean to children and families, in a practical sense.*

4. *Personalize the information*: The information should be adapted to the needs and wishes of the family, and the precise nature of the infant's situation. Many recommendations for antenatal counseling in extreme prematurity demand that information be standardized and that providers describe all the possible complications of prematurity. We disagree that information for these families should be ... [standardized].[53] Parents want much more than standardized information from antenatal counseling[54] – they want information which is directly relevant to their baby, as well as practical parental experiences.[55] This is also true for other conditions, such as trisomy 21, 13, or 18.[56]

5. *Provide balanced information*: Parents should be given an opportunity to ponder what a diagnosis means for them, for their family, for their future; they should be told about the positives as well as the negatives. For example, they should not only hear a list of adverse conditions affecting preterm infants, they should also hear that most extremely preterm babies survive, that most do not have profound disability, that the quality of life of these children (with and without disability) is good. They should also know that the vast majority of families adapt. The example of counseling following a diagnosis of trisomy 21 could be taken as a model, as it has been widely investigated. Parents want information as soon as possible, with balanced facts tailored to the precise situation of their baby.[57] They want to know what life might have in store for them and their baby, and not just to hear the negatives. Parents who have a diagnosis of trisomy 13 and 18 also report desiring balanced information that is relevant and meaningful.[58]

6. *Provide information relative to follow-up programs*: Parents are often not well informed of the reasons for systematic follow-up. Many parents think this is essential to identify potential problems their child may have. They often do not know that this follow-up is important for quality control, to inform future parents, or for clinical research in order to understand/optimize the outcome of neonates like their child. After a long NICU stay, many parents want to "give back" and help the neonatal cause. Coming to neonatal follow-up represents an invaluable way to help their child and all present and future NICU children.

7. *Discuss real-life outcomes*: Providers should have regular interactions with NICU parents about the life trajectory of their child: what is the next step – remove the tube, remove the CPAP, full feeds, transition to oral feeds, oximetry, etc.; what we hope and predict will happen, what we wish will not happen, and how their baby compares to other babies with the same condition. "Real-life" personalized outcomes are different than statistical outcomes.

8. *Normality and normativity*: Avoid the term "normal" when describing babies after NICU discharge. Their tests and imaging may be "normal" or "abnormal," above or below average; but for a family – especially after the NICU experience – these babies are extraordinary.

9. *Empower*: Parents of all NICU children should be able to feel like good parents – doing a good job caring for their child. In the NICU, they should be congratulated when they hold their baby, visit, provide breast milk, read to their child, ask questions, etc. Providers should recognize that while they are the experts of neonatal medical problems, parents are the experts of their children. Parents should be encouraged to engage in goal-setting, in deciding, transitions, and plans for the future – which outcomes are most important to them. When parents feel competent, they engage and can form stronger parent-child relationships.

10. *Inform NICU families of parental support groups or associations that can offer them experiential information about the child/family experience*: It can be very hard for NICU parents to imagine themselves, at home, with a child who is not dependent on technology. Moreover, this connection may enable many families to understand, whatever the outcome – death, survival, disability, medical complexity – that "It won't always be this way," that there is a life after the NICU.

11. *Words are important*: Know the name of the baby and avoid labels: neonates *are not* their condition or their outcome ("the Down's baby" or "the 24 weeker with a grade IV," "the severe BPDer in room 17"). The way we describe babies can have an impact on how parents see their children.

RECOMMENDATIONS FOR RESEARCHERS

1. Research projects should focus on primary outcomes that are of importance to families. Families should be involved in planning research, and in determining which outcomes should be investigated. The incidence of and impacts on

family function of sequelae which are considered to be major or minor should be evaluated and compared.

2. Decreasing the impacts of neonatal critical illness is a vitally important task, given the improved survival of infants with so many different conditions. But unless we investigate which outcomes are truly most important to our patients and their families, we will not be able to progress further.

part five

COMING HOME

Germ-o-phobia

Violette came home in September, with fragile lungs and a cricoid stenosis – that is, part of her trachea (her windpipe) is smaller than the rest, a result of having a tube in her trachea for so long – and her many intubations did not help. She had a month to gain strength before the beginning of the virus season, which lasts seven months. For her, a cold or a runny nose could potentially mean hospitalization again, a respirator again, and maybe more lung damage. We had to stay far away from even the shadow of a virus, and we were obsessed with handwashing. Truly obsessed. We took Axel out of day care, because he caught every bug that came through the place. There were huge disinfectant dispensers everywhere in the house, like in a hospital. We could have been in an ad for Sterigel. We were completely isolated. Axel, Violette, and I stayed in the house almost all day long in our cozy little cocoon. When Keith came home from the hospital, he would go through a decontamination process like a carwash. He would undress in the lobby, taking off his "contaminated" hospital clothing and putting on clean clothes. The toxic clothes would be washed immediately. Then handwashing timed for two minutes under expert supervision. Then the Sterigel.

At sundown, Keith would take Axel to the park, discreetly checking that the place was secure, that there were no children around anymore. Other children (virus vectors) had to be avoided at all costs, as in the movie *Monsters, Inc.* We no longer saw our friends who had children.

For Violette's safety, Axel couldn't see a single friend until he was vaccinated for the flu in December. And when we went for the vaccine, in the waiting room, he shouted, "*Maman* look, there are TILDREN!!!" pointing his finger at all the snot-nosed little patients waiting their turn. At Christmas, we went to my mother's house, and Keith and I took turns upstairs with Violette while the others partied downstairs with their kids.

But it was worth it. Until she was 6 months old, corrected age, Violette didn't catch anything. But then she developed a bad case of laryngitis. I don't know where she could have caught it – none of us were sick. She was having trouble breathing, so we gave her steroids STAT, which we obtained through our "pushers" in the emergency ward. If we hadn't been doctors, she would have been hospitalized in order to be monitored.

And then she had laryngitis or a random virus again, and she had to take more steroids.

And then she had laryngitis or a random virus again, and she had to take more steroids.

And then she had laryngitis or a random virus again, and she had to take more steroids.

The first ten times she had respiratory viruses were the worst. She would gasp for breath, there was terror in her eyes, and her hair was wet with sweat from the effort she was making. Her little joints were white from clinging so hard to us. And I fell back into darkness, crying, my throat tight, my brain on fire, chills down my spine, fear in my belly, ready to scream with desperation. Fortunately, those drugs act fast, and in a few hours she would get better. But those hours were very long. Violette was able to avoid being hospitalized and put on a respirator thanks to regular doses of dexamethasone throughout the winter. Even today, we always have cortisone pills on us wherever we take Violette. A bad case of laryngitis could still kill her.

Families with babies and families without are so sorry for each other.

Ed Howe

Meanwhile, with My Other Kids …

Research shows that having a sick child completely changes parents. Extremely premature babies who survive are often described as victims of exceedingly anxious parents who subject them to constant monitoring: vulnerable child syndrome. That was my case until Violette was eighteen months old, because of her lungs, viruses, and our fears. I overprotected her and indeed treated her like a vulnerable child – and she was one. But I realize now that my other children were the real victims of my stress. And the fact that their mom was a doctor working in intensive care and had in her excellent memory the precise details of all the children she had treated didn't help.

Paediatricians must expect to see children die. And I believe that doctors' children belong to a distinct group. Doctors are not supposed to treat their own children when they're sick. When they're dealing with their own children, some doctors tend to ask for endless tests for a simple sore ankle, because they immediately see it as leukemia or crippling arthritis. Others, like me, trivialize everything that isn't fatal. "Your nose is bleeding? Wipe it." "Your nose is running? Blow it." "You have a fever? That's normal – your body is fighting a virus. Keep having a fever and you'll get better." Kissing it better is also very effective in treating booboos. When children die in our hands, everything else seems relatively unimportant! In fact, before Violette's arrival, we didn't even have a thermometer in the house. When Axel still felt hot after twenty-four hours, we gave him Tylenol. To give him the right dose (15 mg/kg), we referred to what was written on the diaper package; that was how we guessed his weight.

With Violette, everything changed. The main cause of death in the first year of life is prematurity and birth defects, and then, until the age of 42, it's accidents. That's what strikes down most children and young adults. Axel was two years old when Violette was in the NICU. On the paediatricians' recommendation, we didn't give him grapes, or peanuts, or carrots, any foods he could choke on. I've seen children die because of those foods. I've seen children die from swallowing the balloon they were trying to blow up at a birthday party, I've seen kids who've died falling down the stairs, I saw one die from skiing without a helmet. I've seen children die because they were scalded by boiling pasta water. I've seen drowning victims. Every time, it's a loss of a child loved by parents who are not particularly stupid, and yet a loss arising from a stupid accident that could easily have been avoided, like the 18-month-old child found dead with his head in a huge pot of minestrone left outside on the balcony to cool.

When Violette was in the hospital, I was convinced that catastrophes were lying in wait for Axel in the house. At night, I would get up to check the smoke detector. I would make evacuation plans in case a fire broke out between his bedroom and ours. I calculated the distance between our window and the neighbour's window to figure out if we could reach it with a broom handle or a ladder. I've calmed down since then, but not completely. I had Axel take swimming lessons before he could walk so he wouldn't drown. Even after Violette came home, I thought about the mortal dangers that lurk around the kids. I tried to educate Axel: I'd pretend to be choking on a grape, a Christmas tree light (children are especially attracted by the red ones), a peanut, an M&M, a balloon, a piece of sausage, a marble. I would yell, "No, no, boo-boo!" after mimicking choking on each of them. I imagined Axel being raped by a pervert. I imagined cars going through a red light and running over his body. Later, I saw the movie *Run, Lola, Run* and it reminded me of that time. It's a wonderful German film that I highly recommend, starring a marvellous, gorgeous actress with red hair. Several times in the film, Lola stares at a character and that triggers a flash-forward of five seconds, not more, showing how she or he will die. With Axel, I developed a "Run, Lola, Run" syndrome. I would see flashes of all kinds of tragic ends for him, with what would follow: the organ donation, his empty corpse, his extubation from the respirator, the puddle of blood beside the overturned car. All those visions remained very present in my mind. I still have some of them sometimes, but much less than before.

After Violette, I wanted more children. I was well aware that my "incompetent cervix" was truly incompetent: the threat of preterm labour at 23 weeks for Axel, delivery at 24 weeks for Violette. So we decided to close the shop and adopt. I've always wanted four children. Having children was already my dream when I was a little girl. But I never thought that I would adopt. To me, people who adopted were marginal, abnormally generous types, saints like Mother Teresa. At the time, I also wasn't sure if I could love a child I hadn't "made" myself. Life has obviously proven the opposite, and I was completely wrong about adoption. It wasn't a sacrifice when we adopted our adorable Tai (my treasure and my sunshine). I'm the happiest mother in the world, thanks to my kids. He was in critical condition the first time I saw his little dark eyes on my computer screen, on September 28th, 2008, at 11:30 p.m. I immediately fell in love with him: he was already my beloved son. Keith and I knew that he was sick, that he had an ostomy (stools draining into a bag outside his belly) and that something was not right. At 11 months, he weighed just 3.4 kilos. We knew the risks, we knew it was possible he would die. But we didn't want him to die all alone. We wanted to know him. Our families and friends thought we were completely crazy to want to go through all that again, and by "choice"! But I didn't think or feel I had a choice. There are things we must choose to control in order to be able to live with ourselves. We had to go get our son.

I had endless discussions with my friend John, one of my mentors in bioethics, about free choice, free will, and other philosophical questions. As for my mother, she said, "You come to a very high wall and you don't know what's on the other side. You have two options: turn tail and take the easy road, imagining all the problems you might have found on the other side of the wall, or else you jump over it without looking, and you give the best of yourself. I think you want to jump, and Keith also wants to jump. You need to jump, so go for it, jump. I'm with you and I'll always be with you."

I would so much like to tell Tai's first mom that her little boy is doing great, that he no longer needs the bag, that his bowel has been mended, that it took a long time but it finally works, that the burns on his little belly have healed and become scars. We know nothing about her. But I would like it if she could know. Your son is my sun.

Before Violette, I saw all kinds of high walls and I didn't dare go near them. Before each decision I needed to make, I would draw up a list of "pros" and "cons," with lots of "ifs," question marks, and alarm bells. I've changed a lot. I know now that I have more strength in me than I ever would have believed. I know who I am and what kind of person I want to be. I know there are things I don't need to do; I also know that what must be done will be done, whatever happens. Thank you, Violette, for teaching me all that. You're the one who saved Tai's life, not us.

Strangely enough, when they were growing, I was a lot less obsessed with the safety of my two younger children, who were both extremely ill, who both came really close to death. They've gone through enormous ordeals, and they overcame them all. They're my resilient little platinum-plated Teflon kids who can withstand anything. My brain no doubt imagines they are indestructible. But Axel was my obsession, especially when I was at the NICU. The only medical interventions Axel needed were for a urinary tract infection and a sprained wrist, and to correct his molars that were coming in crooked. However, he's also "abnormal," according to my colleagues' criteria, since he wears glasses! So, in spite of myself, I'm waiting to find out what the cosmos has in store for him. I have a feeling he'll end up paying for his good luck, although that's completely irrational.

I don't think there will be a fourth child. For a few years, Keith has been considering a vasectomy, but I'm against it. Our first conversation on the subject went more or less as follows (unfortunately this is not a joke):

"I think it's time I got snipped. No way you're getting pregnant again. We can't have any more biological children. We adopted Tai because we didn't want another child born at 24 weeks."

"And what if we rented a uterus?"

"Annie, I'm not kidding."

"So, because my reproductive organs are screwy, you're the one who has to get sterilized?"

"No. I want a vasectomy because we don't want you to get pregnant again, because it's simpler to shut down the guy than the girl, and I'm a guy. I'm telling you, we don't want another pregnancy."

"Don't worry, you won't get pregnant."

"In any case, I've made my decision, whether you like it or not."

"No, NO! You can't decide by yourself to have a vasectomy. That's a decision for us to make as a couple."

"My body belongs to me. I'll do what I want with it."

"So I could decide to have myself inseminated with exotic sperm. I've always dreamed of having a black baby. Maybe I'd also like an exotic husband. A British husband is kind of ordinary."

"Don't be ridiculous."

"I would rather go for a reversible method. Surgery is radical. We would be surgically sterile."

"That's the whole idea, isn't it? What's the problem, my love? I know you don't want to get pregnant. That's your nightmare. You buy pregnancy tests even when you're having your period: that's extreme!"

" ... "

"What's the matter with you? You look really funny."

"And what if we changed our minds one day?'

"Why would we change our minds?"

"What if one of the children got leukemia?"

"That would be horrible. But why would one of them get leukemia?"

"Because we're unlucky. Axel hasn't had anything wrong yet."

"There's no reason he'll have anything; it's normal to have nothing wrong. And if it were to happen, he would have chemo. Same thing for all of us. And by the way, my sperm wouldn't be very good after chemo."

"You won't get leukemia. It's much more common among children."

"How is that related to a vasectomy, anyway?"

"If the chemo fails, we'll need genetically compatible umbilical cord blood."

"You're crazy. You know that chemo works eight times out of ten. Besides, there are umbilical cord blood banks, and there are bone marrow donors. And we wouldn't get very far with a little 24-week cord, there wouldn't even be enough cells in it to treat a mouse."

"…"

"My darling, I'm telling you, everything will be fine."

"And what if we didn't find a genetically compatible marrow donor? We would have to make one ourselves."

"What? You're losing your mind! Annie, Axel is fine: there's no problem."

"Yes, there is a problem. At least wait until I'm 45."

"What does that change? You'll already be menopausal."

"Not at 45! Wait, maybe we could check if the children are HLA compatible!"

"You want to take samples of their blood and test them to find out if they're compatible in case one of them gets leukemia and the chemo doesn't work. Am I dreaming? Go explain to the hematologists why you would want to carry out such a costly procedure, and we'll have youth protection on our backs. Your case will be called 'Pre-vasectomy HLA compatibility research on healthy children by a paranoid crackpot mother.' Talk about it in your ethics seminars – you'll see how many people are ready to draw children's blood. Contraceptives aren't 100 per cent effective, and that scares me. I'm past that age. We're often on call. Tai still wakes up five times a night. We can't go through that again, Annie."

"You think you're old, but you're not *that* old. If you're young enough to want sex all the time, you're not too old to want more children!"

"There's no connection between sex and children."

"Oh no? I should perhaps ask the people in my ethics seminars if they think there's a link between sex and children. Maybe there'll be a clever theologian in the room who'll find the solution to the puzzle!"

"You know what I mean. I'm tired of being afraid of pregnancy. I don't want to live like that anymore."

"Agreed. But then we would have to freeze sperm and keep it in two different clinics."

"Bloody hell, crazy woman! Let's not talk about it anymore, okay?"

"We've already talked about it! Sperm bank, vasectomy. No sperm bank, no vasectomy! I'll pay for storing the samples."

"The samples. What the hell! Tonight I'll show you my samples. After all, maybe it would be better to give up sex for good, that would spare you a ruptured aneurysm, and me a heart attack. We should buy a trepanation kit, with nitro, an intubator, and a defibrillator, for our bedroom. They would make nice sex toys for us."

"Keith, it's not funny."

"Here's a better idea: from now on, we'll have sex in the hospital. That way, we'll already be on site to deal with any disaster."

There weren't any more children. Keith is right.

Babies control and bring up their families as much as they are controlled by them; in fact … the family brings up baby by being brought up by him.
Erik H. Erikson

Rewriting Your Life

When your baby is admitted to the NICU, your life is never the same. It changes you. Somehow, the Annie that was there before 12 May 2005 is no longer here. I guess being a neonatologist also changes you. When you see many babies dying, when you speak to many parents about what is important in life, about death, about disabilities, it changes you. I think it might be similar for any catastrophic life event. Somehow most people around us are NIs (Normal Inconsiderates): people who are angry at parking tickets, at deadlines, anxious about making lunches for their kids, cross about not getting an article accepted for publication, jealous of the neighbour with the better car/spouse/garden/house/tennis racket ... It is incredible how many people are drowning in ambitions and running on a guinea pig wheel, chasing after a carrot that grows bigger and that they can never bite. So many people do not enjoy life, they run through it, they are stressed about stupid stuff. As my dad used to say, "Tu t'étourdie – pause toi un peu!" (you are dizzying yourself – just land for a while).

Many NIs get really bad news during their lives: a suspicious lump is discovered in their breast, their child has a car accident, their husband is becoming blind. When these moments happen, the world stops. The world as they know it dies. The health care professionals we meet at these moments when we receive bad news will stay with us all our lives.

Neonatologists, fellows, nurse practitioners, residents, you are SOOOOOOO important. Please do not bring your pagers into the room when you give terrible news; turn off your cell phones. Please sit down, speak slowly to the patient, repeat. Please stop talking when both parents are sobbing. Just recognize that what you are doing at this moment is a critical moment in these parents' lives. For you, giving bad news is part of the routine. You see many dying babies. You might not remember having told a family their child was blind or deaf, or had profusely bled in her head. You might not recognize the parents when you see them in the street years later. But this family will remember you all their lives. This is the moment when their life as they knew it stopped and another one started. You are the one who broke their story.

The change from NI to AP (Altered Person) is immediate. A parent in the NICU generally becomes an AP: parking tickets, professional disappointments, deadlines, and many of the ordinary things that stress NIs in their everyday lives will never affect her again in the same way. And routine life becomes much less boring to APs compared to NIs. The routine, simple life, a glass of apple juice in the morning, dressing the kids for school, making lunches, going to work, drinking coffee, seeing babies in the park, coming home to your kids, helping with their homework, slicing carrots for supper, making cookies, bathing the kids, reading to them, talking to a partner, getting ready for bed, and starting again the next day: WHAT A RELIEF! At least once a week, Keith and I have tears in our eyes just watching our kids play, watching them poke the tips of their tongues out when they concentrate to draw a picture, listening to the stories they tell each other, watching them eat and make a mess, and seeing them closely observe an ant for minutes. We are so lucky, we keep repeating, we are so lucky; life is so precious, life is so beautiful, this is such an important moment ... The kids sometimes ask us, "Are you crying because you are happy or because you are sad?" They know we generally cry with happiness. When I was 3, or 5, or 9, I did not know that a person could cry with happiness.

The kids might be tired of my telling them we are lucky to be a family, a family of parents who love each other, who love them, all of us doing okay, in a country where we have enough to eat, where we are not afraid. We are lucky to be healthy. With everything that can go wrong in the human body, health feels like a miracle. I still keep a shoulder half raised and an eye half closed, expecting another blow to come someday, but nothing else has happened. The NICU changed me as a physician, and then it changed me when I became a parent in the NICU with my own baby.

A Mother's Love

Dear Mr M.,

My name is Annie Janvier. I am a member of the team of doctors that took care of your grandson in the NICU. You may not remember me, but I want you to know that your daughter Pamela and your family changed my life, as a doctor, as a person, and as a mother. I have often thought of you all, and I regret that I did not get in touch with you earlier. I often ask for news of you, and today I heard the terrible news of your wife Margaret's death.

I am writing to you because I want to tell you how much your family means to me. There are people and situations that change our lives and make us better people, better doctors. In that regard, your daughter Pamela is part of a truly magical group. The other members of that group are you and her family. I met Pamela under very difficult circumstances. The emergency room had called us to say that a woman who hadn't even known she was pregnant was giving birth there, at that very moment! We rushed to emergency, with the crash cart, just in case. That day, I spent only a few minutes with Pamela. She was so young. She told me that her periods were very rare, and her doctors had thought she was sterile because of her numerous health problems. She never expected to ever get pregnant. If her baby had any chance of survival, she wanted us to seize that chance. Everything was happening very fast, and we didn't have time, under the circumstances, to explain to her in detail the risks for her baby.

Pamela was ready to push, so we hurried to the delivery room. We did a quick ultrasound, which revealed that her child weighed around 750 grams, therefore its gestational age was about 24 weeks. When he was born, he cried and was vigorous. We stabilized him and took him to the NICU. For the first hours of his life, he was stable, but that didn't last. His lungs were very weak and we had difficulty delivering enough oxygen to his body. We had a team meeting and all the neonatologists agreed that we had to warn the parents that there was a high risk that the baby would die, and a significant risk that he would have lasting effects.

I was the one who went to see Pamela. Her son was 48 hours old and there was no improvement in his condition. He was not dying, but his future was uncertain. I went to her room in the hospital. Pamela was really not doing well. They were not able to control her insulin, her cortisol, or her TSH, the hormone that regulates the thyroid. And she had a lot of other problems as well.

She was beautiful, with her sparkling brown eyes! However, she was visibly sick: her very pale skin was yellowish, she was swollen from the birth, or maybe because of the medications. She was wearing red pyjama bottoms with hearts, and a pink T-shirt with a little pink bow. Her room was on the right of the corridor, and her bed was near the window. The setting sun lit the room with a reddish-orange light, giving it a magical, unreal feeling. And she was bathed in that warm light. She insisted that I call her Pamela: "Mrs M. is my mother, not me," she said. In turn, I asked her to call me Annie. And I told her that her baby was very sick, that his lungs were in critical condition, that it was difficult to give him enough oxygen, but that we were managing for the time being. I also told her that babies like her little boy did not always survive. She replied that she knew that but was convinced deep down that he was going to make it. Her son could also be disabled, something we hadn't had time to talk about since her arrival at the hospital. I described to her some of the problems he could develop and told her she was very courageous to hear all that when she was doing so poorly herself. But she wanted to know everything about her son, and we also wanted her to know the risks for him. I told her that, in these circumstances, there were parents who felt it was unreasonable to keep their child in intensive care. We wanted to make sure that, for her, it was not unreasonable to give all that care to her baby with his uncertain future. She knit her brow and asked, "What do you mean?" I was embarrassed. She obviously wasn't prepared for that. There are parents who spontaneously ask us, "Is all this, all the machines, really worth it?" Not Pamela. I explained to her that, given the high risk of death, the condition of her baby's lungs, and the possible disabilities, we wanted to be certain that keeping him alive with our technology was in keeping with her wishes and her values. But I also added that babies like her son, when they do survive, can have a quality of life that the parents consider good, even with disabilities. They can interact with others and bring a lot of joy to their families. That we could decide together, with the baby's dad, with her family. We would be there whatever happened.

She spoke, very slowly, looking at me intently:

You see that window? To let my baby die because of those risks would be like asking me to throw myself out that window. Ever since I was born, I've always been sick. I take huge quantities of drugs. I've been hospitalized more times than I can count. The doctors don't understand what's wrong with me, it's some auto-immune thing, my body is attacking my body, and nobody knows what will happen to me. And yet I'm happy, maybe because that's all I've known, I've never been healthy. I'm happy, because I'm loved, and because I love. The doctors told me I was sterile, and I've had a baby. They didn't even see that I was pregnant when they needed to increase the dosage of my medications and I was swimming in hormones. Not the baby's, but all the others. And then my son landed in my life. It's an ordeal, but at the same time, I'm a mother, and I hadn't thought I would ever be able to say that. I'm a mother. I have a boy.

My parents have taken care of me all my life. They still do. They nurtured me, they took me to all my doctors' appointments, they cried with me when I was in pain, they laughed with me when the news was good. They held me, they supported me, they loved me no matter what. That's what I want for my son, I want him to have parents like mine. My parents moved heaven and earth for me. Always. And that's what I'll do for my boy. If I were facing the same risks as he is, they would take care of me, they would cry at my bedside, they would hold my hand and hope I'd get better. I really hope he'll get better.

And I thought that I myself wished to become a mother like her, a parent like you. I was fighting back tears. I realized that doctors often got things wrong. They think in terms of statistics, while parents think in terms of love and hope. That conversation touched me deeply.

I understand Pamela's words better now that I'm Violette's mother. When I see parents dealing with the same questions, I think back to Pamela, so wise, so serene. I think of her when I see parents exhausted by the ups and downs, the fear and anxiety, the feeling of emptiness that comes with all that. When I find myself in a difficult situation, I think back to the love that inspired her. An unconditional love, in spite of uncertainty, in spite of the possibility of imminent death or disabilities. A love that withstands all the blows of fate. The strength we lack at one moment always ends up coming back, and the great emptiness is always filled.

A few weeks later, I was on duty when I was informed that Pamela had died. I collapsed into a chair in the unit and wept. Unstoppable tears. Normally, I can restrain myself. But that time, I cried all through the rounds, in front of the residents, in front of the parents. Sickness and the world didn't make any sense anymore.

A month later, I took care of her son when he had acute pulmonary failure. Seeing you again, you and your wife, Margaret, moved me to tears. I pulled myself together, I swallowed hard and opened my eyes wide: it's a trick I use to keep from crying. I told myself, "When an unstable baby is placed in your care, Janvier, it's not the time to cry. The grandparents must want to cry too, and yet they're keeping it together." I went and hid in my office to give free rein to my pain. That little boy survived and was being raised by his dad and his grandparents. They were superheroes. They knew everything about him, much more than his medical file, much better than all the doctors working on his "case."

Over the years, I've asked after your grandson from time to time. I knew that, in spite of his difficulties, he was a happy, loved child. His grandmother was passionately protective of him; he was given everything he needed and much more. No one knew him better than she did. His entire extended family took marvellous care of that beloved, happy little boy.

Two weeks ago, I learned that Margaret, the grandmother and adoptive mother, was dying. Cancer. At the age of 52. The heroine, the Amazon, the fighter, the lioness, who had raised several children, two of whom were very sick. A long time ago, I stopped asking myself why these things happen. Sometimes life doesn't make sense.

I am writing to you because I've been thinking a lot about you. I thought that at this difficult time it might be of some comfort to you to know that Pamela and Margaret will always be a great inspiration to me on how to become a better mother, and a better doctor.

Thank you again,

Annie Janvier

The Backpack: The Sequel

The families I provide care to teach me things every day. Sometimes, it's how a candy factory works, or the stress of being a police officer, when that's a parent's job. Sometimes I learn profound things about the meaning of life. Parents and babies have changed my way of being, and my way of seeing things.

Today, I saw Ms Pelletier,* Pascal's* mom, again. I now call her Suzanne,* because, after all the hours we spent together when Pascal was not well, we've become friends. Pascal is two years old now.

"It goes by so quickly!" said Suzanne. She had come to see the urologist. Pascal will probably have to have another operation to relieve pressure on one of his kidneys, because he's been having repeated urinary tract infections. Since he often has problems with his kidneys, you could say he's got a "loyalty card" for the urology and nephrology clinic.

"Do you remember how he was when he was born? We've grown, haven't we?" Who was "we"? I answered that I could see how Pascal had grown, but who else had? Suzanne reminded me of my story about the backpack and the stones you put in it that represent the decisions you have to make in your life.

I met Suzanne when she was 32 weeks pregnant; she had five weeks to go to give birth at full term. When he was at the fetal stage, Pascal had a blockage in his urethra and he wasn't able to eliminate his urine. This is called an obstruction of the posterior urethral valves. Because of the obstruction, urine would accumulate in his urinary tract, putting a lot of pressure on his kidneys. Urine was also accumulating in his body and making his abdomen swell, which was compressing his lungs. During the fetal stage, urine production is very important. The fetus does not breathe air in the uterus. The urine, mixed with the amniotic fluid, which is made by the placenta, enables the lungs to develop and grow. The lungs need to be full of the urine-amniotic fluid. Without fetal urine, the lungs cannot develop. Without lungs, a baby cannot survive at birth. The obstruction in the urethra was an accident of nature, and nothing could have been done to prevent it. There was not enough liquid to do an amniocentesis (taking fluid from the uterine cavity with a needle), which would have shown us if there was also a genetic abnormality. Since there were no other malformations in his body, there were few risks. Pascal was floating in very little amniotic fluid. His lungs had begun to form before the obstruction, but hadn't developed very much. And his abdomen swollen with urine was compressing them even more.

The purpose of my first meeting with Ms Pelletier was to determine what she wanted to do at the time of delivery. My colleague, an obstetrician specializing in high-risk pregnancies, could insert little catheters into Pascal's bladder to relieve the pressure just before childbirth, in preparation for possible drainage, which would facilitate vaginal expulsion of the urine and help the baby's breathing. But the nephrologist (kidney specialist) had said that Pascal would suffer from kidney failure and would have to start dialysis, probably during his childhood, pending a kidney transplant. The possibility of terminating the pregnancy was also mentioned; what awaited Pascal and his family was serious. That could be done by inducing labour or through feticide, a procedure that consists of injecting potassium chloride into the heart of the fetus; the heart stops and labour is triggered. Another option was to drain Pascal's urine out of his bladder through a catheter to relieve the pressure on his kidneys, and wait for the best time to deliver the baby. Pascal would need intensive care starting at birth to manage his breathing and his urine.

Ms Pelletier wanted to know what would happen during the birth and in the NICU. I was on duty that day and I went to see her. Looking at the results of the ultrasound and ascertaining when the blockage had probably occurred, I wasn't able to say whether Pascal's little lungs would work at birth. I was relatively sure that he would need a ventilator, but at what intensity, and for how long? Sometimes, even with our best machines, babies with such small lungs (a condition called pulmonary hypoplasia) do not survive, because the lungs are not big enough to take in sufficient amounts of oxygen. Most babies like Pascal need a ventilator, sometimes for a few days, sometimes for a few weeks. It was clear he wouldn't be able to feed immediately at birth. The urologist would have to place a catheter in his bladder to ensure that the urine was evacuated. Babies with that condition pee enormous quantities, because their kidneys can't concentrate the urine. The quantity of urine evacuated would have to be measured and replaced with the necessary liquid and salts. He would also need a central catheter, an intravenous line installed in a large vein, to allow us to provide him with all the fluids and nutrients he would need.

Pascal's parents asked, "Will he survive?" When babies like Pascal die, it is usually in their first week, because their lungs don't work. However, many have survived in spite of renal or pulmonary problems, but oxygen can damage lungs that are too small. We usually know in the first few days if a baby will survive, depending on the help needed for his lungs and how his kidneys work.

"How would his death occur? Does a baby suffer?" Pascal's parents did not hesitate to ask me for the most explicit details, not just the percentages and physiological concepts. Some parents don't ask so many questions, but others want to know everything. I told them that I was really sorry to be having this conversation with them. At this stage in a pregnancy, parents are usually thinking about the colour of the baby's room, not his death. I would have liked things to be different for them. They were such good parents; they wanted what was best for their son. Babies like Pascal most often die because their lungs are too small; we can't provide them with enough oxygen, even with a respirator. When the lungs aren't capable of exchanging enough oxygen, the baby turns blue and, in the most serious cases, the heart slows down. We make sure the baby is comfortable by giving him medications. The parents can hold their baby in their arms, and we're there for them. Babies in that condition can also die because of an infection, in spite of all the resources of modern medicine. The heart grows weak, as do the lungs. The baby doesn't get enough blood in his organs and he dies. Once again, we're there for the parents and for the baby. We can't always cure an illness or repair small lungs, but we can always assess and treat the pain and make sure the baby is comfortable. We will always be with the parents.

I asked Pascal's parents what they wanted. They both gave the same answer: for their son to survive with the least possible damage to his kidneys. What did they fear most? That Pascal would endure needless suffering, that he would remain on the respirator for weeks and die in the end. They dreaded death, but they were prepared to accept a quick death, the death of the "blue baby whose heart slows down." They could live with kidney failure – they had talked about it with the nephrologist, and, in the waiting room, they had met families with children on dialysis. They looked like normal families, with normal joys and sorrows, despite the many hours spent in the hospital every week. Pascal's parents could live with the possible interventions, they could live with hospitalization in the NICU, if that could bring Pascal home. It was a major ordeal, but it also offered the promise of a future, and the promise of a family. What they weren't ready to accept was if, after having undergone all the procedures of intensive care, Pascal died without knowing life outside the hospital. They feared that their son would suffer too much, too long. I explained to them what happened when a child was dying, that we stopped the respirator, that parents could hold their child in their arms. They had to know what was important to them if Pascal were to die.

I told them the story of the backpack filled with stones representing the decisions one has had to make in one's life. You have to know how to live with yourself, with your regrets, with the need sometimes to rewrite the story you had created for yourself. You have to know what's most important, and how to live with your decisions. Pascal's parents did indeed have a serious decision to make. Some parents can find those interventions excessive in relation to the anticipated results; for them, terminating the pregnancy is the choice to make – not the best one, but the least bad. Some parents want to know how the lungs and the kidneys are doing; they can't resign themselves to death without giving the child a chance. "You apparently belong to that second category of parents," I told them. They replied that they couldn't set a date for their child's death. For them, it was up to nature to decide if his lungs would work or not. They wanted to know at what point they should let nature take its course, and what would happen if the machines were stopped. They made me promise never to lose sight of their child, to always make sure not to inflict too much on him. They repeated that they wanted it to be nature that decided the length of their child's life, not them. Nature, in this case, was Pascal's lungs.

A doctor in a modern intensive care unit is not omnipotent. Even with all the cutting-edge treatments, patients die. The machines don't make us immortal. With some patients, machines indeed extend life, not death.

We don't always have to let "nature" decide. If we just let nature take its course, cancer, minor infections, and appendicitis would kill everyone who had them, and so would many conditions that we can treat very easily. Nature is a real bitch sometimes. It makes terrible mistakes with babies' anatomy, as with Pascal. But we have to ask ourselves what our goal is with all these machines, what the parents' goal is, and what we subject the babies to. I understood what they meant, but it's difficult to accept; health professionals do not all agree when it comes to setting a limit and "letting nature take its course." We have to talk about life and death with parents of babies like Pascal. It's important. And we regularly have to have these conversations when a baby like Pascal is born. And I had to make sure we did not go beyond Pascal's parents' limit.

We always observed Pascal closely for signs of pain and intervened to reduce his discomfort. We were able to limit the pain. His lungs were sick, but he never experienced respiratory failure, he never turned blue, his heart never slowed down. He stayed in the NICU for two long months.

Suzanne pulled me out of my reverie by handing me Pascal, who grabbed my ID badge. "Maybe he wants to become a doctor one day! But something easier than what you do. A dermatologist, for example. You know, I came back to see you because I thought about your backpack story, and about the consequences of our decisions. Yesterday was Pascal's second birthday. When he was blowing out the candles, I thought to myself that I was really the luckiest mom in the world. But there's something not right in your backpack story: it doesn't have an ending. The backpack story has to be concluded."

With her extraordinary strength, that woman could easily carry more than one backpack. I asked her what title she would suggest for the next chapter: The trunk? The container? She had a good laugh.

> "First of all, it's difficult to guess the weight of the stones. When I was pregnant and learned what problems Pascal had, I felt the weight of a mountain on my back. But imagining it and experiencing it are two very different things. And it weighs quite a bit less than I had imagined."

> "But not everyone feels the weight in the same way. Didn't the stone of an unfinished pregnancy seem heavier than the stone of kidney failure?"

"Yes. But usually the stone weighs less and less with time. And you forgot to say that. Maybe to you, it's obvious that by carrying a big backpack, you develop your muscles, and in the long run, the weight becomes easier to carry. Pascal's first months were difficult, but things got better. And now that he's better, we're much better. I guess we got used to them."

"You're right, human beings have a great capacity for adaptation. I should have said that. But there are also people who aren't able to adapt. A minority, but still."

"I haven't encountered that many, and I've spent a lot of time at the hospital, in the waiting rooms, with parents like us. We get weary, and some children are sicker than others. We're regulars at Sainte-Justine, but our families are not so different from others."

"From now on, every time I mention the backpack, I'll tell your story."

"Wait, I haven't finished!"

Suzanne is a passionate woman. At the beginning of the conversation in my office, she was sitting, but at the end she was on her feet, jumping up and down and waving her arms, and I had stood up too, with Pascal in my arms, as if carried by her energy, the two of us were almost dancing. She was on fire, a mother full of joy. What a contrast with our first meeting, when she was so sad, so disheartened!

"The real ending of our backpack story is coming. What I said about carrying the weight and getting stronger is pretty obvious. But in truth, before becoming parents, we weren't very responsible. We didn't have stable jobs and we moved often. We'd party all the time, we'd drink like fish, we didn't care about anything. We were existing, but we weren't living, we were drifting. Well, Pascal made us serious people, and we're proud of it. He changed us. Those stones in our backpacks keep our feet on the ground, they keep us from floating up into the air and being carried off by the wind. Yes, it's sad that we owe that to my son's condition, but that's the way it is. I suppose that his little backpack is pretty full too, but look at him go! I think he has everything he needs to have a very full life, and not an empty, dull existence."

There was nothing to add. I had tears in my eyes. I hugged Suzanne with Pascal sandwiched between us. Maybe I hoped to absorb a little of her energy.

After Violette, Am I a Better Doctor?

I'm often asked if my adventure in the NICU with Violette made me a better doctor. I tend to answer, "Yes, probably." But you don't need to be unlucky to be a good doctor. A psychiatrist doesn't need to be a manic-depressive to be excellent. A good marriage counsellor does not necessarily have to be divorced, and so on. There are lots of good doctors and good nurses who have no children, who've never had a brush with death. That doesn't preclude receptiveness and openness to children and their families.

What is certain is that the experience of meeting parents in the NICU made me a better mother at the bedside of my sick baby. It's hard to explain the mixture of panic, guilt, emptiness, despair, and absurdity that takes over the brain of a parent whose baby is dependent on machines to survive. What I felt was like with an old-fashioned television set when it was between two stations. The sound crackled and the picture was all distorted, and everything came in bursts. My cognitive processes were overwhelmed. In a situation like this, being "reasonable" doesn't have much meaning anymore. Even the word doesn't make sense: as much as I repeated it in my head, it was just noise, like the engine of a machine you don't see. The guideposts aren't clear. It's difficult to accept that your life looks like that now. I would have given a fortune, a leg, or two, for Violette to be able to get off the respirator and leave the NICU in good health. Insomnia and exhaustion don't help either.

My operational brain, which has always served me very well when it comes to thinking, planning, organizing, caring for other babies, going to the most urgent cases, and writing scientific articles or stories, had become a shapeless blob of poutine sauce. I was no longer able to put things in perspective. When Violette was at her worst, I was at my worst. When there was a respite, when she was doing a little better, when the lab results were good, when a day went by without a major drama, I could finally think and focus, and analyse what was happening. My control freak self had lost her independence of mind. My falls were staggering, and my small joys were tremendous. Less fluid in her lungs? YES! A good blood gas test? YES, YES! We can turn down the respirator a little because things are going well? LET'S PARTY! Then, splat! I'd fall on my face again. The damn ups and downs. The least little detail becomes disproportionately important. The tiniest awkward remark by a caregiver can screw up the whole day. Although I believe in the virtues of writing, most of the time my paralysed brain felt only a jumble of panic, chaos, and hope. My capacity to rationally analyse data and possible outcomes was completely swamped.

There are a lot of things I didn't write at those times. You won't find them in the "lived" version of this book. I wasn't capable of it; I was too disorganized. I started a lot of pieces of writing I never finished. During the two first months of Violette's life, between storms and hope, I didn't have the luxury of normal thinking and concentration. After the storms, my brain was usually devastated, drowned, comatose, an inert mass, like a gourd that makes a hollow sound.

Before Violette, I sympathized entirely with parents. Whatever they did, I forgave them. I supported them, even if it was hard, even if it was terribly sad, even if they yelled at me or insulted me. They had a good reason for doing it: their baby was in a plastic box, connected to machines, when it should have been in his mother's arms, surrounded with joy, balloons, and presents. Among bouquets of flowers. Or inside her. Here, parents watch us insert intravenous lines into their child, a child they haven't been able to hold in their arms at birth, a child who often has not yet even cried for the first time.

In my job, you hear a lot of sad stories. During my fellowship, a parent, Andrew,* took a swing at me when I told him his daughter was dying. He had called an ambulance when his wife started having convulsions.

She had eclampsia, a condition that occurs only in pregnant women, in which blood pressure rises to dangerous levels and convulsions occur at the most severe stage; it can lead to death. For the mother to be saved, she has to be no longer pregnant, so you have to get the baby out as quickly as possible. His wife had a C-section under general anaesthesia as soon as she got to the hospital. Andrew arrived a half hour later, after the C-section, while his wife was still unconscious. He saw his tiny daughter very briefly. We had to talk to him; there was no time to spare. The baby, Lauren,* was at 23 weeks and weighed 405 grams. Her lungs were never able to exchange oxygen properly. She was not going to survive. In a situation like that, as a doctor, you know very well when you sit down with the father that with a few words you're going to destroy him, crush his hopes, shatter his family. That feeling of throwing a bomb in a parent's face is horrible. Lauren's dad stood up, took a couple of steps, and then, wham! came his fist. I don't know if it was aimed at me. We talked about it years later and he didn't remember the episode; he only remembered collapsing, falling into a bottomless chasm, feeling sick, stunned, nauseous, suffocated. He thought he was going to die. I managed to duck the blow. His fist made a hole in the wall. The nurse ran out of the room, no doubt to call security. I remember the look of madness in the father's eyes. His fists were clenched, his knuckles white, his lips tight, his legs trembling. The silence was intolerable, but I knew I had to stay with him, look him in the eye, tell him that I was sorry, that I would have wanted Lauren to be better, that she was lucky to have a dad who loved her so much. I felt that by making physical contact with him, I could contain the volcanic eruption. He started sobbing, crying, shouting in my arms. In medical school, no one teaches you how to deal with such distress. What do you do when a father tries to hit you and then collapses in tears in your arms? My left shoulder was wet with his tears; he was panting. I told him we were there for him, for his wife, for Lauren. His wife wasn't in danger. Together, we would give Lauren the best life possible. We would take her to her mother, so she could see her when she woke up.

As a doctor, I've learned a lot from parents; as a parent, that's what saved me. I've developed very strong friendships with some parents. Most of the children regained their health; others died or had lasting effects from their early illness. Sometimes with twins, one child pulls through and the other doesn't. Many parents have seen their child come close to death, come back to life, and then suffer more blows. With time, the feelings of drowning, emptiness, or panic finally fade. When the parents leave the hospital, they usually feel better. The day Violette nearly died, Olivia's mother said to me, "You've lost hope, as I did. But you're speaking as a doctor, not as a mother. You're running away, the way I tried to run away two months ago, when I was told that Olivia might not last the night. Get a grip! You'll get through this. Whatever happens, you'll get through this."

When you go through this kind of crisis as a parent, it's important to be told that things really are going to get better, that you won't always feel like this. It's easy, in hindsight, to tell mothers to hang in there, to tell fathers to keep their heads above water. I may seem insensitive writing this when so many babies in the NICU are hovering between life and death and so many parents are upset. But there is a future. The storm will finally pass – it has to. The life you had imagined for yourself, the plans you had made for your family, may never be fulfilled. Sometimes, you have to imagine and create another story. You have to trust life.

Having been a mother in the NICU certainly helped me to better deal with certain things with parents; there are certain emotions I sense better, appeals for help I understand better. I now have words, better words, to relieve their pain a little, tips I can give them on how to deal with the extended family, with the telephone, with the Others, with the pump. I know how madness threatens us, how guilt eats away at us, and how the Others can hurt us, even when they believe they are doing good. I've stopped telling parents to take things one day at a time. They know that. I've developed a kind of radar to see how deep parents can sink. I ask them if they don't sometimes feel like being put under general anaesthetic for a month. Some parents say no, because they want to spend time with their child. Others look up at me with tearful eyes and ask if it's really possible. I find it upsetting every time. I tell them to imagine their baby in four months, in six months, to visualize her room, with the position of the bed, to imagine their very small baby in her huge bed. I talk to them about the changing of the seasons, the snow melting, the tulips blooming, the summer coming, the little hat and the sunscreen they'll put on her to protect her from the sun, the leaves that fall in the autumn, the smell of a Christmas tree. I tell them to visualize all that, and to hope for all that. There's no harm in hoping. Sometimes you only need a good dose of hope. It's no substitute for general anaesthesia, but it does soothe the pain a little.

I don't want to turn into some kind of Lance Armstrong of neonatology, a strong girl who has survived cancer and thinks that cancer patients just have to do some intensive exercise to heal (without steroids, however). When doctors experience traumatic events themselves, they shouldn't think that everyone will experience things the same way. For example, I feel it's dangerous for a former cancer patient to claim that it was her will that beat the disease. Optimism is not a panacea, and saying that is unfair to people who are terminally ill. The ones who have died are no longer there to tell others how to fight cancer. Just because I myself am the mother of a 24-week baby doesn't mean that my story applies to everyone who finds herself in that situation. Each woman has her own story, each woman lives her own life, each father rewrites it in his own words, and there are very different individuals in the world.

The opposite can be true too. Sometimes it's hard to be a good doctor after having been the mother of a baby in critical condition in the NICU. It could even make me a less good doctor, and I have to remain vigilant. Antoine* was a very small baby boy whose brain had been ravaged by hemorrhages, to such an extent that he had almost no more brain, just blood. What remained of his brain was being crushed by the pressure of the blood. It wasn't anyone's fault; it's something that occurs sometimes when babies like Antoine are born so prematurely at home. We could have installed a drain to evacuate all that blood from his head, but we, the caregivers, all knew that was no longer the best solution for Antoine. He was sick, unstable, very fragile. His lungs were so weak that they might not hold out even as far as the operating room – in any case, not until the next day. If he were to survive, it would be with significant long-term effects. We had to recommend to the parents that we stop intensive care and give their baby comfort care; what we were doing was no longer the most reasonable course of action under the circumstances.

I asked the parents what they wanted for Antoine; I told them they could discuss it with me and tell me if the goals we were pursuing seemed reasonable to them. The medical team felt that a drain was not reasonable under the circumstances. Antoine was not strong enough even for the operating room. The father asked me if I had children. Without giving me a chance to answer, he added that it was clear that I didn't have any, and that to me, as with all the doctors, their son was only a number to get rid of to make room for others and, that way, to make even more money at their expense. He felt we wanted to get rid of all disabled children, that I wanted to create a flawless world in my own image as a successful little entitled doctor. If I had ever had to fear for the life of my child, he said, I would have the decency to install a drain without making a fuss. While he was heaping abuse on me, his wife was sitting in her chair crying.

Before Violette, I would have taken that philosophically. I would have said to myself "The father is angry, he's looking for a scapegoat, and I happen to be here. What he's saying is wounding; maybe I should have presented things differently. I should have avoided talking about the drain, since we don't think it's reasonable to install it. We can't decide anything right now; Antoine can't be taken to the operating room. Did I handle this badly? Let's give them a few hours, and then we'll come back and apologize. We don't mean that Antoine is not worth putting in a drain. And we'll try to repair the damage." After Violette, I still knew that, but it was different.

I told them they didn't know me, they really didn't, and that this was about their baby and not mine. They replied that there was no question of Antoine dying, that they had waited too long for him. His arrival was a miracle, and, for that reason, he should undergo all the surgeries required. But death – never. They threatened us with lawyers. They said I couldn't understand, and, besides, doctors never understood anything. They felt the doctors were there so that their baby would live, not for him to die. It was the first time that my empathy with parents was put to the test. I felt like shouting at them, "Who are you to judge me? My daughter endured everything, and we were ready to let her go when she was dying. Who do you think you are? We can't perform fucking miracles here, even though we dream of it." Basically, those people were suffering because they loved their son. And I had to stay cool, which is what I did. I didn't say anything, I took the mother's hand, I spoke calmly to the father, but it was hard. And sometimes that's what you have to do: simply say nothing. Before Violette, it had never been so difficult.

We made our decisions with the parents and the surgeons. Because Antoine was unstable, we had to wait between twenty-four and forty-eight hours before sending him to the operating room, to give him time to stabilize, otherwise he was likely to die there. His lungs were deteriorating more and more: the machine was pushing the maximum amount of oxygen, but it was no use; Antoine wasn't getting better. His head was swelling; he was having seizures. I gave him morphine and more medication to stop the seizing. His survival might be uncertain, but we could control the pain. I told the parents that their baby wasn't suffering, and that was our priority. He looked comfortable. They organized his baptism. Antoine died thirty-six hours later when I wasn't on duty. And I remember being relieved that it had happened in my absence. Before, I never would have been so cowardly. I sent the parents a card. I wrote that their family had taught me something that made me a better doctor.

I'm always there to help parents, always ready to give everything I have. Maybe those parents, who were ready to do anything in the face of the inevitable, reminded me cruelly that I had been ready to throw in the towel with Violette. We had both got it wrong, in opposite ways. I had been weak in that I hadn't told them clearly that their baby was going to die. And I almost lost my Violette because of my wrong predictions. I was unhappy with myself. I had to overcome that feeling in order to be the good doctor parents really need, one who is able to make decisions with parents, sometimes in uncertainty, and accept the consequences.

And those who were seen dancing were thought to be insane by those who could not hear the music.

Friedrich Nietzsche

This article is the story of Simon, Émile, and their family. In my career, families have often taught me more than textbooks have. This story reflects on the "non-medical" relationships we have with families. Unfortunately, these relationships are increasingly heavily regulated. In some hospital, some clinicians are prevented from having relationships with families outside of the hospital (for example, to go to birthday parties), are not allowed to contact families outside of the medical world (for example, to send a card), cannot "friend" parents or keep in contact with them for non-medical reasons. I practise a more reflective approach, which I find helps both my patients and myself. Often, to speak about tattoos and beer is the only way a father can approach a conversation about death and his fears. My colleague Bonnie Arzuega and I are exploring this empirically. We have published one article[†] and more are to come, if you wish to read further on these topics. Bonnie Arzuega, a great researcher and neonatologist who is the principal investigator in this research, is also examining the perspective of parents on these subjects, so stay tuned!

Tattoos, Beer, and Bow Ties: The Limits of Professionalism in Medicine

Annie Janvier, MD, PhD[‡]

I was at Émile's bedside, one of the newly admitted preemies. I didn't hear anybody enter the room and so was surprised when a boisterous male voice asked, "What's up with the tattoos?"

I turned to see a tall and large man. I wondered when he could possibly have seen my tattoos. At work, my 20 hours of ink job are hidden under my scrubs. Should I ask him where he saw them? Is there a grotesque picture of me half naked in a Jacuzzi, drinking a fluorescent pink cocktail in a crazy glass somewhere on Facebook? Does it have many "likes"? Or worse, no likes at all? Then I remember. I ran to work today in a tank top and shorts. He must have seen me then, before I showered and changed.

"Bonjour! I didn't notice you come in. Are you Émile's papa?"

"Yes," he said with a smile.

"I'm Annie Janvier, the baby doctor who will be taking care of your son for the next 2 weeks."

We shook hands.

"Most parents ask about their baby's health, not their doctor's tattoos. What's up with the tattoo question?"

"Well, doctors don't usually have tattoos. It's unusual."

"Let me go wash my hands to examine Émile and tell you about him."

The familiar scent of an antibacterial mousse soap took my mind off body art. It was a glorious morning. The perfect blue sky clashed with the sickness of the babies, the thick gray clouds above their incubators, the storm in their parents' hearts. Émile had been born 3 days ago, at 26 weeks. His lungs were sick. I was asked to go see him as soon as I arrived on the unit. His lungs were getting worse. Overnight, he'd been switched to an oscillator.

While I was washing my hands, Émile's nurse asked me whether I would answer the tattoo question. She told me about her recent lectures on professionalism and health care professional–patient boundaries: "We learned to tell each other when we see red flags. Is this tattoo question a red flag?" We spoke about the medical/ethical literature, that there were 2 reasons invoked to observe such boundaries: to protect patients and to protect health care professionals. What was the risk of answering the tattoo question?

As I went back to Émile's bedside, the father asked, "What do all of your tattoos mean?"

"They are all about the most important stuff in my life: my kids, nature, family, relationships. Maybe you know what I mean?"

"Yes, I also have a bunch. Some are about my family, here, on my leg."

The nurse almost dropped Émile's chart when the father started rolling up his pants. She looked incredulous.

I sat down next to the father to better see the tattoos he was trying to show me.

"Wow, your whole calf is covered: octopus, sharks, a sea horse, and these huge Maori-style turtles? Are they special turtles?"

"Well, there is papa turtle, me, and mama turtle, my wife Julie. Julie is way smaller than me; I'm a big guy, twice her size ... well, you will understand when you meet her, and then Delphine turtle, our little energizer tornado, and the other one is for Anne."

He paused.

"Anne ... she is not with us anymore."

"Tell me more about Anne."

"She died about 10 years ago. She was very pre-term, too small and fragile to survive. But I wanted the Anne turtle the same size as Delphine's."

"She will be with you always, in your heart. She changed the papa you are."

He nodded. I waited to see if he would say more. He didn't. I asked, "When are you going to get a tattoo for Émile?"

"At some point, when he gets better. You know. What I want is tattoos of living turtles, not dead ones. And Émile is attached to all these tubes everywhere; I can't take it. It hurts me. Watching him, with that tube, makes my throat hurt. My heart hurts too. I am afraid to answer the phone when a confidential number calls the house. But I have to. Julie won't."

"Émile is very sick right now, but he is not dying. He is now on this high-frequency respirator, and he improved."

"When will we know he will be fine?"

"What we are hoping is that his lungs continue to improve. We hope that he will need less oxygen. During the night Émile needed 90% oxygen; the maximum we can give is 100%. Now he is in 60% oxygen. It is still high, and we hope this will decrease. Émile is fragile, his lungs are sick, but many things in his body are working. He is digesting his *maman*'s milk, he did not bleed in his brain, his heart and kidneys work well."

"When the blue saturation numbers go down, I am so powerless, hopeless. I tell Émile he will be OK, but I get really anxious, I feel like a lion in a cage. What can I do?"

"Be there for him, speak to him, hold him. Continue supporting *maman* with pumping; be her milk man! Émile is lucky to have a papa like you, who loves him that much."

"You will tell me when to get an Émile turtle, right?"

"I will."

I got to know Simon much better over the months Émile was hospitalized. We built our relationship on the foundation of that discussion of our tattoos. Simon has generalized anxiety disorder and attention-deficit disorder. He gets agitated rather easily. Simon spoke about his distress through metaphors. He wore a nice shirt and a bow tie on a good day. He wore T-shirts on bad days. A T-shirt was a sign we needed to talk. An old T-shirt was an SOS. There were many T-shirt days. At some point during Émile's hospital stay, Simon needed to optimize his anxiety medication.

Simon is a homebrewer and knows his biology. He understood the microbiome, the prophylactic fluconazole, the probiotics his son was receiving. He taught me about the subtleties of brewing beer, how quickly it can spoil, how to achieve a perfect balance.

After a week with bow ties, I told Simon he should get another turtle tattoo, perhaps a turtle with an extra thick shell.

The "professionalism" movement has had both a positive and negative effect on the practice of medicine and physicians' relationships with patients. Maybe health care professional–patient relationships are safer, now, but only because they have been cleverly sterilized and placed in grids with strict rules of behavior. I'm not sure that this helps patients. Residents are afraid to send cards to parents after a long hospital stay. They hesitate to send condolence notes when a baby dies. Fellows are unsure if it is "professional" to go to a patient's funeral, a baptism, a birthday party, to sit with a parent/patient in the cafeteria. Nurses do not consult patients' medical records after they have been discharged, even when sometimes they have known the family for months. Health care professionals tell patients/parents they cannot exchange email addresses, that this is "the protocol." Many would not approve of my writing this story. Strict policies regarding confidentiality are being adopted in health care centers. Yet, every time I told a family I was thinking of their baby so much during my day and asked permission to tell or write their story, they were touched and honored.

Émile finally left the hospital on oxygen, with 2 smiling parents. Simon brewed "Les brassins d'Émile" with local breweries, and all profits went to support parents of preterm infants. I know about it because Simon, Julie, and I are friends on Facebook. Recently, their family came to my book launch; Simon brought handmade bow ties for my boys and husband.

During a recent night call, I gave a resident an update about Simon's family. He told me about his recent course on "professionalism and social media": "friending ex-patients or parents is not recommended. Some medical schools have very strict rules about this. These rules are also there to help protect us against burnout and provider fatigue." He asked me about the impacts of these "unprofessional" relationships on my life.

Not all parents wear bow ties on good days and T-shirts on bad days; not all parents have metaphors of dead children painted on their bodies. Patients and families express grief in different ways. It is important to get messy and have real conversations in these circumstances, follow a trail, let them decide where to take us. To care for families and practice human medicine, we must sometimes take some risks. This does not have to lead to burnout or fatigue. Not crossing these boundaries may lead to unfinished stories and health care professional emptiness. Breaking boundaries breaks barriers. I could not continue practicing medicine if patients no longer kept me up at night: I need to feel I am part of the story.

26 September

Days of life: no idea

Violette's corrected gestational age: baby

Computer,

I've realized that I haven't been writing directly to you anymore, although we're together every day. I write only when I feel the need, but not about me or Violette. I'm behind with loads of stuff, I haven't answered a single email from the university for my PhD, I haven't gone to the archives to deal with charts that are overdue, and lots of other things that had disappeared have reappeared recently. I can also talk about my inner problems to others besides you! It's my birthday today. I'm 33 years old. So Violette's gestational age is going to be put aside for the day!

I wanted to end our correspondence about Violette, me, and our family on a positive note. You'll find it quite a bit less exciting than the ups and downs of the past months. This morning, for my birthday, Keith bought pastries. A chocolate croissant for Axel, and two raisin rolls for him and me. He knows I like the centre best, so he gave me the two centres and ate the outsides. That's true love!

Damn, it's fun to be back to the ordinary little routines of a mom on maternity leave: you don't get enough sleep, but it's because baby is alive, constantly filling her diapers and spitting up. However, this leave is a little different. We're still having trouble getting used to the fact that Violette isn't hooked up to a monitor, with an alarm and a smiling nurse giving us a pat on the back. We feel like we've been released into the wild.

Violette often chokes when she drinks; we have to be careful and pace her if we don't want her turning purple. We also have to make sure she finishes her bottle (with my milk), even if she plays with the nipple and suckles in empty space. We've started enriching her milk again, because she wasn't gaining enough weight. Sometimes she chokes while drinking, but we know what to do. I mustn't forget to breathe. I mustn't hyperventilate either, or I'm sure to get dizzy spells. Breathe in, breathe out.

Sleep isn't ideal. Although it's recommended that the baby's bed be in the parents' bedroom, I just can't do it. Statistically, it reduces the risk of sudden infant death. Well, yes, we know that. I'm an insomniac at the best of times, even on vacation. I wake up when a fly just thinks of crossing Saint-Joseph Boulevard. We sleep with a fan to mask the outside noise, even in winter, plus I've got earplugs in my ears. Violette's bed in our room? To me, the fact that the doctors made this recommendation after four months of intensive care, to an insomniac, bundle-of-nerves mother is a fucking joke. I can hear my children in their rooms, and that's fine. Yes, even with the fan and the earplugs. But Keith doesn't agree. It's out of the question that his princess get less than optimal care, after everything she's been through. Keith is chair of the Canadian Paediatric Society Fetus and Newborn Committee; he's to some extent responsible for those strict recommendations, so, after all, he has to follow them.

"How would we survive if she suddenly died, knowing that we could have prevented it?" he said.

"I do my job to reduce her risks by giving her my milk. But when it comes to sleeping in the same room at night, I just can't," I replied.

I tried anyway. But after two sleepless nights during which I was up for hours ready to do CPR, punctuated with pumping sessions drenched in tears from yelling at Big Bertha, he reconsidered. Besides, Violette wakes up every three hours, because she's a good little clock programmed by the NICU. So, since her fourth night, Keith sleeps with her in her room, on a mattress on the floor, his hand on her bed. He wakes me up when she's hungry. He is also very anxious and wakes up when she is sleeping, in case she forgot to breathe. He gives her a bottle of mother's milk that has already been pumped, and I draw my milk for the next feeding. Keith is a damn good guy, and an excellent father.

The day goes by quite quickly with my two-year-old Axel, who has too much energy. I'm still a butterball because of lack of exercise and my daily consumption of cake or pastries. Every day at two in the afternoon, while my two darlings are napping, I watch *Sugar* on the Food Network, a wonderful show that explains how to make desserts to women who have absolutely no idea how to do it. She practically spells out F-L-O-U-R so we're sure to grasp what she's talking about. I like it: it's a nice pace for a reintroduction to mental exercise. The beautiful, slender, blonde lady (who, after filming, must throw up the cakes she eats) always has exactly half a cup of flour that magically appears, and all her preparations are creamy or fluffy. I've often been successful with the dessert recipes, but not always. Yesterday the cinnamon rolls were like cement, completely stunted little lumps in the middle of the Pyrex pan. Good for doorstops. They fell – plonk! – right to the bottom of the garbage can after Axel and I scraped off the icing and syrup and put it on vanilla ice cream. I should suggest a new program to them: *Sugar, the Sequel: How to Bounce Back after a Dessert Failure.*

So, Computer, when the children wake up, it's a circus, with the baby bottle and milking the cow. Then I put Violette in her little seat and I make cakes under Axel's nose to make him hungry. As soon as he wakes up from his nap, he asks, "'ake?" Of course, we give Violette a fingertip of icing; it partly replaces the sucrose from the NICU.

What's Your Dream?

In the children's school, there's a charming father, Australian, a bit of a hippie, very cool, artsy, who works in film. He has a nice face and aqua eyes. His children could all be in Benetton ads. His son is in Violette's Grade 1 class. Today, we were both parent volunteers for an outing to the swimming pool. On the bus back, he asked me, "Annie, tell me, what are your dreams?"

"That my children survive and stay healthy. Just for us to be. Simply to exist."

"But Annie, those are not dreams ... they're fears."

I understood that I was in a different category of human beings. I don't dream of winning the lottery, being hired as a photographer for *National Geographic*, or being a gourmet food critic and having regular feasts in three-star restaurants. My dream is not to do the scorpion pose in yoga, bring about world peace, or end the war in Iraq. My dream is for my little nest to stay securely in place on its branch. That's all.

And don't take it away from me. Let me hang on to it. Don't touch us.

22 May 2011

Violette,

You're 7 years old today. There are things I can't tell you now, but one day you'll be able to read them, when you're able to decipher more than a few words and simple sentences. According to the doctors, you're still too small, and your trachea still isn't completely healed, nor are your lungs. School is more difficult for you than for other kids. The results of your last tests weren't perfect. But to us, you're perfect.

My love for my children doesn't depend on the way doctors, speech therapists, optometrists, or psychologists measure and catalogue them. Pain, guilt, stress, and everything have devastated us. Certain moments have marked me permanently. Memories come back when I least expect them, sometimes in the NICU when I hear a mother whisper to her tiny baby, "Sorry, sorry." It's like a punch in the stomach every time, and it takes me back to when I was that mother. Sometimes it's when a baby dies – when I lay my hand on the cold little skull, it sears my mind. Being a parent in the NICU changed me. I'm a lot more patient with people who don't act as quickly as I would like. I tell myself that those people are also their parents' children. My goals have changed. I focus on the most important ones and I concern myself much less with frills, like the grant I was turned down for (again), the insensitive comment of some boor, the article that needs to be rewritten, the paper to be given, what others will think, status.

My heart bled for a long time but, since it has healed, it is twice as big as before. The world is no longer the same. My coffee tastes better than most people's, and the sun shines brighter for me than for others. I hit bottom. I learned how easy it is to fall, and how fast it can happen, and I found out that I could take it. I've often thought I was self-centred, but I know now that I'm also capable of giving my all when the circumstances require it. Thanks to you, Violette, I've discovered things about myself that I would never have learned otherwise. Don't get me wrong: I would have liked for you to be born full-term and not have to be in the NICU. But I know now that I could come to terms with disability, that imperfection is another form of perfection. My couple relationship has become stronger. I knew that your father was the love of my life, that he was loving, charming, brilliant, clever, funny, and sensual, and that he was a genius. Your father is now my hero. When you were sick, he was solid as a rock, while all I could do was snivel. I remember the love and the despair I saw on his face when you came out of me, how he would take you in his arms in the NICU. I hear him talking to you in his sleep. I see him feeding you every night while I pumped my milk. He never stopped supporting you and me; he tried to make me see that everything was going well, to keep me from foundering. He always waited for me to regain my strength before letting himself express his own pain. For six months, he slept on the floor next to you with a hand in your bassinet to make sure nothing would happen to his princess. Even today, every time a baby dies in the unit, he still cries his heart out.

Violette, thanks to you, we're no longer the same doctors. We already cared about the well-being of the families and babies. You turned us into Titans and Amazons. Compromises are no longer possible. Zero tolerance for mediocrity or stupid policies that harm families. We place the babies and their fathers and mothers above everything else, well above our CVs, the reputation of our hospital, and our own reputations. And that will always be so.

We have become particularly intolerant of the way health professionals sometimes talk to parents of babies like you. Some of them feel that parents who embark on an adventure like the one we experienced with you are not acting in the best interests of their children. They feel that those parents don't understand the risks and the handicaps they're exposing their children to. As if they themselves understood! Our culture and our medical system undervalue babies like you. Others think that, in giving their little treasure a chance, parents are playing hero, that they're thoughtless, immature, selfish, masochistic, in complete denial; but those parents are only following their hearts. These health professionals see only handicaps and suffering; they don't understand the positive changes. They talk about statistics; they have only negative conversations about the future of premature babies. They'd like us to just give up and wait to be dealt a better hand. "Better luck next time."

I chose medicine, I decided to be a paediatrician, I worked hard to become a neonatologist. Parents, on the other hand, don't choose to be in the hospital beside their sick child. Our society has no tolerance for chance occurrences, but you taught me to live with uncertainty, to aim for goals other than related to performance. You taught me to distinguish between what is really important and what is not. Sometimes when a baby is sick and you have no control over events, all you can do is go with the current. But, Violette, when something is important, I swim against the current with all the energy my body can muster, for as long as I have to.

At the beginning, I would have wanted to exchange you for another baby, a baby who wasn't sick, who had stayed in my belly longer. I wanted you to be born healthy. I was afraid of handicaps. I would have preferred death to a serious disability. Then I wanted to change the Ungrateful Normals and the Others, who didn't understand what could happen to you and who complained about nothing. I wanted to change society's values. I was afraid you wouldn't be able to live in this fast-moving world where only efficiency and performance are valued. I wanted a better world. Then, at the end of your stay in the hospital, I bargained with nature to keep you alive: "Let her be blind if it must be; just let me take her home." I wanted more than anything to be your mother, for a long time, to take care of you, raise you, feed you, teach you things, tell you stories. I knew I would love you, whatever happened, wherever you led me, and I was ready to go to the ends of the earth for you. I knew I was capable of it, that we all were. And we did it.

After dreaming of changing you, changing society, changing everything and everyone, I finally realized that I was the one who had changed. And for the better. For everything I learned with you, thank you, my child.

This article was written by the POST group (Parents on the Other Side of Treatment). We are a group of providers and researchers who have all had a perinatal and/or neonatal experience. In this article, we have joined our voices together to speak about what we have learned from our NICU experience. We were made more vulnerable by it, but also much stronger. Resilience is rarely investigated in neonatology. This is our balanced view on the lessons parents learn and how they rewrite their story after the NICU.

Stronger and More Vulnerable: A Balanced View of the Impacts of the NICU Experience on Parents

Annie Janvier, MD, PhD, John Lantos, MD, Judy Aschner, MD, Keith Barrington, MB, ChB, Beau Batton, MD, Daniel Batton, MD, Siri Fuglem Berg, MD, PhD, Brian Carter, MD, Deborah Campbell, MD, FAAP, Felicia Cohn, PhD, Anne Drapkin Lyerly, MD, MA, Dan Ellsbury, MD, Avroy Fanaroff, MD, Jonathan Fanaroff, MD, JD, Kristy Fanaroff, MSN, NNP, Sophie Gravel, BNurs, Marlyse Haward, MD, Stefan Kutzsche, MD, PhD, Neil Marlow, DM, FMedSci; Martha Montello, PhD, Nathalie Maitre, MD, PhD, Joshua T. Morris, MDiv, BCC, Odd G. Paulsen, MD, Trisha Prentice, MBBS, Alan R. Spitzer, MD[†]

For parents, the experience of having an infant in the NICU is often psychologically traumatic. No parent can be fully prepared for the extreme stress and range of emotions of caring or a critically ill newborn. Many studies have documented the anxiety, depression, insomnia, grief, and posttraumatic stress symptoms that parents experience.[1] These studies are important because they help us to understand, to empathize, and maybe even to discover ways to improve families' experiences. However, such studies are also incomplete and tell only part of the story. Most are conducted in the first months or years after the NICU hospitalization, when the infants and their parents are still fragile. They generally do not report how parents' feelings, perceptions, and coping mechanisms change over the years.

A different set of studies, from other domains of medicine and pediatrics, has investigated the longer term effects of a critical illness.

These studies show that positive transformations often follow traumatic life-altering events. In the medical literature, these changes are
referred to as posttraumatic growth.[2] They have been reported most
frequently in adults: for example, cancer survivors, trauma victims,
HIV-infected individuals, and those with spinal cord injuries. Recent
investigations, however, have shown that posttraumatic growth also
occurs for children and families after the serious illness of a child.[3]
Many factors are associated with resilience, including socioeconomic
status, the nature and permanence of the health condition, patient/
parent psychological state, and family/social/societal support. Unfortunately, investigations relating to positive family transformations
after neonatal hospitalizations are scarce. They have been described
for parents of children with Down syndrome, trisomy 18, trisomy 13,
and cerebral palsy.[4] However, positive effects of the NICU experience
can be found in abundance outside of the medical literature, from
first-person reports in books, memoirs, and parental blogs.[5] Clinicians and researchers must be mindful that the negative impacts of
the NICU experience are only 1 side of the story.

As health care providers familiar with the NICU, we thought that
we understood the impact of the NICU on parents. But we were not
prepared to see the children in our own families as NICU patients.
We were not ready for the ways in which the medical jargon could
be alienating to us when used to describe "our" infants.[6] We were
not ready for the lack of control that accompanies a typical NICU
stay. Even if we are highly rational and organized individuals as providers, as parents we often gave consent for interventions with our
heart, not our heads.[7] We had trouble when health care professionals attempted to be honest with us and to help us develop realistic
expectations about the future. Neonatal intensive care providers
were often perceived as negative and pessimistic, especially at times
when we needed hope. We came to a new appreciation regarding
the delicate balance that health care providers must seek between
honesty and compassion, between realism and optimism.

The experience of having an infant in the NICU altered both
our professional and our personal lives in profound and permanent ways. We had to slowly reinvent ourselves to be a new parent with a fragile infant, instead of the healthy infant that we had
hoped for and dreamed about.

Here are some of the lessons our NICU experience has taught us. We offer them in the hope of helping health care professionals consider a balanced view of the NICU's impact on families. Despite sharing similar experiences in our professional lives, our perinatal and NICU experiences were different. We all rewrote our life stories to include parts we were not prepared for; some of us had to write a chapter about being the parent of a dead child, others about being the parents of children with lifelong disabilities. Our children have grown. Some are now 1 year old; others are >30 years old. We are not the same people nor the same providers we were before being parents in the NICU. For many, these are a series of small transformations. All of us had to rebuild ourselves after our challenging perinatal and NICU experiences that, to some degree, destroyed who we were. We share our perspective of a life transformation rather than a "posttraumatic growth." We did not grow. We are stronger and yet more vulnerable. Families' reports of positive transformations outside of the medical literature resonate with our experiences. All families have unique and different experiences, but many will learn similar lessons.

GRATITUDE

Gratitude for the gift of life, for simple and important things in life. Gratitude for our families and friends, for skilled professionals, for the kindnesses of strangers. We understand every day, with our heart, that we have much to be grateful for.

PERSPECTIVE

Learning to not sweat the small stuff and to recognize what is truly precious. We now pay less attention to things that are not worth fussing over and fight like hell for the things that are. We now see that perfection is in many places where we could not see it before. Perfection does not necessarily equate with percentages, excellence, performance, high grades, beauty, speed, or quantity.

LACK OF CONTROL

One of the most difficult things for a parent to recognize is that many things are beyond our control. We now focus on controlling the things that we can but recognize when there are things that we cannot. We no longer plan and predict what may happen with every possible decision. Often, life does not follow our predictions.

DECIDING WITH THE HEART

We have experienced the limitations of informed consent, statistics, probabilities, and predictions. We know that being informed repeatedly that something bad may happen to X% of infants does not help much; parents do not have 100 infants. We have gained a new appreciation of uncertainty, of the role of emotions in decision-making. We know that vulnerability and emotions are sources of strength. They allow us to connect with our passion and purpose, to become happier, more compassionate, and more hopeful as human beings and as providers.

CONNECTEDNESS

In whole new ways, we have come to understand the importance of family and relationships and the need to nurture precious connections. In the most difficult moments in life, some people held us while others disappeared. The NICU experience reminds us how important it is to be there for those who matter in our lives.

RESILIENCE

We learned that we are stronger than we think. We now know it is possible to see our hopes, dreams, and plans totally destroyed and then to rewrite our story with a new plotline. We can adapt.

We can experience a "freedom from fear" when dealing with life challenges or with the imperfections of the health care system. We rarely look backward and regret.

HUMILITY

We are more humble about the powers of science. As providers, we had thought about what we would do as parents if tragic things happened to our children. We were convinced we knew what we would do. However, faced with reality, we often did not act in ways we thought we would: more important thoughts came through our heads, more important values we did not predict. We now have a much greater respect for how to act in unexpected scenarios, in situations of uncertainty. We are more flexible.

FORGIVENESS

Having a sick infant is often associated with parental guilt or grief. The ability to "move on" not only takes time but requires forgiveness. Forgiveness for ourselves, for what we perhaps could have, should have, done or been. For those of us whose child dies, we must forgive ourselves when, in time, we realize that life goes on. Forgiveness for those who disappeared when we needed them, for real and perceived human failings of our families or friends or providers. We have learned that forgiveness is a journey and apply that understanding to other spheres of our lives.

DEDICATION

We are more dedicated to excellence in clinical care. We witnessed the pure beauty of bedside clinical excellence, which we sometimes found in unexpected places and with all types of health care providers. We learned the power of small gestures, the deep impact of an extra effort, a genuine smile, or a kind word.

We also met some less competent people. We are now intolerant of mediocrity and uncompromising with regard to patient care.

RECOMMENDATIONS TO CLINICIANS AND RESEARCHERS

1. Be aware that parents experience both negative and positive impacts after a NICU experience. Researchers examining these outcomes should investigate both sides of the story. Communications with parents should be balanced.
2. Remain humble. Avoid sentences such as "Parents don't understand" or "If I were in their situation, I would not …" Too often, it is providers who do not understand.
3. Tell parents that they did not choose the misfortunes that are happening to their infant, that there is nothing they could have done to prevent this. Remind them often that their infant is lucky to have parents who love him or her.
4. Let parents know that positive transformations are possible.
5. Temper discussions about risks with words about something good happening, such as resilience, love, and the chances of healing.
6. Help parents prioritize their energy and recognize what they can and cannot control. Encourage them to let go where they can.
7. Inform parents that life will not always be like this, that the roller coaster will become a train with a known destination. That one day, it will be better. That they are stronger than they think. That they have to believe it.
8. We can be there for parents at tough moments or avoid them. Be there.

These lessons do not in any way attempt to sugarcoat or diminish the difficult and bitter reality of having an infant in the NICU. However, parental NICU experiences may be improved by balancing the cold, hard facts, bleak outcomes, and psychological toll with the insights we offer. Most parents are resilient. They advocate for their child in ways they cannot or would not advocate for themselves. The realization of their own strength and resilience will lead to "life transformations" that allow the world to make sense again and their families to rebuild themselves and write a new story.

MORE ON THE POST GROUP AUTHORS (IN ALPHABETICAL ORDER) AND THEIR "NICU CHILDREN"

Judy Aschner (neonatologist) is the mother of Nadav, who was born at 31 weeks after rupture of membranes at 21 weeks' gestational age (GA).

Beau Batton (neonatologist) is the father, and Daniel Batton (neonatologist) is the grandfather, of Charlie, who was born with a univentricular heart.

Siri F. Berg (anesthesiologist) and Odd G. Paulsen (anesthesiologist and emergency physician) are the parents of Evy Kristine, who was born with trisomy 18 and died of cardiac failure.

Deborah Campbell (neonatologist) is the mother of Courtney Alexis, born at 27 weeks during a pregnancy complicated by pre-eclampsia and massive abruption. Courtney died at 28 days of age.

Brian Carter (neonatologist, palliative care physician, and clinical ethicist) is the father of Sean, who was born at 34 weeks' GA.

Felicia Cohn (clinical ethicist) is the mother of Amanda, who was born with transposition of the great vessels.

Dan Ellsbury (neonatologist) is the father of Codey, Kyle, and Hope. Codey and Kyle were born at 28 weeks' GA. Kyle died of complications of prematurity and Beckwith-Wiedemann syndrome. Hope was born with hypoplastic left heart syndrome.

Jonathan Fanaroff (neonatologist and bioethicist) and Kristy Fanaroff (neonatal nurse practitioner) are the parents of Mason, who was born at 32 weeks' GA. Avroy Fanaroff (neonatologist) is the grandfather of Mason and the father of Jonathan, who was critically ill at birth with meconium aspiration syndrome.

Sophie Gravel (chief NICU nurse) is the mother of Roxanne, who was born with in utero volvulus at 29 weeks.

Marlyse Haward (neonatologist and bioethicist) is the mother of Charlie, who was diagnosed in utero with congenital anomalies. He is now doing well.

Annie Janvier (neonatologist and clinical ethicist) and Keith Barrington (neonatologist) are the parents of Violette, who was born at 24 weeks' GA.

Stefan Kutzsche (neonatologist and anesthesiologist) is the grandfather of Jakob and Vegard, twins who were born at 25 weeks' GA.

John Lantos (pediatrician and clinical ethicist) and Martha Montello (clinical ethicist) are the grandparents of Sam and Will, who were born at 23 weeks' GA. Sam died of complications of prematurity.

Anne Drapkin Lyerly (obstetrician and bioethicist) is the mother of Will, who was born at term with an intra-abdominal mass.

Nathalie Maitre (neonatologist, follow-up physician, and researcher) is the mother of Leo, who was born at 27 weeks' GA, and Lucas, who was born at 36 weeks' GA.

Neil Marlow (neonatologist) is the father of Tom and Simon, who were born at 30 weeks' GA.

Joshua T. Morris (pediatric hospital chaplain) is the father of Isaac, who was born at 28 weeks' GA.

Trisha Prentice (neonatologist and doctoral candidate) is the mother of Jordain, who was born at 28 weeks' GA.

Alan R. Spitzer (neonatologist and researcher) is the grandfather of Jacob, Matthew, Alexandra, and Shaun, born at 29, 36, 35, and 35 weeks' GA, respectively.

Survival Guide for Parents

1. Do Not Try to Find a Guilty Party

It's not your fault, or the fault of your job, or the fault of your partner. Usually it's not the fault of the health care system. Mom, there is nothing you could have done to prevent what is happening to your baby. Stop replaying the movie of the past few weeks. This search for the guilty party drains you of the little energy you have available and that's needed in this intensely stressful situation. Nothing can change what has happened or what is happening now. By spending too much time brooding, we neglect what is really important to us and our families.

Sometimes men feel they have let their partner down and have failed to protect them. Some men feel guilty for initiating sexual relations. Others blame themselves for letting their wives work while pregnant, when they feel they should have insisted on a little more rest, as they think a man, a husband, should do. In a situation like this, both parents suffer and feel guilty. But talking about it can bring couples closer together. It can be a good start to say "I wish I had done something to prevent this. I feel like I didn't do what I should have done for you and our child." But, in reality, there's nothing you could have done. Doctors should inform the parents or the spouse of this fact in order to reassure them and free them from guilt. Regret and guilt are heavy burdens to bear. And they've never healed anyone.

Occasionally, a partner can become a toxic Other: he needs to find a guilty party. Since the situation is intolerable, there has to be a reason for it, a cause, and it's too hard for him to question his own behaviour. In addition, it's the mother who carries the child. And the role of the mother is to be a perfect-pregnant-woman-who-does-not-drink-tea-or-coffee-who-does-not-eat-salmon-or-tuna-sushi-contaminated-with-mercury-who-avoids-chocolate-who-does-not-do-too-much-exercise-who-does-not-go-in-the-bath-or-jacuzzi-with-the-water-too-hot-who-does-not-stay-standing-too-long-just-enough-to-not-put-on-too-much-weight-who-consumes-nothing-artificial-only-organic-but-who-can-still-have-sex-because-men-want-it. Sometimes, even when a woman is "normal" – that is, amazing, like 99 per cent of pregnant women – her spouse thinks it's because of her that their baby is sick. And that's an additional burden for the woman.

Partners, please don't do that. If you absolutely must find a guilty party, blame nature, blame medical research, which is unable to prevent premature births, birth defects, pre-eclampsia, and everything else, blame the Lord of term pregnancies, blame the spaghetti monster, blame angels and demons, blame whomever you like, but not the mother of your baby.

On rare occasions, there really is a culprit (inadequate medical care, a car accident, etc.). In these cases, you have to try to turn the page on this unfortunate cause. You can go back to it later when you have more energy. For example, if the medical care was inadequate (or you think it was), write down the facts and try to address the situation briefly (meeting with the doctor or sending a letter to the director of professional services at the hospital or the College of Physicians) in order to move on to the important things. It's counterproductive to try to accuse, attack, and/or sue while managing to be the parent of a sick baby in the NICU. Write it down, do the first steps, and you can sue later. But be with your baby now.

2. Find a Spokesperson

When your baby is in the NICU, you receive tons of calls, texts, emails, visits, and cards. You spend so much time informing others that it's exhausting. When Violette was one week old, a mom in the NICU recommended that I designate someone to keep friends and family informed. Excellent advice! My mother was chosen for the job. She was the town crier who made proclamations in the public square. You want news? Go to the town crier.

Find yourself a spokesperson, a trusted person who really wants to help and whom you like to talk to. A person who will act as town crier and spread the news. Some people find more than one: the grandma updates the family; two colleagues provide brief information to people at work.

Here's a list of tips I collected by speaking with parents in the NICU. These suggestions should be adapted according to your situation and preferences:

- Make a list of all the people who ask for news and give it to the spokesperson. Some parents give the spokesperson carte blanche, full discretion. Others write down or dictate the information to be passed along. I've even met parents who established a code: green means they can tell them everything; yellow, that they can say a lot, but should be careful about prying questions; and red means that they give only cursory information. The spokesperson can also notify certain people of the birth of the sick baby (the other children's school or soccer coach, work colleagues, etc.) without providing exhaustive detail.
- Make a list of people to thank if you receive presents or other signs of affection, and give instructions to the spokesperson (what to print on the thank-you card or birth announcement, who to send a note, a card, an email).
- Create a Facebook page and update it yourself or with the help of the spokesperson(s). Direct people there when they ask for news.
- Start a blog for yourself, to keep people informed, and for the baby later.
- Leave a welcome message in your voicemail box with the phone number of the spokesperson or the address of the Facebook page or blog.

3. Learn to Deal with the Others

When something difficult happens, you quickly realize who is there for you. Some people become closer, sometimes in surprising ways. Others who should have been part of your life disappear. Too busy? Too sensitive? Too far away? Too little experience with death or disease, especially the sickness of a child? Maybe you discouraged them? Maybe they thought or felt you didn't want to see them? Maybe they aren't wrong. These events reveal people's true nature.

Many people will try to provide encouragement, but they don't always know how. To remain sane, you have to develop strategies to quickly get out of painful conversations or situations. You've got enough stress as it is. Avoid all other irritants! Conserve your energy; spend a minimum amount of time with toxic people.

For example, the Others usually start a conversation with "How are you?" It's a convention. "How do you think I am, for fuck sakes, when my baby is in intensive care, hooked up to a respirator?!" When I was depressed, I found that question very tough. So I'd answer in a neutral way – "I'm managing," "I'm getting by," "As good as I can be under the circumstances," "Okay, I guess."

A better question is "Is today a good or a bad day?" A mom in the NICU once asked me, "What did you get today, a rose or a kick in the teeth?" I liked that.

Some parents find it helps to replace one-on-one meetings with group meetings. Two-person conversations can be draining. When there are several people, the conversations are often more varied. Other parents replace long telephone conversations or meetings in restaurants, cafés, or bars with a soccer game, a bike ride, a walk or a run, an outing to the swimming pool. Often, when you're doing something together, you can be with friends and family without needing to talk. It's sometimes better to avoid words – it's easier, it prevents awkward situations, and it hurts less. It also lets you get the bad stuff out and it increases your endorphins while burning fat!

Among the Others, there's a subcategory of super-toxic jerks, and they are often women. In these circumstances, the words of a toxic woman often cause more hurt than those of a toxic man. These women are instant self-proclaimed epidemiology experts on prematurity, congenital anomalies, and infections. They carry out an investigation. The guilty party must be found. Of course, all the causes they list never apply to themselves. If they don't work outside the home, they're convinced it's because you do. If they have jobs and you have a home day care, it's because you've lifted too many 18-month-old babies. If you like Pepsi and they like Coke, it's the Pepsi's fault. If they drink caffeine-free Pepsi and you drink the kind with caffeine, it's the fault of the caffeine. If you drink Diet Pepsi and they drink regular Pepsi, it's the fault of the aspartame. If you take the pill and they don't, it's the fault of the pill. If you travel and they don't, it's the airplane's fault.

It's hard being a woman these days because of all the choices we have to make. When women didn't have the right to vote, didn't have degrees, and stayed home to take care of the children and make dinner for their husbands, did they show more solidarity with each other? Today women have to make choices: if and when to have children, when to work outside the home, whether to stop working, when to use contraceptives, and how many children to have. Sometimes they decide to have children without a spouse. All these choices make life wonderful, but complicated.

All the women I know have moments of despair when one of their choices turns out badly or at normal low points in life. Women who decide to be stay-at-home moms have to deal with stomach upsets and crises, and sometimes miss the days when they "had a brain" and wore high heels. Women who go back to work may miss being at home and may think to themselves, "I can't believe I'm in a boring meeting instead of being with my kids. Why am I sweating blood to earn money while somebody else is raising my children in my place?" At these difficult times, most women feel powerless and guilty, and some fall apart. In my work as a neonatologist and ethics researcher, and also in my life as a mother, I often see women confront women who've made different choices than they have with regard to all kinds of things: infertility, fetal anomalies, prematurity, autism, behavioural problems, dyslexia, harassment, sexuality, and son on. I'm grateful as a woman to be born where I am and in this time in history, but it's still difficult, because all the choices we have to make can have impacts on our children and families. More choices also mean more potential regrets. But these choices do not cause your baby to be sick. So, mothers, don't listen to toxic people.

4. Get the Bad Stuff Out

It is essential to be able to switch your brain off at times, or else you rot, you smother, you explode. I provide long list of ways to "disconnect" in the chapter "Getting the Bad Stuff Out" below. Please, let me know about any other liberating activity you have so that it can be included in another edition or, who knows, a future blog entry (anniejanvier@hotmail.com).

5. Familiarize Yourself with the NICU

Every NICU is different. Most have their way of letting parents know their ABCs. The important things to clarify when the baby is admitted are the following:

- *What are the visiting hours for parents?* Generally speaking, parents can visit twenty-four hours a day, seven days a week. In some units, parents are not allowed to visit during specific short periods, such as shift changes, for example.
- *Who can come to the NICU with you, when, and how many people at a time?* Every unit has a different schedule for visitors. Some units have a different policy for children. Visits by children can also vary according to their age and the time of year (sometimes visits are limited for young children and during the winter months, because of the risk of infections).
- *Who are all these people?* There are so many people in the NICU, it's hard to know who's who. There's not just a single person caring for your baby, but a whole team. You are now part of this team. And it's important to know the other members, who are all there for your baby. The stars of the NICU, the cornerstone of care, are the staff nurses. They are close to your baby and take care of the baby every hour of the day and night. The neonatologist is the doctor responsible for your child's medical care. This doctor is a paediatrician (doctor for children) who is a specialist in the care of sick babies. The medical team may also include the following individuals: medical students, paediatric residents (doctors who are specializing to become paediatricians), residents in other specialties, and/or fellows (paediatricians who are specializing to become neonatologists). Nurse specialists are valuable assets in the NICU; they are specialized in acute care of newborns, continuity of care, and relations with families. Pharmacists manage prescriptions for medications and intravenous nutrition, and their participation greatly

reduces the risk of errors. Respiratory therapists optimize the baby's breathing and are the masters of the machines that help babies breathe. Lactation consultants support mothers in breastfeeding. Many other people are essential to the functioning of the teams: physiotherapists, occupational therapists, social workers, spiritual advisers, psychologists, clerks, support staff, laboratory technicians, radiology technicians, and so on. You have the right to know who is who, and what their role is on the team taking care of your baby. Don't hesitate to ask.

- *What are all those machines?* It can be a shock to see your baby all hooked up. The baby usually has a cardiorespiratory monitor (to monitor the baby's heartbeat and breathing: three electrodes stuck to the baby's torso and belly), a saturometer (to monitor the level of oxygen in the baby's blood and adjust it if necessary: a red light on the foot or hand), a temperature sensor (to regulate the temperature around the baby and keep it at the optimal level: the sensor is on the baby's skin). The baby may also need help breathing, by means of nasal cannulas (little tubes that carry oxygen) or a respirator. The respirator may only provide pressure (in this case, CPAP: continuous positive airway pressure) or it may assist breathing. If the baby is intubated, it means there's a breathing tube in the trachea, or windpipe. All these gizmos have alarms, and you shouldn't be surprised if they ring. They may even ring when things are going too well – for example, when your baby is getting too much oxygen (in this case, the oxygen is turned down).

- *What can you do to care for your baby?* Parents can do a lot: give the baby a bath, change diapers, bring milk, give the baby milk, hold the baby (skin to skin), and many, many other things. You can help your baby heal and you will help brain development. You can also ask when the medical rounds take place (when the medical team discusses your baby and makes decisions), so that you can attend. That's usually a good time to get information.

It's important to know that it's not essential to understand everything and know everything about the functioning of all the machines, what all the numbers from the blood tests mean, and what are all the possible consequences of prematurity. This information is helpful to some parents, but is not for others. It calms some parents to know what all the medical gibberish means, but it may cause others stress. Many parents have told me that extensive information from big books on premature babies, detailing all the potential problems faced by these babies, has been upsetting for them. It's important to go at your own pace and respect your limits. The staff nurses are a source of valuable information and can answer your questions about the machines in an individualized way. Even when you know everything about the world of the NICU and all the science, you still feel lost when your baby is hooked up to machines – and I say that as a neonatologist! Sometimes, medical and technical information doesn't help. Sometimes too much information is as bad as not enough. Sometimes we get hooked on numbers and lose perspective of what really counts or what is valuable to us. Sometimes you have to let go. The percentages don't mean much: your baby is ONE baby, not a hundred babies.

Parents who come through it best are those who quickly realize what they can control and what cannot be controlled. You can't control everything, but you can still control many things. It's important to remember that you can make a big difference for your baby.

6. Remember That It's Normal to Find Things Hard

Having a sick baby in the NICU is challenging. It's the supreme punch in the solar plexus. In our performance-oriented society, with its emphasis on efficiency and goals, you suddenly find yourself in a world of uncertainty where it's impossible to plan things in advance. A world where life usually triumphs, but death constantly lurks. This experience brings out the best and the worst in people. It can sometimes expose personality defects that are well hidden and controlled in everyday life. The skeletons in the closets knock on doors, poorly mended hearts bleed profusely, fragile seams split open and the stuffing bursts out. It's normal to feel incapable of dealing with it all. It's normal to be a shadow of your former self. It's normal for a loudmouth to be unable to utter a word. It's normal for a mild-mannered person to scream and freak out. When you feel that way, the best thing to do is to tell yourself that you're normal. It's not insanity: it's hard to be where you are, to endure what you're going through, and to do what you're doing.

BUT, it's *not* normal to think you would be better off dead, to think about ending your life or to want to kill someone. Post-partum depression and psychological problems are very real. If you are obsessed with such thoughts, talk about them with a health professional or someone you trust. Your baby needs you; you are important.

7. Do Not Lose Hope

It can be difficult to keep your hopes up, especially with all the ups and downs. Yes, you often feel like you're in a game of snakes and ladders. But you mustn't lose hope. That your baby will live, that she will be happy, that he will have a good quality of life. That you will finally be home together as a family. The story can also be sad, infinitely sad, so sad that you start thinking there's no more hope. But you have to hang onto hope, always. Sometimes hopes are adjusted. The hope of seeing your baby survive will be replaced by the hope that she will not suffer and that her short life will be as full as possible, the hope that you will heal from this sadness, the hope of continuing as a family, with your baby in your heart forever.

It won't always be like this. You have to really believe that: it won't always be like this. It is almost unthinkable that one day you will be able to breathe normally, but you have to believe that it will happen, and repeat that often. You are the parent of a sick baby, and you are there for that baby. You are stronger than you think – you have to believe that, too. Yes, even though you've been flattened like a pancake. You go on with your life, you go see your baby in the hospital, you cope with your new reality, and you keep it together. You're stronger than you think. Really.

8. Find an Alternative to "One Day at a Time!"

When Violette was sick, if I'd had a dollar for every time someone told me to take things "one day at a time," I could have retired. Yes, it's true that things can change quickly – that everything can collapse in an instant and that things can also get better in an instant. In order to put things in perspective, it can be useful for you to ask the following questions:

"How do you find my baby?"

"How does my baby's condition compare to that of other babies born at X weeks (or with whatever problem your baby has), on average?"

"Are there things that my baby does better than average for comparable babies? Things she does less well?"

"What is the next step for the baby? What do you anticipate for her, according to your experience with sick babies like her?"

"When do you think she will be able to breathe without the respirator? When does that happen with babies who have lungs like hers?"

"What sign would encourage you, or worry you in the next few days or weeks?"

It's best to be specific. Doctors are often afraid to give an opinion with regard to time. With a doctor who doesn't want to take a position, you can ask, "When you tell me you can't predict when you'll take the baby off the respirator, that doesn't help me. I don't know anything about that. Is it realistic to think she'll no longer be on the respirator in one week, two weeks? Could she still be on the respirator in six months? I know you don't have a crystal ball, but roughly, according to your experience and my daughter's condition, what do you think is the average time, approximately, that she'll need the respirator?"

Ask questions about the life trajectory of babies like yours – what the average is, what the doctors fear, what they hope for. It's easier that way. Don't ask for your baby's discharge date on the day of his admission. That kind of question is impossible to answer – we can only give ranges. But a good clinician should be able to inform you about the next step in your baby's life (and in yours): for example: taking out the central line, extubating the baby, trying to breastfeed, placing the baby in a bed, and so on.

9. Avoid Reading Parents' Magazines

Magazines for parents are everywhere. They drive me crazy. All NICU parents who come across specialized magazines on pregnancy or parenthood should be told "Don't read them! Don't even look at them!" They do talk about the real discomforts that make pregnancy difficult for many women: hemorrhoids, swollen breasts, aching joints, blemishes on the skin, stretch marks, reflux. But very often, they have nothing about premature babies, even though they represent approximately 8 per cent of births, or about neonatal intensive care, about birth defects, about the serious diseases some babies are exposed to (apart from runny noses), about fatal accidents, and so on. The worst thing is that these magazines are everywhere parents have to take their sick children: in hospitals and paediatric clinics. I understand that, for the majority of parents outside the NICU, this information would be useless and probably traumatic. At a minimum, for parents who are in such exceptional situations, the stuff about runny noses, diaper absorbency, colic, and hemorrhoids is annoying.

I met my friend Maria, who is Moroccan, in the NICU. I took care of her son Jeremy. We have remained friends. She's a marvellous woman. Jeremy was born with malformations, and he died from an acute infection after eight months in the NICU. He was an adorable baby, with big chocolate-brown eyes and incredibly long, curly eyelashes. Maria hated (and still hates) the magazine for new parents that's distributed free at the hospital entrance. When Violette was a few months old, Maria came back from Morocco. She called to say she would come by the house to see us. That was a delight, because Maria is great and lifts my spirits. She also brought me a small Moroccan ottoman to stuff. But before coming to my place, she had to swing by the hospital. "We'll have fun," she promised. I wondered what she needed to pick up there. In fact, she went to raid the free magazines on motherhood. She brought a big box full. "I took them all!" We had a great time tearing out the pages, crumpling them up, and stuffing them in the ottoman. It was the best time I'd had since Violette's birth.

10. Individualize the Care of Your Baby (and Your Family)

Parents have different realities and different schedules. Babies need different care depending on their condition. It's often very good for parents to establish a routine in the NICU early on. Who comes to visit, and when? How is the care provided, and when can you do something to help your baby (or yourself!)? When is the best time for kangaroo care? Your baby's nurse can tell you the times of the medical rounds, the baby's bath, diaper changing, eye examinations, vaccinations, transfusions, or feedings.

It's useful to organize your schedule with the nurse of your baby. It's not essential for you to be there all the time. You also need to rest and see your family (and sometimes, unfortunately, work). You can establish a routine and a schedule. That at least is something you can control: when you hold your baby, when you're present for rounds, when to read the baby a book or talk to him, and so on. When your baby starts to feed by mouth (bottle or breast), it's a good idea to make detailed plans and schedules with the doctor and the nurse so as to avoid contradictory messages.

All parents are different. Some want to be notified of any change in their baby's condition. Others want to be called only for emergencies. Some parents write up a little card indicating their preferences as soon as their baby is admitted. For example, one family recently wrote this on a little plasticized sheet of paper stuck to their child's incubator: "We are Daniel Renard* and Dominique Pelletier,* David's* parents. We are at David's bedside from 9 a.m. to 12 p.m. and from 6 p.m. to midnight. Grandma comes from 2 p.m. to 4 p.m. with Mom. David has twin brothers who are 18 months old, Romain and Rafael, so Mom is often with them during the day. We are nervous parents, and we panic when the phone rings! Please call us only if there's an emergency. Please tell us anything we can do for our little boy. Thank you for taking care of him." There were photos of the parents, the twins, and the tiny baby at the bottom of the page.

Another card I read recently went something like this:

"Welcome to the kingdom of my baby, Arthur. I've been at his side 16 hours a day since his birth more than two months ago. Arthur is learning to drink and it's not easy, but he's slowly improving. I've been sleeping at Cachou† since his birth and I want to be here to feed him. If Arthur looks awake and seems to want to suckle, please call me. NO, you won't be disturbing me. I'll come right over! Thank you for helping us!" This little card was written in pink, with lots of highlighting and stickers of silver cows.

---

† A "hotel" for parents of hospitalized children at Sainte-Justine Hospital.

Although there's a great deal of uncertainty, there are still a lot of things you can control in the NICU: your visiting hours, generally, what you say (or sing) to your baby, the information you receive, how many times you pump your milk during the day (or if you pump, too), your personal hygiene practices, and so on.

You can also do extra little things that can go a long way with respect to infections and comfort. The clinicians all have to wash their hands before touching your baby. Infections are one of the main causes of mortality in the NICU, and many infections come from caregivers' hands. Health professionals don't always get exceptional grades when it comes to hand-washing. It can be difficult to remind a doctor you'll be seeing for weeks to wash his hands. I have a hint for handling that: say "Dr X (a doctor in the NICU) told me I should remind caregivers to wash their hands before they touch Jacob." A good caregiver will reply, "Thanks for reminding me."

In most NICUs, we carry out a systematic evaluation of your baby's comfort or pain. It's usually the nurse who does this. For example, it is essential that interventions (such as intubations or lumbar punctures) be carried out with analgesia (pain medication). You can make sure your baby receives this medication. Also sucrose (sugar solution) greatly reduces the discomfort related to minor interventions such as drawing blood. Even in a unit where the protocol exists, it can happen that the sucrose is forgotten (I raged about it with Violette). You can do something about it. You can be there during blood drawing and emphasize the importance of sucrose to reduce pain. (You could say "Usually they give sucrose. Violette desaturates a lot less during blood drawing with it," and not "Is this a joke? Not again! Where's the fucking sucrose? Do I have to draw you a picture?") As a matter of fact, a picture can sometimes help! A dad once put up a big fluorescent yellow sticker of a smiley face with the words, "I love my sucrose and I want it!" on his baby's incubator. If you find that your baby doesn't look well, talk about it with your nurse. Don't be afraid. Yes, it's your role as a parent to ask these questions. The nurses are champions of the babies' comfort. And even in a world of ups and downs, you can step up as a parent if you want to.

Every baby is different. You'll get to know yours with time. Some babies digest their milk well but take respiratory pauses to drink. Others always need more oxygen after their feeding. Some like to lie on their belly,‡ others in anti-reflux position (head higher than the body). Some

‡ Only in the NICU. At home, it's back on the back.

babies like being patted on their back. Some take their milk without too many problems; others need the nipple to be withdrawn every twenty seconds because they're choking. In short, you are going to discover your baby: what makes her stable, what he finds unpleasant, what helps her. The older your baby, the more you've been there, the more you'll recognize his unique qualities and needs. Here, too, a card at the baby's bedside can contribute to personalizing her care.

Here are a few examples of cards I've seen recently in the NICU:

Hello, my name is Charlie. I was born at 26 weeks, two months ago. My breathing is good, except when I've just eaten. My mom calls me her vomit machine! Please: Don't examine my belly for an hour after my feedings. Thank you!

My daughter Mélissa LIKES:
Being held by us or caregivers during feedings.
Being patted on her back, even energetically, after her feedings; she often burps 2 or 3 times!
Silence, songs, and soft words.
An extra dose of morphine when she's uncomfortable; her signs of discomfort are usually faster breathing, accelerated pulse, clenched fists, and frowning.
She DOESN'T LIKE:
Being fed in her bed.
Too much noise, especially when she's sleeping; Mélissa has a lot of trouble falling asleep, especially since her last surgery.
Being on her back, although it's necessary; she should be well positioned on her back because she arches her spine and tenses. The best position to place her in is this one (photo).
SHE WILL LIKE: Going home with Mom, Dad, and her sister! Thank you for helping her reach that dream with us!

I can't repeat it enough: *each family and each baby is different.* It can sometimes be hard to avoid comparing yourself with other parents (who come more often, who nurse better, who seem to always be smiling) and making yourself miserable. It's also hard, sometimes, not to analyse the other babies. "Why has Rémi, who was born the same time as Violette, been off the respirator for three weeks, dammit?" "Chloé died yesterday, and I'm freaking out!" "This mom does skin-to-skin three times a day, I am useless." "That mother is so slender and healthy-looking, with her gallon of milk every day. What the heck is my problem?"

A word of advice: forget the others, look at your baby!

part six

NEONATOLOGY INFORMATION FOR
PARENTS, FAMILIES, CLINICIANS, AND
ALL THOSE WHO CARE ABOUT BABIES

Getting the Bad Stuff Out

Having a baby in the NICU means trying to build a routine under stress: going to see your baby, drawing milk, taking your other kids to day care, putting labels on the containers of milk, thinking about the baby. All this can drive you crazy. You have to be able to let off steam, get the pus and the shit out of your body. No one ever told me that when I was with Violette in the NICU. Not in so many words. But I think that's the kind of words you have to use (maybe a little more polite with some parents); and those are the words I would have needed. When the nurse tells you, "Take care of yourself," that's what it means. You really have to disconnect.

Yes, alcohol, drugs, an economy-size container of Coaticook caramel ice cream, and a general anaesthetic are quick ways to flip the switch off, but they're not very good for your health – especially in the long term! Sometimes you have to give yourself a swift kick in the ass to disconnect. It's hard, you often feel guilty, but it's important to release the pressure, or else you go around in circles, you spin your wheels, you get discouraged, and you explode. You have to be able to sometimes get your head out of the hole.

Here are some ways to get the bad stuff out. I put together this list over recent years by asking parents what they do to disconnect. Some of the activities are surprising, and I would have liked to think of them myself. Others are not for everyone. Please, parents, tell me of any that I've forgotten!

1. Exercise

Exercise is great. Not only does it keep you in shape, but it also increases your endorphins. Many studies on mood disorders have shown that regular exercise helps as much as antidepressants. That's why I'm putting it first. I know it's hard and sometimes unpleasant to get moving, but putting physical activity on your agenda is the best thing you can do for your physical and mental health.

Some parents, such as Pierre Lavoie (of the Pierre Lavoie Great Challenge),[1] even started doing physical activity when their baby was in the hospital, and were "liberated" through exercise. I admire that inspiring man, although he sometimes makes me feel like a clumsy oaf on my bicycle!

2. Sensory Activities

Listening and Watching

Listen to music. Some parents say they crank up the music and have a wild time dancing. Others sit quietly and reflect or weep while listening to their favourite classical piece: the point is to listen to something that strikes a chord in you, to switch off.

Play music. I started playing drums two years ago; it would have helped when Violette was sick.

Watch movies and TV series, whether serious, funny, or stupid. Our favourite series while Violette was sick were *Chef!* and *The Thin Blue Line*, with a glass of wine. We were able to laugh, even during the most difficult times. To my surprise, some parents watch horror movies or ones with a lot of violence: it helps them unwind and makes them feel that their life is still relatively calm. It takes all kinds to make a world.

Go to a show: anything, anywhere.

Read a book, a graphic novel, a detective story, anything the helps you unwind.

Write, in an organized way, or spontaneously, without thinking. A diary or a "Dear Computer." (More about writing below.)

Taste

Cook, alone or with others. Chocolate has a place of honour here. Or a nice piece of meat. One dad told me he started going to the butcher when his baby was sick, so he could cook the best steaks for his wife, who was anemic; it became a habit. For me, it was red gelatin candies of all shapes and sizes. For Jessica and Jean-François, it was a fancy chocolate out of a precious box every day.

Eat out. Even if it's in a windowless cafeteria at the hospital, you can sometimes find a little pleasure. A mother once confessed to me that her perfectly sunny-side-up egg prepared at the hospital cafeteria every morning, after pumping her milk, was the little pleasure of her day. She would close her eyes and try to forget everything else.

Drink. If it's alcohol, not too much. If it's coffee, not too much either – it causes anxiety. Except for premature babies, who get a daily dose of caffeine. And a lot of moms take out their juicers and concoct exotic drinks for themselves.

Touch

Massage (by others or by yourself), applying body lotion, massaging your children (including the baby in the NICU). Sexual relations, which are also in the realm of touch, are in a separate category below, the "sensory potpourri."

Smell

Smelling flowers, perfume, body lotion, and so on, makes you feel good. Your baby also has a pleasant smell. Violette smelled a little like yogurt with honey, although for the first weeks of her life, she often smelled like disinfecting alcohol or the benzoin used to secure her tube.

Sensory Potpourri

Sexual relations. Among other things, sex has the advantage of increasing your endorphins. You can have pleasure with your partner or by yourself. You may not be in the mood, but it's like getting back on a bicycle after a long time. It can also be a good way of communicating with your partner. When your baby is sick, you're tense, you often say the wrong thing. Sometimes, you don't know how to talk to each other anymore or what to say. Making love can open up the channels of communication (no pun intended).

Talk

Talk if you can. Talk with the people who are important in your life. Talk about everything and nothing. Even if the psychologist you know (or the pseudo-psychologist in your family) says it's essential to talk about your feeeeelings, to vent them, it's not necessarily true. If you need it and it helps you, go ahead, but you don't need to force it.

3. Creative Activities

Writing: a diary, a blog, an email, a book, letters, or a Facebook page. In my case, I wrote to my computer, in English. Writing greatly reduced the size of the lump I had in my throat. I wouldn't have been able to say it at the time, but I felt the need, and, while I was writing, I was no longer in the present, I was somewhere else, letting go. I was probably not even capable of thinking about writing a diary. Nor would I have been capable of letting go if I had written in French: writing those things in my mother tongue would have made me too sad and miserable. In English, I could clear my mind; in French, I would have gone around in circles. English allowed me to put some distance between myself and my words, and to free myself. You have to find what works for you.

Drawing, painting, making things with the kids. One mom made a mobile with all the caps (from bottles of sterile water, commercial formula, etc.) that would have been thrown away in the NICU. It was an exorcism for her and a great project for her 5-year-old son, who felt a connection with his brother in the NICU. Every day, they added pieces to their work.

Play

Games. Board games, video games. One very quiet, reserved dad recently confessed that he got out his negative energy by playing violent video games. He didn't play often, or for very long each time, but his wife was really critical of it. She was afraid he would become violent in the NICU. My message here is that it's important to realize we don't all unwind in the same way. When I spoke with those parents, the dad finally told his wife, "You don't understand. I don't attack anyone here because I get my craziness out with those stupid games! I'm going to throw them all out when our little guy comes home. You can even destroy them yourself if it'll make you feel good." Many parents have told me about "build and destroy" activities: make a Lego project, a house of cards, a tall tower of blocks, a jigsaw puzzle, and then destroy it. Someone should do a study on that, maybe there's a symbol hidden in it! Keith and I played Carcassonne and Rummikub like crazy. Playing Settlers of Catan with friends was also a release. Thank you to all those who were our game partners during that period (special wink to Annabelle and Jean). I think there were days when you probably even let me win, your trades were too generous – come on, one sheep for three rocks!

5. Relaxation Activities

Sleep. It's good to take a nap whenever you have a minute. When you're asleep, you really get away from it all.

Meditation. It's not for everyone. Personally, I find that it bugs me, but it helps lots of people, so don't follow my example.

Yoga of all kinds, from yoga-on-steroids, as my sister-in-law calls the kind I do, to calmer forms.

Tidying up. Yes, it's an activity described by quite a few moms, often before the baby's discharge: throw out all the stuff you don't need anymore. I would never have had the energy to do it. But for some people, making room in their homes makes room in their heads.

Gardening, playing outside. One mom "got over her bummer of the day" (those are her words) by going to pick apples with her older girl. They made 30 litres of applesauce; the whole day, between milk-pumping sessions, did her good.

6. Additional Tactics

There are all kinds of tactics that help you unwind in more regular or effective ways.

Signing up for an activity often helps you actually do it.

Doing an activity with another parent from the NICU (eating in the cafeteria, going for a walk or a run, etc.) is also often beneficial: that person is in the same boat as you.

If there are activities for parents in the unit, try them. They may not be your kind of thing, but you may be surprised. And if they are not, you tried and you don't need to go back.

Try a new activity (I started doing yoga while Violette was sick), one in which you can only improve.

Being with positive people in any group activity that helps you unwind is a big plus.

Seven Don'ts for Families and Friends Helping Parents

1. Don't Ignore the Parents' Feelings

Often there are Others who can't help saying that "everything will be fine," even at the worst times. The staff inform parents as tactfully as possible, but it isn't easy. Families organize things as best they can to be with their child in her final moments. And then an Other shows up. I once saw an extreme case: a baby was dying, and a real jerk, a close relative of the family, said, "He's great. He'll come out of this just fine!" I wanted to throw him out the window. A little later, I saw the death certificate on the counter. I would have liked that jerk to choke on that certificate.

This doesn't mean you should be systematically pessimistic. At times when the parents feel that things are going well, avoid discouraging them by saying that their baby is still at risk. Let them enjoy their day of happiness.

So what should you say? It's simple. Ask the parents "Is it is good of a bad day?" Listen to them. If it's a bad day, just say "I wish things were better for Violette"; "It's sad that it's not going better"; "I hope things will be better tomorrow." If it's a good day, "I'm glad it's a good day"; "I hope the good days will continue."

Sometimes you need to shake up parents who seem to be stuck in their pessimism or unrealistic optimism. But only sometimes.

2. Don't Mention Famous Personalities Who Were Born Prematurely

"How are you?"

"As well as possible, under the circumstances. Today, it's not going too badly, it seems." (Ambiguous answer to fend off the potential recommendation to remain cautious or positive.)

"Hey! Did you know that Isaac Newton was born prematurely? 1.3 kilograms! That's more than Violette, but at the time, science wasn't what it is today. When we heard that at the Planetarium, we said, 'Wow! We'll have to tell Annie!' That's good news for Violette."

"But there are also all the premature babies who died, who didn't live long enough to become famous."

"Don't be so negative. But wait! You yourself told us President Kennedy had a son born prematurely who died shortly after birth, which raised public awareness and made it possible to put more money into neonatology research and care! You can see very well that he had time to become famous! What was his name anyway?"

"Patrick Kennedy. But we're not the Kennedys. And we don't … Thank you for calling, it's very kind of you. I have to leave you now. I need to pump my milk."

"Don't hesitate … uh, I'm thinking of you. Call whenever you like."

It's a real obsession among the Others to talk about celebrities who were born prematurely. It bugs me so much that I finally went on the internet to check which stars were born prematurely, and I made a list. Another way to put the Others in their place is to quickly show them that you already know these things, so they can talk about something else.

- Albert Einstein: born three weeks prematurely. They also say, to reassure those who have or who know an autistic child, that he was an "intelligent autistic child," with an IQ of 160.

- Victor Hugo: we don't know exactly how premature he was, but they put him in an oven when he was born. That's what they did in 1802 to keep babies warm. His mother apparently said he was no longer than a knife when he was born and she ordered a coffin for him.
- Mark Twain was born two months early in 1835 (at 32 weeks).
- Stevie Wonder was born at 34 weeks, in 1950. He's blind because, at that time, they gave premature babies too much oxygen, and he had the most severe form of retinopathy of prematurity.

In my career, I've seen quite a few babies die. They did not become famous. And I have seen many survive and do very well, without becoming famous either. I didn't give a damn whether Violette became famous. I just wanted her to come home. I just wanted her to be my daughter, in my arms, far from the hospital.

3. Don't Name All the People You Know Who Were in the NICU and Are "Doing Well"

There's always an Other who knows a baby born very prematurely or who had a congenital anomaly, who spent months in the hospital, and who today is doing very well: his neighbour, the son of a cousin, the little newspaper boy. Wonderful! Good for the child, good for the parents. But we're not in competition to see who can name the most premature babies. We're not playing "Where's Waldo, the former 26-week premature baby with glasses"!

Approximately 8 per cent of children are born prematurely in Canada; in the United States, it's 12 per cent. So everyone necessarily knows at least one person who was premature. Many children also had congenital anomalies at birth. What of it? It's like when you travel abroad and someone proudly announces to you that he knows Bob in Canada. Sometimes, an Other will get mixed up and say that his boss was born at 19 or 20 weeks, and that he became an accountant. Yeah, right! And if he had been taken out when he was a giant clot stuck to an extra-absorbent tampon and implanted in an artificial uterus, he would have won a Nobel Prize.

4. Don't Make Analogies to War

People sometimes say that sick babies are "fighters." But the babies don't decide to fight – they didn't sign up for a boxing match or a karate course. They are simply unlucky and they needed medical intervention to survive. There are even some nurses who call premature babies fighters! Yet they should know, since they're the ones who prick them, take their vital signs, feed them, and change their diapers, that no fighter would let himself be messed around with like that! To me, Violette was not a fighter. If there's an analogy to war that could be applied to her, it would be that of a soldier who hesitates to get up again after being knocked down. Violette always got up again. Babies' bodies are often built strong.

The Others will never say a child is "fighting cystic fibrosis," "fighting muscular dystrophy," or "fighting Down syndrome." And yet we say "fighting cancer." That's stupid too; as if survival depended only on adopting a warrior attitude. Health professionals shouldn't use such simplistic expressions. They know very well that patients do the best they can to keep going during chemo.

Sick babies don't "fight" prematurity or heart defects. Quite the contrary! They endure more than they fight. In fact, we want them to get through the adversity of the NICU without having to suffer and fight. We fight pain. We want babies to be comfortable. There are parents who call their child their "little boxer," or their "acrobat," or their "fighter." That's their right. But when the Others use their own warrior metaphors, it's often annoying.

5. Don't Tell Stories about Your Own Pregnancies and Children unless the Parents Ask You

The Others often complain about the "problems" they had during their pregnancy or with their child. "I'm tired too; Billy wakes up constantly at night." "Nursing is killing me. My breasts hurt. Are your breasts smaller when you pump milk for a smaller baby?" "I can't take it anymore, I can't sleep, I'm too fat! I still have two weeks to endure. Couldn't the baby come out now? Violette should show him how to come out faster!" "Édith has caught the worst cold – she's really not doing well. She spent the whole night in bed with us, sniffling and coughing on us. I can't concentrate on my work; I'm exhausted." It is not useful for you to talk about your previous miscarriages. If your child died very young, you do not need to bring it up: parents are focused on their baby.

I hated the mothers with big flabby bellies who'd just given birth to a huge monster and were complaining about lack of sleep or their kid's snotty nose. Meanwhile, the nurses had to wake up my Violette to aspirate her secretions or draw blood. I hated the mothers who complained about their engorged breasts. I had two babies: my Violette and a super pump. Both of them needed electricity in order to work. I had no patience for the little problems of mothers outside the NICU. No, I was not amused.

6. Don't Give Unsolicited Advice

The Others always have advice to give: what to do to relax, what to eat to be healthy, how to produce more milk. How to produce more milk – wow, I could write a book with all that advice: eat cabbage leaves, massage yourself with almond oil, don't use an electric pump, sleep on your belly, and so on. Expressing your milk is already hard enough as it is – mothers don't need more information and instructions. They especially don't need to be criticized! The advice we get from lay people or pseudo-experts is often ridiculous. It's incredible the kind of things mothers hear. Some of them aren't familiar with any empirical data, and so they listen to those stupidities. They sometimes believe them and try to put them into practice. We should tell mothers in the NICU with their sick babies that they know much more than the Others about their milk, maintaining their pumps, and their little babies' bowels.

Sometimes we get unsolicited advice on how to get through the difficult times or how to "take it easy." It's good to try to help parents, but you mustn't insist. Yes, propose things for parents and try to get them moving, but don't badger them. Meditation is always in the top three recommendations to vulnerable people. And if you're reluctant, the Other has to add, "You absolutely have to meditate." ENOUGH ALREADY! No, it's not a question of training; I don't need to learn to like it. I've already tried many times, I've even taken part in retreats and meditation weekends;

I know the tricks, yes, even the stuff about mindfulness. Don't push it. That causes me stress. I don't like it, so stop bugging me about it. Yes, I know, it works for a lot of people, but not for me. Without actually making me aggressive, every time someone tells me to meditate to relieve stress, it causes me even more stress. The problem isn't meditation. The problem is people who insist on and prescribe recipes. Making suggestions is nice. When you insist, it ends up being oppressive.

It's also practically impossible to go through a crisis in life without somebody talking about yoga. Leave me alone. I can immediately reply that I've been doing it since Violette was born. And not just any yoga – Ashtanga, a form of yoga in which you don't do too much navel gazing, and they don't bother you too much about meditation. I started when Violette was one week old, and it's true that it did me good. No doubt because I was very bad at it, and I needed all my concentration to breathe properly and not break my neck. Today still, it empties my head and body. For ninety minutes, I manage to turn the "existential crisis" switch off. Unbelievable. After a while, I feel like I have my head in the clouds, but my feet solidly on the ground. I become rooted and regain my strength. And then everything makes sense again. Then there's a lack of sense. While Violette was sick, the Others were so delighted: "Bravo! That will help you; you see, you can do something."

In fact, I started yoga, not on the unsolicited advice of the Others, but thanks to a formidable mom I met in the NICU, long before Violette arrived. A woman with an amazing presence, energy, and radiance, who stood up remarkably well to all the shit in the unit. I even thought at the time that if one day I had a child in the NICU, I would like to be like her. I told her I wanted to move and do some cardio, but that yoga, until then, had not given me much satisfaction. She, Jessie, was the one who told me about Ashtanga yoga, an intense activity that makes you sweat a lot. I wrote "Ashtanga Yoga Montreal – Jessie & Eugene" on a Post-it note that I stuck on the wall of my office. When Violette was three days old, I went to my office at one point and cried my eyes out. It was then that I happened to glance at the Post-it note. I thought back to Jessie and Eugene. I wondered if Jessie had ever felt as powerless as I did, and I wanted to talk to her. Maybe if I gave my heart a workout it would keep it from exploding? Maybe if I went to see Jessie and Eugene at their studio, I would burst into sobs, but at the very least, I would do some exercise?

Once again, it was the NICU parents who helped me, the neonatologist, to defeat my demons. Yoga really did me good – Ashtanga yoga, the kind taught at the studio I go to. But that's me.

Not all parents are alike. I met many NICU parents before becoming one. What I conclude from all these encounters is that it's important to de-stress, or to "get the bad stuff out," as a father said to me one day. All kinds of activities can help you de-stress and it's okay to suggest some. What's hard for parents is when people insist on one thing and won't let it drop.

7. Don't Play the Epidemiologist

There were a lot of non-health care provider know-it-alls around me, supposed experts on prematurity, intensive care, and childhood diseases. They would analyse my case and come up with all kinds of hypotheses to explain my premature delivery and the reasons Violette was in such a fix. I had enough problems of my own to deal with! Leave me alone!

Parents spend enough time trying to understand what is happening to them – they don't need others for that. I knew rationally that there was nothing that could have been done to prevent all this, but, in spite of myself, I was looking for the cause. An incompetent cervix, that was one, but why did I have to have an incompetent cervix? What could I have done to delay the birth? I had to repeat to myself again and again, "THERE WAS NOTHING YOU COULD HAVE DONE." I had to convince myself of that to keep from going crazy. But sometimes it takes more than that to convince the Others. They too have to find the reason for it.

"I've just heard the news, I'm really sorry. She came so early; it must be terrible!" (At least that's a good start to a conversation,)

"Yes, 24 weeks. She's small, but she's hanging in there. We're hopeful."

"Why did you give birth prematurely?"

"Because my cervix, the lower part of the uterus, opened up too early. It can happen to anyone. I was unlucky."

"But if it opened up too early, maybe it's because you stayed standing too long? Your job is hard, you know."

"I stayed standing a maximum of forty minutes a day. Thank you for calling; it's very kind of you. I've got to go. I need to pump my milk."

"Don't hesitate … uh, I'm thinking of you. Call whenever you want."

These conversations were usually followed by fits of tears and by a resurgence of the feeling that I could have done better as a mom. The pseudo-experts in epidemiology come up with all kinds of explanations for prematurity. As a neonatologist, I've heard them all, from parents, spouses, and friends. You mustn't waste your time with those stupid questions. You have to stay focused on what needs to be done at the moment. And above all, support the parents.

The Best Ways to Help Parents in the NICU

Show up. Don't run away. Don't be afraid; don't hide.

Just be there; that's usually enough.

Listen to the parents, and accept them as they are. You can happen on a bad day or a better day. If the parents are quiet, tolerate their silence. If they're crying, give them a hug.

Don't look for what could have caused their baby's condition (malformation, premature birth, infection). Never suggest that they could have done things differently. If the parents feel guilty about something, you can talk about it with the nurse or doctor. They'll provide advice on how to handle the subject. They can help.

Tell parents that their baby is lucky to have them. Give them positive reinforcement by emphasizing everything they're doing right: visits to the NICU, the pump, the arrangements they make at work in order to be with their child, the calm they manage to maintain under the circumstances, and all they're doing to make their other children feel cared for, and so on.

Get ready for a shock when you visit the baby. Seeing a sick baby can be upsetting. Don't hesitate to tell the parents that their baby is wonderful, if that's what you think.

Be helpful: bake them a pie, mow their lawn, babysit their children and help them with their homework, pay for their parking at the hospital, pay their bills, bring them a snack in the NICU. Surprise them with a gift: a book, skin cream, a poem, flowers, a nice frame for a photo of the baby, a pack of Bubblicious, a book to write and vent in, anything that will give them pleasure. And know that helping doesn't always mean visiting. You need to understand that no means no. There are parents who prefer to be alone.

If you can, offer to be their spokesperson. If you can't, help them find the right person to handle news, calls, email, and Facebook.

Offer to take photos of the parents, with or without the baby. Parents sometimes forget to take photos because they have other things on their minds, because they don't realize they're living through a time they'll want to remember. But one day, the baby may want to know the story of her birth. The photos will then be useful in recounting the first chapter of her life.

Parents don't have an easy time! The NICU can bring out the best and the worse in people. If a parent gives you a hard time, don't take it personally (not always, in any case!).

This article was written by the POST group. We realized that when parents feel less cared for in the NICU, it is often not because the clinicians made mistakes or lacked medical or nursing knowledge; rather, it was often because of a lack of "basic etiquette" in care. The aim of this article is to describe an easy framework for clinicians to work with in order for families to feel well cared for.

Ethics and Etiquette in Neonatal Intensive Care[†]

Annie Janvier, MD, PhD; John Lantos, MD; for the POST Investigators[‡]

Many of the ethical controversies in neonatology reflect problems in communication between health care professionals and parents. Policy statements and pedagogy alike urge health care professionals to be empathetic, compassionate, honest, and caring. However, these theoretical concepts are generally endorsed without practical suggestions for how to achieve these goals. Empathy, compassion, and caring are hard to fake.

All of the authors of this article are health care professionals who regularly communicate with parents of sick children and who have had a sick child or grandchild of their own in the neonatal intensive care unit (NICU).[1] Some have experienced the death of their child. Our collective experience gives us insight into what it is like to be on the other side of these interactions.

Having a critically ill child is always a challenging experience. Being a parent in the NICU presents unique challenges. Parents are grieving the loss of their hope for a healthy pregnancy, delivery, and term newborn. The sickness of their child is preceded immediately by pregnancy and the major impact that a high-risk delivery entails. Parents are often still trying to understand what it feels like to be a parent and to process the responsibility of that role as they establish an intimate relationship with this new life. Furthermore, most of the babies in the NICU depend on life-sustaining interventions, making bonding more complex. This bonding may be complicated by the fact that many parents do not know how much time they will have with their child, whether minutes, days, weeks, or years. When a newborn survives, the acute crisis of the first days is followed by many "ups and downs" and a seeming normalcy of the crisis/comfort situation. This is often referred to as a "roller coaster" by many parents. When parents have a baby in the NICU, life as they knew it comes to an end. Health care professionals sometimes may not comprehend how disorienting this experience can be.

When families voice their dissatisfaction with the NICU, it is often not because they think their baby has not received good medical care. Instead, it is because the parents' needs have not been acknowledged and addressed. For instance, we sometimes observe health care professionals speaking to each other about a sick baby without acknowledging the parents at the bedside, as if they were invisible. We often see confused parents who think the resident is a nurse or the attending physician a psychologist. We meet parents who feel that their baby is a "number in the system" or that health care professionals do not see their child as fully human. When we witness these encounters, each of us flashes back to the time when we were parents of a child in the NICU, similarly lost, despite all our medical knowledge. These negative encounters for parents are not about the caregivers' technical expertise or knowledge. They reflect a failure in a different domain.

We often hear that some medical professionals are "good with people." This seems like a gift, something that some people just have and others do not. We disagree. We believe that anyone can learn simple techniques to express their compassion in ways that help parents navigate the difficult experience of having a baby in the NICU. Often we have our trainees read stories written by parents, interact with simulated parents, and speak with parents who have been through a NICU experience. These are useful exercises. But what we most need is a rapid way to teach health care professionals how to interact with families in a uniformly empathetic, helpful way.

In an article on etiquette-based medicine, Kahn[2] suggested that physicians can learn simple behaviors that convey empathy and respect. Even when they are unable to fully understand patients'

suffering, he writes, they "can nevertheless behave in certain specified ways that will result in [their] feeling well treated." He provides a checklist of behaviors that are easily taught and practiced
and efficiently evaluated. The checklist is a guideline for good
manners. Kahn stresses that the checklist "does not address the
way the doctor feels, only how he or she behaves; it provides guid-
ance for [those] … whose bedside skills need the most improvement." From Kahn's valuable guidelines, we have developed a
more robust etiquette-based approach to communication with
families in the NICU. We hope these specific and practical recommendations will help physicians help parents as they go through
a challenging NICU stay. They may even prevent some ethical
dilemmas from arising.

Here are 10 essentials of etiquette-based neonatal care from the
parents' perspective:

1. Say my baby's name, regardless of how odd or misspelled it
   may be to you. Know my baby's sex.
2. Don't label my baby. My baby is not a diagnosis. She is
   not the "T-18," the "23-weeker," the "tiny critter," or the
   "horribleBPDerinroom8."
3. Say your name. Tell us who you are, what your profession
   is, and why you are here. Don't assume we know and don't
   assume we remember.
4. Listen to me. When you enter my baby's bedside, acknowledge my presence. Sit down if you can. Ask me how I think
   my baby is doing. Embrace silence. Expect us to be upset.
   Don't take it personally.
5. Speak my language. Every parent is different. Some of us
   want numbers, predictions, and statistics. Others don't. We
   generally want to know whether our baby's course is comparable with other babies with similar conditions or gestational
   age. Adapt your language to fit our needs.
6. Speak with one voice. We are overwhelmed with health care
   team members – nurses, students, residents, advanced practice nurses, respiratory therapists, and more. Limit the number of providers attending deliveries, difficult conversations,

and code situations. Limit the number of people who examine my baby. Communicate with us in a consistent way.

7. Know my baby. We expect you to know everything about our baby. Take ownership and be responsible. Give us the results that are important to us the same day. Know the facts. Never tell us "I'm just covering for today."

8. Acknowledge my role. I contribute to my baby's care too. I spend hours at the bedside; I pump my breastmilk. I may be juggling a job or other children, operating on little sleep, and exercising continuous worry. Please understand and acknowledge this. Your acknowledgment of me in the role of a caring parent strengthens my resolve to be that good parent.

9. Don't label me. Remember you are meeting me under the worst of circumstances. What is routine to you may be the greatest stress I've encountered in my life. Avoid the expression "difficult parents." Instead, talk about "parents in a difficult situation." If you feel the need to complain about my family, do so in private.

10. Know how important you are to me. I am placing my child's life in your hands. Do not underestimate how important you are to our family.

Conclusions

Although these guidelines may seem like common sense, simple rules of etiquette are not always applied in a busy NICU or in the hospital at large. A physician who can remember a patient's hemoglobin level can remember a patient's name. These guidelines do not require the system to change; they require us to change.

Notes

Foreword

1 Aleksandar Hemon, "The Aquarium," *New Yorker*, 6 June 2001, https://www
.newyorker.com/magazine/2011/06/13/the-aquarium
2 A.H. Hawkins, "Pathography: Patient Narratives of Illness," *Western Journal of Medicine* 171, no. 2 (1999): 127–9.

End-of-Life Decisions for Extremely Low-Gestational-Age Infants

† *Seminars in Perinatology* 38, no. 1 (February 2014): 31–7. DOI: http://dx.doi
.org/10.1053/j.semperi.2013.07.006. © 2014 Elsevier Inc. All rights reserved.
1 T. Moore, E.M. Hennessy, J. Myles, et al., "Neurological and Developmental
Outcome in Extremely Preterm Children Born in England in 1995 and 2006: The
EPICure Studies," *British Medical Journal* 345 (2012): e7961.
2 A.L. Jefferies and H.M. Kirpalani, "Canadian Paediatric Society FaNC: Counselling
and Management for Anticipated Extremely Pre-term Birth," *Paediatrics and Child
Health* 17, no. 8 (2012): 443; J.A. Gerrits-Kuiper, R. de Heus, H.A. Bouwers, G.H.
Visser, A.L. den Ouden, and L.A. Kollee, "At the Limits of Viability: Dutch Referral
Policy for Premature Birth Too Reserved," *Nederlands Tijdschrift Geneeskunde* 152,
no. 7 (2008): 383–8; Nuffield Council on Bioethics, *Neonatal Medicine: Critical
Care Decisions in Fetal and Neonatal Medicine: Ethical Issues* (2007).
3 Jefferies and Kirpalani, "Canadian Paediatric Society FaNC"; J.W. Kaempf, M.
Tomlinson, C. Arduza, et al., "Medical Staff Guidelines for Periviability Pregnancy
Counseling and Medical Treatment of Extremely Premature Infants," *Pediatrics*
117, no. 1 (2006): 22–9; F.A. Chervenak, L.B. McCullough, and M.I. Levene,

"An Ethically Justified, Clinically Comprehensive Approach to Periviability: Gynaecological, Obstetric, Perinatal and Neonatal Dimensions," *Journal of Obstetrics and Gynaecology* 27, no. 1 (2007): 3–7.

4 Gerrits-Kuiper et al., "At the Limits of Viability."

5 P. Sladkevicius, S. Saltvedt, H. Almstrom, M. Kublickas, C. Grunewald, and L. Valentin, "Ultrasound Dating at 12–14 Weeks of Gestation: A Prospective Cross-Validation of Established Dating Formulae in In-vitro Fertilized Pregnancies," *Ultrasound in Obstetrics and Gynaecology* 26, no. 5 (2005): 504–11; U.B. Wennerholm, C. Bergh, H. Hagberg, B. Sultan, and M. Wennergren, "Gestational Age in Pregnancies after in Vitro Fertilization: Comparison between Ultrasound Measurement and Actual Age," *Ultrasound in Obstetrics and Gynaecology* 12, no. 3 (1998): 170–4; W. Lee, M. Balasubramaniam, R.L. Deter, et al., "New Fetal Weight Estimation Models Using Fractional Limb Volume," *Ultrasound in Obstetrics and Gynaecology* 34, no. 5 (2009): 556–65.

6 J.E. Tyson, N.A. Parikh, J. Langer, C. Green, and R.D. Higgins, "Intensive Care for Extreme Prematurity: Moving Beyond Gestational Age," *New England Journal of Medicine* 358, no. 16 (2008): 1672–81.

7 Moore et al., "Neurological and Developmental Outcome."

8 Ibid.; B. Andrews, J. Lagatta, A. Chu, S. Plesha-Troyke, M. Schreiber, J. Lantos, et al., "The Nonimpact of Gestational Age on Neuro-Developmental Outcome for Ventilated Survivors Born at 23–28 Weeks of Gestation," *Acta Paediatrica* 101, no. 6 (2012): 574–8; L. Schlapbach, M. Adams, E. Proietti, et al., "Outcome at Two Years of Age in a Swiss National Cohort of Extremely Preterm Infants Born between 2000 and 2008," *BMC Pediatrics* 12, no. 1 (2012): 198.

9 N. Marlow, E.M. Hennessy, M.A. Bracewell, D. Wolke, and Group ftES, "Motor and Executive Function at 6 Years of Age after Extremely Preterm Birth," *Pediatrics* 120, no. 4 (2007): 793–804.

10 M. Hack, H.G. Taylor, D. Drotar, et al., "Poor Predictive Validity of the Bayley Scales of Infant Development for Cognitive Function of Extremely Low Birth Weight Children at School Age," *Pediatrics* 116, no. 2 (2005): 333–41; B. Schmidt, P.J. Anderson, L.W. Doyle, et al., "Survival without Disability to Age 5 Years after Neonatal Caffeine Therapy for Apnea of Prematurity," *Journal of the American Medical Association* 307, no. 3 (2012): 275–82, http://refhub.elsevier.com/S0146 -0005(16)30081-7/sbref21

11 B. Latal, "Prediction of Neurodevelopmental Outcome after Preterm Birth," *Pediatric Neurology* 40, no. 6 (2009): 413–19.

12 L.J. Schneiderman, "Defining Medical Futility and Improving Medical Care," *Journal of Bioethical Inquiry* 8, no. 2 (2011): 123–31.

13 L.J. Schneiderman, N.S. Jecker, and A.R. Jonsen, "Medical Futility: Its Meaning and Ethical Implications," *Annals of Internal Medicine* 112, no. 12 (1990): 949–54.

14 Express Group, "Incidence of and Risk Factors for Neonatal Morbidity after Active Perinatal Care: Extremely Preterm Infants Study in Sweden (EXPRESS)," *Acta Paediatrica* 99, no. 7 (2010): 978–92.

15 Schneiderman, "Defining Medical Futility."

16 A. Janvier, K.J. Barrington, K. Aziz, and J. Lantos, "Ethics Ain't Easy: Do We Need Simple Rules for Complicated Ethical Decisions?" *Acta Paediatrica* 97, no. 4 (2008): 402–6.

17 "Part 2: Ethical Aspects of CPR and ECC," *Resuscitation* 46, nos. 1–3 (2000): 17–27.

18 J.F. Lucey, C.A. Rowan, P. Shiono, et al., "Fetal Infants: The Fate of 4172 Infants with Birth Weights of 401 to 500 Grams: The Vermont Oxford Network Experience (1996–2000)," *Pediatrics* 113, no. 6 (2004): 1559–66.

19 K.J. Barrington, and S. Saigal, "Long-Term Caring for Neonates," *Paediatrics and Child Health* 11, no. 5 (2006): 265–6.

20 A. Janvier and J.D. Lantos, *Variations of Practice in the Care of Extremely Preterm Infants* (Cambridge: Cambridge University Press, 2011).

21 Gerrits-Kuiper et al., "At the Limits of Viability"; Nuffield Council on Bioethics, *Neonatal Medicine*; Janvier and Lantos, *Variations of Practice*; M.S. Pignotti, and G. Donzelli, "Perinatal Care at the Threshold of Viability: An International Comparison of Practical Guidelines for the Treatment of Extremely Preterm Births," *Pediatrics* 121, no. 1 (2008): e193–8; D.G. Batton and Committee on the Fetus and Newborn, "Antenatal Counseling Regarding Resuscitation at an Extremely Low Gestational Age," *Pediatrics* 124, no. 1 (2009): 422–7; Ethics DCO, *Extreme Prematurity: Ethical Aspects* (Copenhagen: Danish Council of Ethics, 1995); Y. Kono, J. Mishina, T. Takamura, et al., "Impact of Being Small-for-Gestational Age on Survival and Long-Term Outcome of Extremely Premature Infants Born at 23–27 Weeks' Gestation," *Journal of Perinatal Medicine* 35, no. 5 (2007): 447–54; B. Salle and C. Sureau, "Le préma de moins de 28 SA, sa réanimation et son avenir," *Bulletin de l'Académie nationale de médecine* 190 (2006): 1261–74.

22 J.M. Lorenz, N. Paneth, J.R. Jetton, L. den Ouden, and J.E. Tyson, "Comparison of Management Strategies for Extreme Prematurity in New Jersey and the Netherlands: Outcomes and Resource Expenditure," *Pediatrics* 108, no. 6 (2001): 1269–74.

23 Janvier and Lantos, *Variations of Practice*.

24 Kaempf et al., "Medical Staff Guidelines"; J.D. Lantos and W. Meadow, "Variation in the Treatment of Infants Born at the Borderline of Viability," *Pediatrics* 123, no. 6 (2009): 1588–90.

25 Jefferies and Kirpalani, "Canadian Paediatric Society FaNC."

26 A. Janvier, K. Barrington, and B. Farlow, "Communication with Parents Concerning Withholding or Withdrawing of Life Sustaining Interventions in Neonatology," *Seminars in Perinatology* 38, no. 1 (2014): 39–47.

27 Schlapbach et al., "Outcome at Two Years of Age."

28 A. Janvier and S.R. Leuthner, "Chronic Patients, Burdensome Interventions and the Vietnam Analogy," *Acta Paediatrica* 102, no. 7 (2013): 669–70.

29 Jefferies and Kirpalani, "Canadian Paediatric Society FaNC"; J.E. Tyson, N.A. Parikh, J. Langer, C. Green, and R.D. Higgins, "The National Institute of Child Health and Human Development Neonatal Research Network: Intensive Care for

Extreme Prematurity – Moving Beyond Gestational Age," *New England Journal of Medicine* 358, no. 16 (2008): 1672–81.

30 Janvier and Leuthner, "Chronic Patients, Burdensome Interventions."

31 S. Saigal, B.L. Stoskopf, D. Feeny, et al., "Differences in Preferences for Neonatal Outcomes among Health Care Professionals, Parents, and Adolescents," *Journal of the American Medical Association* no. 21 (1999): 1991–7; H.S. Lam, S.P.S. Wong, F.Y.B. Liu, H.L. Wong, T.F. Fok, and P.C. Ng, "Attitudes toward Neonatal Intensive Care Treatment of Pre-term Infants with a High Risk of Developing Long-Term Disabilities," *Pediatrics* 123, no. 6 (2009): 1501–8.

32 S. Saigal, P.L. Rosenbaum, D. Feeny, et al., "Parental Perspectives of the Health Status and Health-Related Quality of Life of Teen-Aged Children Who Were Extremely Low Birth Weight and Term Controls," *Pediatrics* 105, no. 3 (2000): 569–74.

33 H. Harrison, "Making Lemonade: A Parent's View of 'Quality of Life' Studies," *Journal Clinical Ethics* 12, no. 3 (2001): 239–50.

34 J.E. Pless, "The Story of Baby Doe," *New England Journal of Medicine* 309, no. 11 (1983): 664.

35 K.B. Sheets, R.G. Best, C.K. Brasington, and M.C. Will, "Balanced Information about Down Syndrome: What Is Essential?" *American Journal of Medical Genetics* 155A, no. 6 (2011): 1246–57; B.G. Skotko, "Prenatally Diagnosed Down Syndrome: Mothers Who Continued Their Pregnancies Evaluate Their Health Care Providers," *American Journal of Obstetrics and Gynaecology* 192, no. 3 (2005): 670–7.

36 S. Turner and A. Alborz, "Academic Attainments of Children with Down's Syndrome: A Longitudinal Study," *British Journal of Educational Psychology* 73, Pt. 4 (2003): 563–83.

37 N. Marlow, D. Wolke, M.A. Bracewell, M. Samara, and the EPICure Study Group, "Neurologic and Developmental Disability at Six Years of Age after Extremely Preterm Birth," *New England Journal of Medicine* 352, no. 1 (2005): 9–19.

38 S. Saigal, B. Stoskopf, D. Streiner, et al., "Transition of Extremely Low-Birth-Weight Infants from Adolescence to Young Adulthood: Comparison with Normal Birth-Weight Controls," *Journal of the American Medical Association* 295, no. 6 (2006): 667–5; A. Janvier, B. Farlow, and B.S. Wilfond, "The Experience of Families with Children with Trisomy 13 and 18 in Social Networks," *Pediatrics* 130, no. 2 (2012): 293–8.

39 S. Saigal, "Quality of Life of Former Premature Infants during Adolescence and Beyond," *Early Human Development* 89, no. 4 (2013): 209–13.

40 D. Van Dyke, "Clinical Management Considerations in Long-Term Survivors with Trisomy 18," *Pediatrics* 85 (1990): 753–9.

41 L. Singer, M. Davillier, P. Bruening, S. Hawkins, and T. Yamashita, "Social Support, Psychological Distress, and Parenting Strains in Mothers of Very Low Birthweight Infants," *Family Relations* 45 (1996): 343–50.

42 Skotko, "Prenatally Diagnosed Down Syndrome"; B.G. Skotko, S.P. Levine, and R. Goldstein, "Having a Brother or Sister with Down Syndrome: Perspectives from Siblings," *American Journal of Medical Genetics* 155A, no. 10 (2011): 2348–59.

43 B.G. Skotko, S.P. Levine, and R. Goldstein, "Having a Son or Daughter with Down Syndrome: Perspectives from Mothers and Fathers," *American Journal of Medical Genetics* 155A, no. 10 (2011): 2335–47; K. Sheets, B. Crissman, C. Feist, et al., "Practice Guidelines for Communicating a Prenatal or Postnatal Diagnosis of Down Syndrome: Recommendations of the National Society of Genetic Counselors," *Journal of Genetic Counseling* 20, no. 5 (2011): 432–41.

44 A. Janvier, J.M. Lorenz, and J. Lantos, "Antenatal Counseling for Parents Facing an Extremely Preterm Birth: Limitations of the Medical Evidence," *Acta Paediatrica* 101, no. 8 (2012): 800–4.

45 Singer et al., "Social Support, Psychological Distress, and Parenting Strains."

46 L. Caeymaex, C. Jousselme, C. Vasilescu, et al., "Perceived Role in End-of-Life Decision Making in the NICU Affects Long-Term Parental Grief Response," *Archives of Disease in Childhood: Fetal and Neonatal Edition* 98, no. 1 (2013): F26–31.

47 American Academy of Pediatrics, *Neonatal Resuscitation Program (NRP) Textbook*, 6th ed. (Elk Grove Village, IL: American Academy of Pediatrics, 2010).

48 Jefferies and Kirpalani, "Canadian Paediatric Society FaNC"; Janvier, Barrington, et al., "Ethics Ain't Easy"; A. Janvier, J. Lantos, M. Deschenes, E. Couture, S. Nadeau, and K.J. Barrington, "Caregivers Attitudes for Very Premature Infants: What If They Knew?" *Acta Paediatrica* 97, no. 3 (2008): 276–9; A. Janvier, I. Leblanc, and K.J. Barrington, "Nobody Likes Premies: The Relative Value of Patients' Lives," *Journal of Perinatology* 28, no. 12 (2008): 821–6; A. Janvier, K.L. Bauer, and J.D. Lantos, "Are Newborns Morally Different from Older Children?" *Theoretical Medicine and Bioethics* 28, no. 5 (2007): 413–25; A. Janvier, I. Leblanc, and K.J. Barrington, "The Best-Interest Standard Is Not Applied for Neonatal Resuscitation Decisions," *Pediatrics* 121, no. 5 (2008): 963–9; T.W. Hansen, A. Janvier, O. Aasland, and R. Forde, "Ethics, Choices, and Decisions in Acute Medicine: A National Survey of Norwegian Physicians' Attitudes," *Pediatric Critical Care Medicine* 14, no. 2 (2013): e63; M.S. Fontana, C. Farrell, F. Gauvin, J. Lacroix, and A. Janvier, "Modes of Death in Pediatrics: Differences in the Ethical Approach in Neonatal and Pediatric Patients," *Journal of Pediatrics* 162, no. 6 (2013): 1107–11; K. Armstrong, C.A. Ryan, C.P. Hawkes, A. Janvier, and E.M. Dempsey, "Life and Death Decisions for Incompetent Patients: Determining Best Interests – The Irish Perspective," *Acta Paediatrics* 100, no. 4 (2011): 519–23; N. Laventhal, M.B. Spelke, B. Andrews, L.K. Larkin, W. Meadow, and A. Janvier, "Ethics of Resuscitation at Different Stages of Life: A Survey of Perinatal Physicians," *Pediatrics* 127, no. 5 (2011): e1221–9.

49 R. Carbajal, A. Rousset, C. Danan, et al., "Epidemiology and Treatment of Painful Procedures in Neonates in Intensive Care Units," *Journal of the American Medical Association* 300, no. 1 (2008): 60–70; V. Losacco, M. Cuttini, G. Greisen, et al., "Heel Blood Sampling in European Neonatal Intensive Care Units: Compliance

with Pain Management Guidelines," *Archives of Disease in Childhood: Fetal and Neonatal Edition* 96, no. 1 (2011): F65–8; C. Johnston, K.J. Barrington, A. Taddio, R. Carbajal, and F. Filion, "Pain in Canadian NICUs: Have We Improved over the Past 12 Years?" *Clinical Journal Pain* 27, no. 3 (2011): 225–32.

50 Carbajal et al., "Epidemiology and Treatment of Painful Procedures"; Johnston et al., "Pain in Canadian NICUs."

51 Janvier, Barrington, et al., "Ethics Ain't Easy."

52 Fontana et al., "Modes of Death in Pediatrics."

53 Lantos and Meadow, "Variation in the Treatment of Infants."

54 Janvier, Leblanc, and Barrington, "Nobody Likes Premies"; Laventhal et al., "Ethics of Resuscitation at Different Stages of Life."

55 Ibid.

56 A. Janvier, and M.R. Mercurio, "Saving vs Creating: Perceptions of Intensive Care at Different Ages and the Potential for Injustice," *Journal of Perinatology* 33 (2013): 333–5.

57 Janvier, Barrington, et al., "Ethics Ain't Easy."

58 Janvier, Lorenz, and Lantos, "Antenatal Counseling for Parents."

Difficult Decisions

1 Daniel Kahneman, *Thinking, Fast and Slow*. New York: Farrar, Straus and Giroux, 2011.

2 Annie Janvier, "How Much Emotion Is Enough?" *Journal of Clinical Ethics* 18 (2007): 362–5.

3 Louis C. Charland. "Is Mr Spock Mentally Competent? Competence to Consent and Emotion," *Philosophy, Psychiatry, and Psychology* 5, no. 1 (1998): 67–81. https://muse.jhu.edu/

4 Martha Nussbaum, *The Upheavals of Thought: The Intelligence of Emotions* (Cambridge: Cambridge UP, 2003).

Naming

1 Peter Ubel, *You're Stronger Than You Think: Tapping into the Secrets of Emotionally Resilient People* (New York: McGraw-Hill, 2006).

2 Saroj Saigal, *Preemie Voices* (self-published, 2014). See also https://vimeo.com/111486911

Personalized Decision Making: Practical Recommendations for Antenatal Counseling for Fragile Neonates

† J.D. Lantos, "Ethical Problems in Decision Making in the Neonatal ICU," *New England Journal of Medicine* 379, no. 19 (November 2018): 1851–60.

‡ *Clinics in Perinatology* 44, no. 2 (June 2017): 429–45. DOI: http://dx.doi.org/10.1016/j.clp.2017.01.006. 0095-5108/17/© 2017 Elsevier Inc. All rights reserved.

1 A.G.S. Philip "The Evolution of Neonatology," *Pediatric Research* 50, no. 4 (2005): 799–815, http://refhub.elsevier.com/S0095-5108(17)30009-X/sref1

2 Ibid.; M.E. Avery, "A 50-Year Overview of Perinatal Medicine," *Early Human Development* 29, nos. 1–3 (1992): 43–50, http://refhub.elsevier.com/S0095 -5108(17)30009-X/sref2

3 Committee on Hospital Care, "Family Centered Care and the Pediatrician's Role," *Pediatrics* 112, Pt 1–3 (2003): 691–6. http://refhub.elsevier.com/S0095 -5108(17)30009-X/sref3; American Academy of Pediatrics, "Patient and Family Centered Care and the Pediatrician's Role: Policy Statement," *Pediatrics* 129, no. 2 (2012): 394–404, http://refhub.elsevier.com/S0095-5108(17)30009 -X/sref4

4 L. Davis, H. Mohay, and H. Edwards, "Mothers Involvement in Caring for Their Premature Infants: An Historical Overview," *Journal Advanced Nursing* 42, no. 6 (2003): 578–86, http://refhub.elsevier.com/S0095-5108(17)30009-X/sref5

5 Philip, "The Evolution of Neonatology"; Davis et al., "Mothers' Involvement in Caring for Their Premature Infants."

6 M.J. Barry and S. Edgman-Levitan, "Shared Decision-Making: The Pinnacle of Patient Centered Care," *New England Journal of Medicine* 366, no. 9 (2012): 780–1, http://refhub.elsevier.com/S0095-5108(17)30009-X/sref6

7 President's Commission for the Study of Ethical Problems in Medicine and Biomedical and Behavioral Research, *Deciding to Forego Life-Sustaining Treatment: A Report on the Ethical, Medical and Legal Issues in Treatment Decisions* (Washington, DC: The Commission, 1983), http://refhub.elsevier.com/S0095 -5108(17)30009-X/sref7

8 A. Gilmore, "Sanctity of Life versus Quality of Life: The Continuing Debate," *Canadian Medical Association Journal* 130, no. 2 (1984): 180–1, http://refhub .elsevier.com/S0095-5108(17)30009-X/sref8

9 Committee on Hospital Care, "Family Centered Care and the Pediatrician's Role"; Barry and Edgman-Levitan, "Shared Decision-Making"; National Research Council, *Crossing the Quality Chasm: A New Health Care System for the 21st Century* (Washington, DC: National Academies Press, 2001), http://refhub.elsevier .com/S0095-5108(17)30009-X/sref9

10 Committee on Hospital Care, "Family Centered Care and the Pediatrician's Role."

11 E. Emmanuel and L. Emanuel, "Four Models of the Physician-Patient Relationship," *Journal of the American Medical Association* 262, no. 16 (1992): 2221–6, http://refhub.elsevier.com/S0095-5108(17)30009-X/sref10; C. Charles, A. Gafni, and T. Whelan, "Shared Decision-Making in the Medical Encounter: What Does It Mean? (Or It Takes at Least Two to Tango)," *Social Science and Medicine* 44, no. 5 (1997): 681–92, http://refhub.elsevier.com/S0095-5108(17)30009 -X/sref11

12 H. MacDonald, the American Academy of Pediatrics, and the Committee on the Fetus and Newborn, "Perinatal Care at the Threshold of Viability," *Pediatrics* 110, no. 5 (2002): 1024–7, http://refhub.elsevier.com/S0095-5108(17)30009-X/sref12;

J.E. Tyson and B.J. Stoll, "Evidence-Based Ethics and the Care and Outcome of Extremely Premature Infants," *Clinical Perinatology* 30, no. 2 (2003): 363–87, http://refhub.elsevier.com/S0095-5108(17)30009-X/sref13

13 Charles et al., "Shared Decision-Making in the Medical Encounter."

14 MacDonald et al., "Perinatal Care at the Threshold of Viability"; D.G. Batton, the American Academy of Pediatrics, and the Committee on the Fetus and Newborn, "Clinical Report: Antenatal Counseling Regarding Resuscitation at an Extremely Low Gestational Age," *Pediatrics* 124, no. 1 (2009): 422–7, http://refhub.elsevier.com/S0095-5108(17)30009-X/sref14; J. Cummings, the American Academy of Pediatrics, and the Committee on the Fetus and Newborn, "Antenatal Counseling Regarding Resuscitation and Intensive Care before 25 Weeks of Gestation," *Pediatrics* 136, no. 3 (2018): 588–95, http://refhub.elsevier.com/S0095-5108(17)30009-X/sref15; K.J. Griswold and J.M. Fnanaroff, "An Evidence-Based Overview of Prenatal Consultation with a Focus on Infants Born at the Limits of Viability," *Pediatrics* 125, no. 4 (2010): e931–7, http://refhub.elsevier.com/S0095-5108(17)30009-X/sref16

15 Cummings et al., "Antenatal Counseling Regarding Resuscitation and Intensive Care."

16 Ibid.

17 M.F. Haward, and A. Janvier, "An Introduction to Behavioural Decision-Making Theories for Paediatricians," *Acta Paediatrica* 104, no. 4 (2015): 340–5, http://refhub.elsevier.com/S0095-5108(17)30009-X/sref17; S. Bogardus, E. Holmboe, and J. Jekel, "Perils, Pitfalls and Possibilities in Talking about Medical Risk," *Journal of the American Medical Association* 281, no. 11 (1999): 1037–41, http://refhub.elsevier.com/S0095-5108(17)30009-X/sref18; C.B. Renjilian, J.W. Womer, K.W. Carroll, et al., "Parental Explicit Heuristics in Decision-Making for Children with Life-Threatening Illnesses," *Pediatrics* 131, no. 2 (2013): e566–72, http://refhub.elsevier.com/S0095-5108(17)30009-X/sref19

18 A.A. Kon, "The Shared Decision-Making Continuum," *Journal of the American Medical Association* 304, no. 8 (2010): 903–4, http://refhub.elsevier.com/S0095-5108(17)30009-X/sref20; M.A. de Vos, A.P. Bos, F.B. Plotz, et al., "Talking with Parents about End-of-Life Decisions for Their Children," *Pediatrics* 135, no. 2 (2015): e465–76, http://refhub.elsevier.com/S0095-5108(17)30009-X/sref21

19 A. Janvier, J.M. Lorenz, J.D. Lantos, "Antenatal Counselling for Parents Facing an Extremely Preterm Birth: Limitations of the Medical Evidence," *Acta Paediatrica* 101, no. 8 (2012): 800–4, http://refhub.elsevier.com/S0095-5108(17)30009-X/sref22; A. Janvier, K. Barrington, and B. Farlow, "Communication with Parents Concerning Withholding or Withdrawing of Life Sustaining Interventions in Neonatology," *Seminars in Perinatology* 38, no. 1 (2014): 38–46, http://refhub.elsevier.com/S0095-5108(17)30009-X/sref23

20 A. Payot, S. Gendron, F. Lefebvre, et al., "Deciding to Resuscitate Extremely Premature Babies: How Do Parents and Neonatologists Engage in the Decision?" *Social Science and Medicine* 64, no. 7 (2007): 1487–500, http://refhub.elsevier.com/S0095-5108(17)30009-X/sref24; L. Caeymaex, M. Speranza, C. Vasilescu, et al.,

"Living with a Crucial Decision: A Qualitative Study of Parental Narratives Three Years after the Loss of Their Newborn in the NICU," *PLoS One* 6, no. 12 (2001): e28633, 1–7, http://refhub.elsevier.com/S0095-5108(17)30009-X/sref25

21 Kon, "The Shared Decision-Making Continuum"; Caeymaex et al., "Living with a Crucial Decision."

22 J.E. Tyson, N.A. Parikh, J. Langer, C. Green, and R.D. Higgins for the The National Institute of Child Health and Human Development Neonatal Research Network, "Intensive Care for Extreme Prematurity: Moving Beyond Gestational Age," *New England Journal of Medicine* 358 (April 2008): 1672–81; B. Lemyre, T. Daboval, S. Dunn, et al., "Shared Decision-Making for Infants Born at the Threshold of Viability: A Prognosis Based Guideline," *Journal of Perinatology* 36, no. 7 (2016): 503–9, http://refhub.elsevier.com/S0095-5108(17)30009-X/sref27; A. Dupont-Thibodeau, K.J. Barrington, B. Farlow, et al., "End of Life Decisions for Extremely Low-Gestation-Age Infants: Why Simple Rules for Complicated Decisions Should Be Avoided," *Seminars in Perinatology* 38, no. 1 (2014): 31–7, http://refhub.elsevier.com/S0095-5108(17)30009-X/sref28

23 H.P. Robinson, "Sonar Measurement of Fetal Crown-Rump Length as Means of Assessing Maturity in First Trimester of Pregnancy," *British Medical Journal* 4, no. 5883 (1973): 28–31, http://refhub.elsevier.com/S0095-5108(17)30009-X/sref29; F.A. Chervenak, D.W. Skupski, R. Romero, et al., "How Accurate Is Fetal Biometry in the Assessment of Fetal Age?" *American Journal of Obstetrics and Gynaecology* 178, no. 4 (1998): 678–87, http://refhub.elsevier.com/S0095-5108(17)30009-X /sref30; C.D. Lynch and J. Zhang, "The Research Implications of the Selection of a Gestational Age Estimation Method," *Paediatric and Perinatal Epidemiology* 21, Suppl 2 (2007): 86–96, http://refhub.elsevier.com/S0095-5108(17)30009-X/sref31; S. Salvedt, H. Almstron, M. Kublickas, et al., "Ultrasound Dating at 12–14 or 15–20 Weeks of Gestation? A Prospective Cross-Validation of Established Dating Formulae in a Population of In-vitro Fertilized Pregnancies Randomized to Early or Late Dating Scan," *Ultrasound in Obstetrics and Gynaecology* 24, no. 1 (2004): 42–50, http://refhub.elsevier.com/S0095-5108(17)30009-X/sref32

24 Tyson et al., "The National Institute of Child Health and Human Development Neonatal Research Network."

25 Dupont-Thibodeau et al., "End of Life Decisions for Extremely Low-Gestation-Age Infants"; M.F. Haward, N.W. Kirshenbaum, and D.E. Campbell, "Care at the Edge of Viability: Medical and Ethical Issues," *Clinical Perinatology* 38, no. 3 (2011): 471–92, http://refhub.elsevier.com/S0095-5108(17)30009-X/sref33

26 Express Group, "Incidence of and Risk Factors for Neonatal Morbidity after Active Perinatal Care: Extremely Preterm Infants Study in Sweden (EXPRESS)," *Acta Paediatrica* 99, no. 7 (2010): 978–92, http://refhub.elsevier.com/S0095 -5108(17)30009-X/sref34

27 Ibid.

28 J. Perlbarg, P.Y. Ancel, B. Khoshnood, et al., "Epipage-2 Ethics Group: Delivery Room Management of Extremely Preterm Infants: The EPIPAGE-2 Study," *Archives*

of Disease in Childhood: Fetal and Neonatal Edition 101, no. 5 (2016): F384–90, http://refhub.elsevier.com/S0095-5108(17)30009-X/sref35; A. Janvier and J. Lantos, "Delivery Room Practices for Extremely Preterm Infants: The Harms of the Gestational Age Label," *Archives of Disease in Childhood: Fetal and Neonatal Edition* 101 (2016): F375–6, http://refhub.elsevier.com/S0095-5108(17)30009-X/sref36

29 M.S. Pignotti and R. Berni, "Extremely Preterm Births: End-of-Life Decisions in European Countries," *Archives of Disease in Childhood: Fetal and Neonatal Edition* 95, no. 4 (2010): F273–6, http://refhub.elsevier.com/S0095-5108(17)30009-X /sref37; R. de Leeuw, M. Cuttini, M. Nadai, et al., "Treatment Choices for Extremely Preterm Infants: An International Perspective," *Journal of Pediatrics* 137, no. 5 (2000): 608–15, http://refhub.elsevier.com/S0095-5108(17)30009-X/sref38; L. Taittonen, P.H. Korhonen, O. Palomäki, et al., "Opinions on the Counselling, Care and Outcome of Extremely Premature Birth among Healthcare Professionals in Finland," *Acta Paediatrica* 103, no. 3 (2014): 262–7, http://refhub.elsevier.com /S0095-5108(17)30009-X/sref39; R.A. Khan, L. Burgoyne, M.P. O'Connell, et al., "Resuscitation at the Limits of Viability: An Irish Perspective," *Acta Paediatrica* 98, no. 9 (2009): 1456–60, http://refhub.elsevier.com/S0095-5108(17)30009-X /sref40; M. Rysavy, L. Li, E. Bell, et al., "Between-Hospital Variation in Treatment and Outcomes in Extremely Preterm Infants," *New England Journal of Medicine* 372, no. 19 (2015): 1801–11, http://refhub.elsevier.com/S0095-5108(17)30009-X /sref41; J.D. Lantos and W. Meadow, "Variation in the Treatment of Infants Born at the Borderline of Viability," *Pediatrics* 123, no. 6 (2009): 1588–90; I. Seri and J. Evans, "Limits of Viability: Definition of the Gray Zone," *Journal of Perinatology* 28, suppl. 1 (2008): S4–8, http://refhub.elsevier.com/S0095-5108(17)30009-X /sref43; K. Itabashi, T. Hiriuchi, S. Kusuda, et al., "Mortality Rates for Extremely Low Birth Weight Infants Born in Japan in 2005," *Pediatrics* 123, no. 2 (2009): 445–50, http://refhub.elsevier.com/S0095-5108(17)30009-X/sref44; A.A.E. Verhagan and P.J.J. Sauer, "End of Life Decisions in Newborns: An Approach from The Netherlands," *Pediatrics* 116, no. 3 (2005): 736–9, http://refhub.elsevier.com /S0095-5108(17)30009-X/sref45; W. Meadow and J. Lantos, "Moral Reflections on Neonatal Intensive Care," *Pediatrics* 123, no. 2 (2009): 595–7, http://refhub.elsevier .com/S0095-5108(17)30009-X/sref46; A. Janvier, J. Lantos, and POST Group Investigators, "Stronger and More Vulnerable: A Balanced View of the Impacts of the NICU Experience on Parents," *Pediatrics* 138, no. 3 (2016): e20160655, http:// refhub.elsevier.com/S0095-5108(17)30009-X/sref47

30 Cummings et al., "Antenatal Counseling Regarding Resuscitation and Intensive Care."

31 Dupont-Thibodeau et al., "End of Life Decisions for Extremely Low-Gestation-Age Infants."

32 Charles et al., "Shared Decision-Making in the Medical Encounter."

33 Haward and Janvier, "An Introduction to Behavioural Decision-Making Theories."

34 MacDonald et al., "Perinatal Care at the Threshold of Viability"; Batton et al., "Clinical Report"; Cummings et al., "Antenatal Counseling Regarding Resuscitation and Intensive Care"; Griswold and Fnanaroff, "An Evidence-Based Overview of

Prenatal Consultation"; W.H. Yee, and R. Sauve, "What Information Do Parents Want from Antenatal Consultation?" *Paediatrics and Child Health* 12, no. 3 (2007): 191–6, http://refhub.elsevier.com/S0095-5108(17)30009-X/sref48; D. Paul, S. Epps, K. Leef, et al., "Prenatal Consultation with a Neonatologist Prior to Preterm Delivery," *Journal of Perinatology* 21, no. 7 (2001): 431–7, http://refhub.elsevier.com/S0095 -5108(17)30009-X/sref49; J.E. Brazy, B.M. Anderson, P.T. Becker, et al., "How Parents of Premature Infants Gather Information and Obtain Support," *Neonatal Network* 20, no. 2 (2001): 41–8, http://refhub.elsevier.com/S0095-5108(17)30009-X/sref50

35 Payot et al., "Deciding to Resuscitate Extremely Premature Babies"; Caeymaex et al., "Living with a Crucial Decision"; Yee and Sauve, "What Information Do Parents Want?"; Paul et al., "Prenatal Consultation with a Neonatologist"; Brazy et al., "How Parents of Premature Infants Gather Information."

36 Cummings et al., "Antenatal Counseling Regarding Resuscitation and Intensive Care"; U.O. Kim and M.A. Basir, "Informing and Educating Parents about the Risks and Outcomes of Prematurity," *Clinical Perinatology* 41, no. 4 (2014): 979–91, http://refhub.elsevier.com/S0095-5108(17)30009-X/sref51

37 M.F. Haward, R.O. Murphy, and J.M. Lorenz, "Message Framing and Perinatal Decisions," *Pediatrics* 122, no. 1 (2008): 109–18, http://refhub.elsevier.com/S0095 -5108(17)30009-X/sref52

38 D.J. Malenka, J.A. Baron, S. Johanson, et al., "The Framing Effect of Relative and Absolute Risk," *Journal of General Internal Medicine* 8, no. 10 (1993): 543–8, http://refhub.elsevier.com/S0095-5108(17)30009-X/sref53; D.J. Mazur and D.H. Hickman, "Patients' Interpretations of Probability Terms," *Journal of General Internal Medicine* 6, no. 3 (1991): 237–40, http://refhub.elsevier.com/S0095 -5108(17)30009-X/sref54

39 Janvier, Lorenz, and Lantos, "Antenatal Counselling for Parents Facing an Extremely Preterm Birth"; Janvier, Barrington, and Farlow, "Communication with Parents Concerning Withholding or Withdrawing of Life Sustaining Interventions"; A. Bowling and S. Ebrahim, "Measuring Patients' Preferences for Treatment and Perceptions of Risk," *Quality Health Care* 10, Suppl. 1 (2001): i2–8, http://refhub.elsevier.com/S0095-5108(17)30009-X/sref55

40 Renjilian et al., "Parental Explicit Heuristics in Decision-Making."

41 C. Holmber, E.A. Water, K. Whitehouse, et al., "My Lived Experiences Are More Important Than Your Probabilities: The Role of Individualized Risk Estimates for Decision-Making about Participation in the Study of Tamoxifen and Raloxifene (STAR)," *Medial Decision Making* 35, no. 8 (2015): 1010–22, http://refhub.elsevier .com/S0095-5108(17)30009-X/sref56

42 Haward and Janvier, "An Introduction to Behavioural Decision-Making Theories"; S. Plous, *The Psychology of Judgment and Decision-Making* (New York: McGraw-Hill, 1993), http://refhub.elsevier.com/S0095-5108(17)30009-X/sref57

43 A. Aleszewski and T. Horlink-Jones, "How Can Doctors Communicate Information about Risk More Effectively?" *BMJ* 327, no. 7417 (2003): 728–31, http://refhub.elsevier.com/S0095-5108(17)30009-X/sref58; C. Cox and Z. Fritz,

"Should Non-disclosures Be Considered as Morally Equivalent to Lies within the Doctor-Patient Relationship?" *Journal of Medical Ethics* 42, no. 10 (2016): 632–5, http://refhub.elsevier.com/S0095-5108(17)30009-X/sref59

44 U. Guillen, S. Suh, D. Munson, et al., "Development and Pretesting of a Decision-Aid to Use When Counseling Parents Facing Imminent Extreme Premature Delivery," *Journal of Pediatrics* 160, no. 3 (2012): 382–7, http://refhub.elsevier.com /S0095-5108(17)30009-X/sref60; V. Kakkilaya, L. Groome, D. Platt, et al., "Use of a Visual Aid to Improve Counseling at the Threshold of Viability," *Pediatrics* 128, no. 6 (2011): e1511–19, http://refhub.elsevier.com/S0095-5108(17)30009-X/sref61; A.D. Muthusamy, S. Leuthner, C. Gaebler-Uhung, et al., "Supplemental Written Information Improves Prenatal Counseling: A Randomized Trial," *Pediatrics* 129, no. 5 (2012): e1269–74, http://refhub.elsevier.com/S0095-5108(17)30009-X/sref62

45 Guillen et al., "Development and Pretesting of a Decision-Aid."

46 Kakkilaya et al., "Use of a Visual Aid to Improve Counseling."

47 Ibid.

48 Janvier, Lantos, and Post Group, "Stronger and More Vulnerable"; W. Godolphin, "The Role of Risk Communication in Shared Decision-Making," *BMJ* 327, no. 7417 (2003): 692–3, http://refhub.elsevier.com/S0095-5108(17)30009-X/sref63.

49 Janvier, Lorenz, and Lantos, "Antenatal Counselling for Parents Facing an Extremely Preterm Birth."

50 Caeymaex et al., "Living with a Crucial Decision"; Yee and Sauve, "What Information Do Parents Want?"

51 Caeymaex et al., "Living with a Crucial Decision."

52 Janvier, Barrington, and Farlow, "Communication with Parents Concerning Withholding or Withdrawing of Life Sustaining Interventions"; P. Slovic, ed., *The Feeling of Risk* (London: Earthscan, 2001), http://refhub.elsevier.com/S0095 -5108(17)30009-X/sref64; J. Walter and L.F. Ross, "Relational Autonomy: Moving Beyond the Limits of Isolated Individualism," *Pediatrics* 133, Suppl 1 (2014): S16–23, http://refhub.elsevier.com/S0095-5108(17)30009-X/sref65.

53 Payot et al., "Deciding to Resuscitate Extremely Premature Babies."

54 Caeymaex et al., "Living with a Crucial Decision."

55 Ibid.; Guillen et al., "Development and Pretesting of a Decision-Aid"; E. Young, E. Tsai, and A. O'Riordan, "A Qualitative Study of Predelivery Counselling for Extreme Prematurity," *Paediatrics and Child Health* 17, no. 8 (2012): 432–6, http:// refhub.elsevier.com/S0095-5108(17)30009-X/sref66

56 Slovic, *The Feeling of Risk.*

57 C. Lerman, M. Daly, W. Walsh, et al., "Communication between Patients with Breast Cancer and Health Care Providers Determinants and Implications," *Cancer* 72, no. 9 (1993): 2612–20, http://refhub.elsevier.com/S0095-5108(17)30009-X/sref67

58 A. Bechara, D. Tranel, and H. Damasio, "Characterization of the Decision-Making Deficit of Patients with Ventromedial Prefrontal Cortex Lesions," *Brain* 12, pt. 11 (2000): 2189–202, http://refhub.elsevier.com/S0095-5108(17)30009-X/sref68

59 Walter and Ross, "Relational Autonomy."

60 Janvier, Barrington, and Farlow, "Communication with Parents Concerning
    Withholding or Withdrawing of Life Sustaining Interventions."
61 Janvier, Lorenz, and Lantos, "Antenatal Counselling for Parents Facing an
    Extremely Preterm Birth."
62 N. Gaucher and A. Payot, "From Powerlessness to Empowerment: Mothers Expect
    More Than Information from the Prenatal Consultation for Preterm Labour,"
    Paediatrics and Child Health 16, no. 10 (2011): 638–42, http://refhub.elsevier.com
    /S0095-5108(17)30009-X/sref69
63 Gaucher and Payot, "From Powerlessness to Empowerment."
64 Ibid.; N. Gaucher, S. Nadeau, A. Barbier, et al., "Personalized Antenatal
    Consultations for Preterm Labor: Responding to Mothers' Expectations,"
    Journal of Pediatrics 178 (2016): 130–4, e7, http://refhub.elsevier.com/S0095
    -5108(17)30009-X/sref70
65 Payot et al., "Deciding to Resuscitate Extremely Premature Babies"; Gaucher and
    Payot, "From Powerlessness to Empowerment"; Gaucher et al., "Personalized
    Antenatal Consultations for Preterm Labor."
66 H.E. McHaffie, I.A. Laing, M. Park, et al., "Deciding for Imperilled Newborns:
    Medical Authority or Parental Autonomy?" *Journal Medical Ethics* 27, no. 2 (2001):
    104–9, http://refhub.elsevier.com/S0095-5108(17)30009-X/sref71
67 Janvier, Barrington, and Farlow, "Communication with Parents Concerning
    Withholding or Withdrawing of Life Sustaining Interventions."
68 M.F. Haward, A. Janvier, J.M. Lorenz, et al., "Speaking to Parents before Premature
    Birth: Whose Agenda?" Paper presented at Pediatrics Academic Societies meeting,
    Baltimore, MD, 4 May 2016.
69 B. Bohnhorst, T. Ahl, C. Peter, et al., "Parents' Prenatal Onward and Postdischarge
    Experiences in Case of Extreme Prematurity: When to Set the Course for a
    Trusting Relationship between Parents and Medical Staff," *American Journal
    of Perinatology* 32, no. 13 (2015): 1191–7, http://refhub.elsevier.com/S0095
    -5108(17)30009-X/sref73
70 D.M. Post, D.J. Cegala, and W.F. Miser, "The Other Half of the Whole: Teaching
    Patients to Communicate with Physicians," *Family Medicine* 34, no. 5 (2002):
    344–52, http://refhub.elsevier.com/S0095-5108(17)30009-X/sref74
71 Caeymaex et al., "Living with a Crucial Decision"; J. Paling, "Strategies to Help
    Patients Understand Risks," *BMJ* 327, no. 7417 (2003): 745–8, http://refhub.elsevier
    .com/S0095-5108(17)30009-X/sref75; R. Smith, "Communication Risk: The Main
    Work of Doctors," *BMJ* 327, no. 7417 (2003), http://refhub.elsevier.com/S0095
    -5108(17)30009-X/sref76
72 Janvier, Barrington, and Farlow, "Communication with Parents Concerning
    Withholding or Withdrawing of Life Sustaining Interventions."
73 Ibid.; Payot et al., "Deciding to Resuscitate Extremely Premature Babies"; Gaucher
    and Payot, "From Powerlessness to Empowerment"; Gaucher et al., "Personalized
    Antenatal Consultations for Preterm Labor."
74 Payot et al., "Deciding to Resuscitate Extremely Premature Babies"

75 Ibid.
76 Gaucher and Payot, "From Powerlessness to Empowerment"; Gaucher et al., "Personalized Antenatal Consultations for Preterm Labor."
77 Ibid.
78 Payot et al., "Deciding to Resuscitate Extremely Premature Babies."
79 Ibid.; Gaucher et al., "Personalized Antenatal Consultations for Preterm Labor."
80 Gaucher and Payot, "From Powerlessness to Empowerment."
81 Gaucher et al., "Personalized Antenatal Consultations for Preterm Labor."
82 Ibid.
83 L. Arnold, A. Sawyer, H. Rabe, et al., "Parents' First Moments with Their Very Preterm Babies: A Qualitative Study," *BMJ* 3, no. 4 (2013): e002487, http://refhub .elsevier.com/S0095-5108(17)30009-X/sref77
84 Payot et al., "Deciding to Resuscitate Extremely Premature Babies"; F. Miquel-Verges, S.L. Woods, S.W. Aucott, et al., "Prenatal Consultation with a Neonatologist for Congenital Anomalies: Parental Perceptions," *Pediatrics* 124, no. 4 (2009): e573–9, http://refhub.elsevier.com/S0095-5108(17)30009-X/sref78; R.D. Boss, N. Hutton, L.J. Sulpar, et al., "Values Parents Apply to Decision-Making for High-Risk Newborns," *Pediatrics* 122, no. 3 (2008): 385–9, http://refhub.elsevier.com/S0095 -5108(17)30009-X/sref79
85 Payot et al., "Deciding to Resuscitate Extremely Premature Babies"; Gaucher et al., "Personalized Antenatal Consultations for Preterm Labor"; Boss et al., "Values Parents Apply to Decision-Making."
86 R.B. Deber, "Physicians in Health Care Management: 8. The Patient-Physician Partnership: Decision-Making, Problem Solving and the Desire to Participate," *Canadian Medical Association Journal* 151, no. 4 (1994): 423–7, http://refhub .elsevier.com/S0095-5108(17)30009-X/sref80
87 Bogardus et al., "Perils, Pitfalls and Possibilities in Talking about Medical Risk"; Caeymaex et al., "Living with a Crucial Decision."
88 Payot et al., "Deciding to Resuscitate Extremely Premature Babies"; Godolphin, "The Role of Risk Communication," Deber, "Physicians in Health Care Management"; N.B. Perlman, J.L. Freedman, A. Abramovitch, et al., "Informational Needs of Parents of Sick Neonates," *Pediatrics* 88, no. 3 (1991): 512–18, http:// refhub.elsevier.com/S0095-5108(17)30009-X/sref81; M.W. Doron, K.A. Veness-Meehan, L.H. Margolis, et al., "Delivery Room Resuscitation Decisions for Extremely Premature Infants," *Pediatrics* 102, no. 3 (1998): 574–82, http://refhub .elsevier.com/S0095-5108(17)30009-X/sref82
89 Caeymaex et al., "Living with a Crucial Decision"; H.T. Keenan, M.W. Doron, and B.A. Seyda, "Comparison of Mothers' and Counselors' Perceptions of Predelivery Counseling for Extremely Premature Infants," *Pediatrics* 116, no. 1 (2005): 104–11, http://refhub.elsevier.com/S0095-5108(17)30009-X/sref83
90 V.N. Madrigal, K.W. Carroll, K. Hexem, et al., "Parental Decision-Making Preferences in the Pediatric Intensive Care," *Critical Care Medicine* 40, no. 10 (2012): 2876–82, http://refhub.elsevier.com/S0095-5108(17) 30009-X/sref84

91 Bohnhorst et al., "Parents' Prenatal Onward and Postdischarge Experiences";
L. Caeymaex, C. Jousselme, C. Vasilescu, et al., "Perceived Role in End-of-Life
Decision Making in the NICU Affects Long-Term Parental Grief Response,"
Archives of Disease of Childhood: Fetal and Neonatal Edition 98, no. 1 (2013):
F26–31, http://refhub.elsevier.com/S0095-5108(17)30009-X/sref85

92 Madrigal et al., "Parental Decision-Making Preferences in the Pediatric Intensive
Care."

93 Haward and Janvier, "An Introduction to Behavioural Decision-Making Theories";
Bogardus et al., "Perils, Pitfalls and Possibilities in Talking about Medical Risk";
Renjilian et al., "Parental Explicit Heuristics in Decision-Making for Children";
Janvier, Lorenz, and Lantos, "Antenatal Counselling for Parents Facing an
Extremely Preterm Birth"; Janvier, Barrington, and Farlow, "Communication with
Parents Concerning Withholding or Withdrawing of Life Sustaining Interventions."

Pepperoni Pizza and Sex

† Payot and K.J. Barrington, "The Quality of Life of Young Children and Infants with
Chronic Medical Problems: Review of the Literature," *Current Problems in Pediatric
and Adolescent Health Care* 41, no. 4 (April 2011): 91–101. DOI: 10.1016/j
.cppeds.2010.10.008.

‡ *Current Problems in Pediatric and Adolescent Health Care* 41 (April 2011): 106–8.

Measuring and Communicating Meaningful Outcomes in Neonatology

† *Acta Paediatrica* 108, no. 6 (June 2019): 1067–73. DOI: 10.1111/apa.14634.

1 W.A. Silverman, "Overtreatment of Neonates? A Personal Retrospective," *Pediatrics*
90, no. 6 (1992): 971–6, http://refhub.elsevier.com/S0146-0005(16)30081-7/sbref1

2 K. Staub, J. Baardsnes, N. Hebert, M. Hebert, S. Newell, and R. Pearce, "Our
Child Is Not Just a Gestational Age: A First-Hand Account of What Parents Want
and Need to Know before Premature Birth," *Acta Paediatrica* 103, no. 10 (2014):
1035–8, http://refhub.elsevier.com/S0146-0005(16)30081-7/sbref2; R. Pearce and J.
Baardsnes, "Term MRI for Small Preterm Babies: Do Parents Really Want to Know
and Why Has Nobody Asked Them?" *Acta Paediatrica* 20, no. 6 (2012): 436–41,
http://refhub.elsevier.com/S0146-0005(16)30081-7/sbref3; A. Janvier and B.
Farlow, "The Ethics of Neonatal Research: An Ethicist's and a Parents' Perspective,"
Seminars in Fetal and Neonatal Medicine 20, no. 6 (2015): 436–41, http://refhub
.elsevier.com/S0146-0005(16)30081-7/sbref4

3 All the authors of this article are parents who had a sick neonate, with varying
experiences and outcomes, including death. Two of the authors (Barrington and
Janvier) are also neonatologists and clinical researchers.

4 C.J. Morley, P.G. Davis, L.W. Doyle, L.P. Brion, J.M. Hascoet, and J.B. Carlin,
"Nasal CPAP or Intubation at Birth for Very Preterm Infants," *New England
Journal of Medicine* 358, no. 7 (2008): 700–8. http://refhub.elsevier.com/S0146
-0005(16)30081-7/sbref5

5 W.A. Carlo, N.N. Finer, M.C. Walsh, et al., "Target Ranges of Oxygen Saturation in Extremely Preterm Infants," *New England Journal of Medicine* 362, no. 21 (2010): 1959–69, http://refhub.elsevier.com/S0146-0005(16)30081-7/sbref6

6 B. Schmidt, P. Davis, D. Moddemann, A. Ohlsson, R.S. Roberts, and S. Saigal, "Long-Term Effects of Indomethacin Prophylaxis in Extremely-Low-Birth-Weight Infants," *New England Journal of Medicine* 344, no. 26 (2001): 1966–72, http://refhub.elsevier.com/S0146-0005(16)30081-7/sbref7

7 G. Tomlinson, and A.S. Detsky, "Composite End Points in Randomized Trials: There Is No Free Lunch," *Journal of the American Medical Association* 303, no. 3 (2010): 267–8, http://refhub.elsevier.com/S0146-0005(16)30081-7/sbref8; V.M. Montori, G. Permanyer-Miralda, I. Ferreira-Gonzalez, et al., "Validity of Composite End Points in Clinical Trials," *British Medical Journal* 330, no. 7491 (2005): 594–6, http://refhub.elsevier.com/S0146-0005(16)30081-7/sbref9

8 A. Jefferies, H. Kirpalani, the Canadian Paediatric Society, and the Fetus and Newborn Committee, "Counselling and Management for Anticipated Extremely Preterm Birth," *Paediatrics Child Health* 17, no. 8 (2012): 443, http://refhub.elsevier.com/S0146-0005(16)30081-7/sbref10

9 Schmidt et al., "Long-Term Effects of Indomethacin Prophylaxis"; Tomlinson and Detsky, "Composite End Points in Randomized Trials."

10 Janvier and Farlow, "The Ethics of Neonatal Research."

11 Early Treatment for Retinopathy of Prematurity Cooperative Group, "The Incidence and Course of Retinopathy of Prematurity: Findings from the Early Treatment for Retinopathy of Prematurity Study," *Pediatrics* 116, no. 1 (2005): 15–23, http://refhub.elsevier.com/S0146-0005(16)30081-7/sbref11

12 Morley et al., "Nasal CPAP or Intubation at Birth."

13 Y.E. Vaucher, M. Peralta-Carcelen, N.N. Finer, et al., "Neurodevelopmental Outcomes in the Early CPAP and Pulse Oximetry Trial," *New England Journal of Medicine* 367, no. 26 (2012): 2495–504, http://refhub.elsevier.com/S0146-0005(16)30081-7/sbref12.

14 A. Corbet, R. Bucciarelli, S. Goldman, M. Mammel, D. Wold, and W. Long, "Decreased Mortality Rate among Small Premature Infants Treated at Birth with a Single Dose of Synthetic Surfactant: A Multicenter Controlled Trial," *Journal of Pediatrics* 118, no. 2 (1991): 277–84, http://refhub.elsevier.com/S0146-0005(16)30081-7/sbref13

15 J. Lagatta, M. Uhing, and J. Panepinto, "Comparative Effectiveness and Practice Variation in Neonatal Care," *Clinical Perinatology* 41, no. 4 (2014): 833–45, http://refhub.elsevier.com/S0146-0005(16)30081-7/sbref14

16 J.E. Tyson, N.A. Parikh, J. Langer, C. Green, and R.D. Higgins, "The National Institute of Child Health and Human Development Neonatal Research Network: Intensive Care for Extreme Prematurity – Moving beyond Gestational Age," *New England Journal of Medicine* 358, no. 16 (2008): 1672–81, http://refhub.elsevier.com/S0146-0005(16)30081-7/sbref15

17 Montori et al., "Validity of Composite End Points in Clinical Trials"; A. Dupont-Thibodeau, K.J. Barrington, B. Farlow, and A. Janvier, "End-of-Life Decisions for Extremely Low-Gestational-Age Infants: Why Simple Rules for Complicated Decisions Should Be Avoided," *Seminars in Perinatology* 38, no. 1 (2014): 31–7, http://refhub.elsevier.com/S0146-0005(16)30081-7/sbref16

18 Lagatta et al., "Comparative Effectiveness and Practice Variation in Neonatal Care."

19 J. Einarsdottir, "Emotional Experts: Parents' Views on End-of-Life Decisions for Preterm Infants in Iceland," *Medical Anthropology Quarterly* 23, no. 1 (2009): 34–50, http://refhub.elsevier.com/S0146-0005(16)30081-7/sbref17

20 Janvier and Farlow, "The Ethics of Neonatal Research."

21 G. Roberts, P.J. Anderson, and L.W. Doyle, "The Stability of the Diagnosis of Developmental Disability between Ages 2 and 8 in a Geographic Cohort of Very Preterm Children Born in 1997," *Archives of Disease in Childhood* 95 (2010): 786–90, http://refhub.elsevier.com/S0146-0005(16)30081-7/sbref18; M. Hack, H.G. Taylor, D. Drotar, et al., "Poor Predictive Validity of the Bayley Scales of Infant Development for Cognitive Function of Extremely Low Birth Weight Children at School Age," *Pediatrics* 116, no. 2 (2005): 333–41, http://refhub.elsevier.com/S0146-0005(16)30081-7/sbref19

22 Roberts et al., "The Stability of the Diagnosis of Developmental Disability."

23 Einarsdottir, "Emotional Experts."

24 Roberts et al., "The Stability of the Diagnosis of Developmental Disability."

25 M.M. Spencer-Smith, A.J. Spittle, K.J. Lee, L.W. Doyle, and P.J. Anderson, "Bayley-III Cognitive and Language Scales in Preterm Children," *Pediatrics* 135, no. 5 (2015): e1258–65, http://refhub.elsevier.com/S0146-0005(16)30081-7/sbref20

26 B. Schmidt, P.J. Anderson, L.W. Doyle, et al., "Survival without Disability to Age 5 Years after Neonatal Caffeine Therapy for Apnea of Prematurity," *Journal of the American Medical Association* 307, no. 3 (2012): 275–82, http://refhub.elsevier.com/S0146-0005(16)30081-7/sbref21

27 C. Limperopoulos, H. Bassan, N.R. Sullivan, et al., "Positive Screening for Autism in Ex-preterm Infants: Prevalence and Risk Factors," *Pediatrics* 121, no. 4 (2008): 758–65, http://refhub.elsevier.com/S0146-0005(16)30081-7/sbref22

28 M.A. Pritchard, T. de Dassel, E. Beller, et al., "Autism in Toddlers Born Very Preterm," *Pediatrics* 137, no. 2 (2016): 1–8, http://refhub.elsevier.com/S0146-0005(16)30081-7/sbref23

29 T.M. Luu, B.R. Vohr, W. Allan, K.C. Schneider, and L.R. Ment, "Evidence for Catch-Up in Cognition and Receptive Vocabulary among Adolescents Born Very Preterm," *Pediatrics* 128, no. 2 (2011): 313–22, http://refhub.elsevier.com/S0146-0005(16)30081-7/sbref

30 Limperopoulos et al., "Positive Screening for Autism in Ex-preterm Infants."

31 L.J. Woodward, P.J. Anderson, N.C. Austin, K. Howard, and T.E. Inder, "Neonatal MRI to Predict Neurodevelopmental Outcomes in Preterm Infants," *New England*

Journal of Medicine 355, no. 7 (2006): 685–94, http://refhub.elsevier.com/S0146 -0005(16)30081-7/sbref

32 Luu et al., "Evidence for Catch-Up in Cognition and Receptive Vocabulary"; B. Sklöld, B. Vollmer, B. Bohm, et al., "Neonatal Magnetic Resonance Imaging and Outcome at Age 30 Months in Extremely Preterm Infants," *Journal of Pediatrics* 160, no. 4 (2012): 559–66.e1, http://refhub.elsevier.com/S0146-0005(16)30081-7/sbref

33 Luu et al., "Evidence for Catch-Up in Cognition and Receptive Vocabulary."

34 Pearce and Baardsnes, "Term MRI for Small Preterm Babies."

35 Ibid.

36 G. Donley, S.C. Hull, and B.E. Berkman, "Prenatal Whole Genome Sequencing," *Hastings Center Report* 42, no. 4 (2012): 28–40, http://refhub.elsevier.com/S0146 -0005(16)30081-7/sbref

37 K.B. Sheets, R.G. Best, C.K. Brasington, and M.C. Will, "Balanced Information about Down Syndrome: What Is Essential?" *American Journal of Medical Genetics* 155A, no. 6 (2011): 1246–57, http://refhub.elsevier.com/S0146-0005(16)30081-7/sbref; B.G. Skotko, G.T. Capone, P.S. Kishnani, and the Down Syndrome Diagnosis Study Group, "Postnatal Diagnosis of Down Syndrome: Synthesis of the Evidence on How Best to Deliver the News," *Pediatrics* 124, no. 4 (2009): e751–8, http://refhub.elsevier.com /S0146-0005(16)30081-7/sbref; A. Janvier, B. Farlow, and B.S. Wilfond, "The Experience of Families with Children with Trisomy 13 and 18 in Social Networks," *Pediatrics* 130, no. 2 (2012): 293–8, http://refhub.elsevier.com/S0146-0005(16)30081-7/sbref

38 T. Ho, D. Dukhovny, J.A. Zupancic, D.A. Goldmann, J.D. Horbar, and D.M. Pursley, "Choosing Wisely in Newborn Medicine: Five Opportunities to Increase Value," *Pediatrics* 136, no. 2 (2015): e482–9, http://refhub.elsevier.com/S0146 -0005(16)30081-7/sbref

39 A. Janvier, and B. Farlow, "Arrogance-Based Medicine: Guidelines Regarding Genetic Testing in Children," *American Journal of Bioethics* 14, no. 3 (2014): 15–16, http://refhub.elsevier.com/S0146-0005(16)30081-7/sbref

40 Pearce and Baardsnes, "Term MRI for Small Preterm Babies"

41 S.R. Jadcherla, M. Wang, A.S. Vijayapal, and S.R. Leuthner, "Impact of Prematurity and Co-Morbidities on Feeding Milestones in Neonates: A Retrospective Study," *Journal of Perinatology* 30, no. 3 (2010): 201–8, http://refhub.elsevier.com/S0146 -0005(16)30081-7/sbref

42 N. Rommel, A.M. De Meyer, L. Feenstra, and G. Veereman-Wauters, "The Complexity of Feeding Problems in 700 Infants and Young Children Presenting to a Tertiary Care Institution," *Journal of Pediatric Gastroenterol Nutrition* 37, no. 1 (2003): 75–84, http://refhub.elsevier.com/S0146-0005(16)30081-7/sbref

43 D.M. Smith, G. Loewenstein, A. Jankovic, and P.A. Ubel, "Happily Hopeless: Adaptation to a Permanent, But Not to a Temporary, Disability," *Health Psychology* 28, no. 6 (2009): 787–91, http://refhub.elsevier.com/S0146-0005(16)30081-7/sbref

44 P. Ubel, *You're Stronger Than You Think: Tapping into the Secrets of Emotionally Resilient People* (New York: McGraw-Hill, 2006), http://refhub.elsevier.com/S0146 -0005(16)30081-7/sbref

45 P. Raina, M. O'Donnell, P. Rosenbaum, et al., "The Health and Well-Being of Caregivers of Children with Cerebral Palsy," *Pediatrics* 115, no. 6 (2005): e626–36, http://refhub.elsevier.com/S0146-0005(16)30081-7/sbref

46 M. Seear, A. Kapur, D. Wensley, K. Morrison, and A. Behroozi, "The Quality of Life of Home-Ventilated Children and Their Primary Caregivers Plus the Associated Social and Economic Burdens: A Prospective Study," *Archives of Disease in Childhood* (2016). PMID: 26940814 [Epub ahead of print], http://refhub.elsevier .com/S0146-0005(16)30081-7/sbref

47 Spencer-Smith et al., "Bayley-III Cognitive and Language Scales in Preterm Children"; Sheets et al., "Balanced Information about Down Syndrome."

48 J. Guon, B.S. Wilfond, B. Farlow, T. Brazg, and A. Janvier, "Our Children Are Not a Diagnosis: The Experience of Parents Who Continue Their Pregnancy after a Prenatal Diagnosis of Trisomy 13 or 18," *American Journal of Medical Genetics* 164A, no. 2 (2014): 308–18, http://refhub.elsevier.com/S0146-0005(16)30081-7 /sbref

49 Rommel et al., "The Complexity of Feeding Problems."

50 S. Saigal, J. Pinelli, D.L. Streiner, M. Boyle, and B. Stoskopf, "Impact of Extreme Prematurity on Family Functioning and Maternal Health 20 Years Later," *Pediatrics* 126, no. 1 (2010): e81–8, http://refhub.elsevier.com/S0146-0005(16)30081-7/sbref

51 K. Scorgie and D. Sobsey, "Transformational Outcomes Associated with Parenting Children Who Have Disabilities," *Mental Retardation* 38, no. 3 (2000): 195–206, http://refhub.elsevier.com/S0146-0005(16)30081-7/sbref

52 M.E. Redshaw and M.E. Harvey, "Explanations and Information-Giving: Clinician Strategies Used in Talking to Parents of Preterm Infants," *BMC Pediatrics* 16, no. 1 (2016): 1–13, http://refhub.elsevier.com/S0146-0005(16)30081-7/sbref

53 Tyson et al., "The National Institute of Child Health and Human Development Neonatal Research Network."

54 N. Gaucher and A. Payot, "From Powerlessness to Empowerment: Mothers Expect More Than Information from the Prenatal Consultation for Preterm Labour," *Paediatrics Child Health* 16, no. 10 (2011): 638–42, http://refhub.elsevier.com /S0146-0005(16)30081-7/sbref

55 Staub et al., "Our Child Is Not Just a Gestational Age."

56 Seear et al., "The Quality of Life of Home-Ventilated Children."

57 Skotko et al., "Postnatal Diagnosis of Down Syndrome."

58 Janvier et al., "The Experience of Families with Children with Trisomy 13 and 18."

Tattoos, Beer, and Bow Ties: The Limits of Professionalism in Medicine

† B.H. Arzuaga, C. Petty, and A. Janvier, "The Therapeutic Space and Doctor-Parent Relationship in Paediatrics: Trainees' Experiences and Perspectives," *Acta Paediatrica* 108, no. 6 (June 2019): 1067–73. DOI: 10.1111/apa.14634.

‡ JAMA Pediatrics, online 6 June 2016. DOI: 10.1001/jamapediatrics. I thank Simon Vaillancourt and Julie Lévis for optimizing this narrative and granting permission

to publish this information. Simon specified on the patient permission form, "This story is about my family, my dead child and my two surviving heroes. This article is a tribute to them and we do not wish it to be published under a false name."

Stronger and More Vulnerable: A Balanced View of the Impacts of the NICU Experience on Parents

† *Pediatrics* 138, no. 3 (September 2016). DOI: 10.1542/peds.2016-0655.
1 W.J. Kim, E. Lee, K.R. Kim, K. Namkoong, E.S. Park, and D.W. Rha, "Progress of PTSD Symptoms Following Birth: A Prospective Study in Mothers of High-Risk Infants," *Journal of Perinatology* 35, no. 8 (2015): 575–9.
2 P.A. Linley, and S. Joseph, "Positive Change Following Trauma and Adversity: A Review," *Journal of Traumatic Stress* 17, no. 1 (2004): 11–21.
3 J.A. Picoraro, J.W. Womer, A.E. Kazak, and C. Feudner, "Posttraumatic Growth in Parents and Pediatric Patients," *Journal of Palliative Medicine* 17, no. 2 (2014): 209–18.
4 K. Scorgie, and D. Sobsey, "Transformational Outcomes Associated with Parenting Children Who Have Disabilities," *Mental Retardation* 38, no. 3 (2000): 195–206; A. Janvier, B. Farlow, and B.S. Wilfond, "The Experience of Families with Children with Trisomy 13 and 18 in Social Networks," *Pediatrics* 130, no. 2 (2012): 293–8; B.G. Skotko, S.P. Levine, E.A. Macklin, and R.D. Goldstein, "Family Perspectives about Down Syndrome," *American Journal of Medical Genetics* 170A, no. 4 (2016): 930–41.
5 March of Dimes, "2 Here 2 in Heaven," *What My Children Have Taught Me*, http://share.marchofdimes.org/blog/b/weblog18812/archive/2007/04/20/what-my-children-have-taught-me#.Vr40lvnhAgs; P. Thiele, S.F. Berg, and B. Farlow, "More Than a Diagnosis," *Acta Paediatrica* 102, no. 12 (2013): 1127–9; A. Janvier, "Ces choses que Violette m'a apprises" in *Respire, bébé, respire! Prématurités et naissances difficiles* (Montreal: Québec Amérique, 2015).
6 Thiele et al., "More Than a Diagnosis."
7 F. Cohn, "Suddenly 'I' Was a 'Them.'" *Current Problems in Pediatric and Adolescent Health Care* 41, no. 4 (2011): 111–12.

Getting the Bad Stuff Out

1 For information on Pierre Lavoie, see https://fr.wikipedia.org/wiki/Pierre_Lavoie

Ethics and Etiquette in Neonatal Intensive Care

† JAMA Pediatrics 168, no. 9 (September 2014): 857–8. DOI: 10.1001/jamapediatrics.2014.527.
‡ The POST investigators are Judy Achner, MD, Albert Einstein College of Medicine, New York, New York; Keith Barrington, MB, ChB, Université de Montréal, Quebec;

Beau Batton, MD, Southern Illinois University School of Medicine Health Care, Springfield; Daniel Batton, MD, Southern Illinois University School of Medicine Health Care, Springfield; Siri Fuglem Berg, MD, PhD, Sykehuset Innlandet Hospital Trust, Brumunddal, Norway; Brian Carter, MD, University of Missouri-Kansas City School of Medicine, Kansas City; Felicia Cohn, PhD, University of California, Irvine; Dan Ellsbury, MD, Mercy Medical Center, Des Moines, Iowa; Avroy Fanaroff, MD, Case Western Reserve University, Cleveland, Ohio; Jonathan Fanaroff, MD, JD, Case Western Reserve University, Cleveland, Ohio; Kristy Fanaroff, NNP, Rainbow Babies and Children's Hospital, Cleveland, Ohio; Sophie Gravel, BSN, Hôpital Sainte-Justine, Montreal, Quebec; Annie Janvier, MD, PhD, Hôpital Sainte-Justine, Montreal, Quebec; Stefan Kutzsche, MD, PhD, Oslo University, Oslo; John Lantos, MD, Children's Mercy Hospital, University of Missouri-Kansas City School of Medicine, Kansas City; Anne Drapkin Lyerly, MD, MA, University of North Carolina, Chapel Hill; Neil Marlow, MBBS, University College London Hospitals, London, England; Martha Montello, PhD, University of Missouri-Kansas City School of Medicine, Kansas City; Odd G. Paulsen, MD, Sykehuset Innlandet Hospital Trust, Brumunddal, Norway.

1   A. Janvier, "I'm Only Punching In," *Archives of Pediatrics and Adolescent Medicine* 161, no. 9 (2007): 827; P. Thiele, S.F. Berg, B. Farlow, "More Than a Diagnosis" *Acta Paediatrica*, 16 September 2013, doi:10.1111/apa.12411; M. Montello, "Being There," *Current Problems in Pediatric and Adolescent Health Care* 41, no. 4 (2011): 109–10; F. Cohn, "Suddenly 'I' Was a 'Them,'" *Current Problems in Pediatric and Adolescent Health Care* 41, no. 4 (2011): 111–12; B. Batton, "A Piece of My Mind: Healing Hearts," *Journal of the American Medical Association* 304, no. 12 (2010): 1303–4; B.S. Carter and C.A. Carter, "The NICU Experience in Retrospect," *Clinical Pediatrics* 27, no. 9 (1988): 450.

2   M.W. Kahn, "Etiquette-Based Medicine," *New England Journal of Medicine* 358, no. 19 (2008): 1988–9.

Glossary of Common Abbreviations Used in the NICU

ABG   (arterial blood gas): ABG is measured to determine how well the lungs and gas exchange are working in the body; for an ABG test, blood is drawn from the arteries.

BP   (blood pressure): A measure of the pressure in the blood vessels, which usually is an indication of how the heart is doing.

BPD   (broncho pulmonary dysplasia): A chronic lung condition many premature babies have due to their immature lungs and the use of a respirator and oxygen.

CBC   (complete blood count): A count of the blood constitutents: red blood cells, while blood cells, and platelets.

CBG   (capillary blood gas): CBG is measured to determine how well the lungs and gas exchange are working in the body; for a CBG test, blood is drawn, generally through pricking the heel.

CNS   (central nervous system): The brain and spinal cord; how the baby is moving gives a sense of the health of the CNS.

CPAP   (continuous positive airway pressure): A way to give oxygen or air to babies, using a mask or prongs inserted in the nose. The baby breathes on his or her own with a CPAP. The CPAP is attached to a respirator (breathing machine) or another mechanism that delivers the pressure.

CPR   (cardiopulmonary resuscitation): Also known as resuscitation, which in the NICU usually include intubation (placing a tube down the trachea/windpipe) and cardiac massage. A way to get the heart and lungs to start working again when they have stopped or slowed a lot.

d/c   (discontinue): To stop something (for example, d/c medication PO); can also be used for discharge ("d/c home").

ETT   (endotracheal tube): A breathing tube that goes in the trachea (windpipe). It is inserted through the mouth or the nose.

g, kg   (gram), (kilogram): The measures used for babies' weight in the NICU: 100 grams is about 3.5 ounces; 1 kilogram is 2.2 pounds.

HFV   (high-frequency ventilator) also HFO (high-frequency oscillator): A "super respirator" that gives many breaths per second, making babies vibrate.

IV   (intravenous): Given in the veins.

IV   A tiny, flexible, hollow plastic tube (catheter) that is inserted in a vein.

IVH   (intraventricular hemorrhage): A bleed in the middle of the brain; premature infants are at higher risk of IVH, especially in the first week of life, but not after 2 weeks.

LP   (lumbar puncture): A test done to examine the liquid around the spinal column, to determine if the baby has meningitis. A small needle is inserted between two vertebrae at the bottom of the back to obtain the fluid.

mL   (millilitre): A unit of volume, usually used to describe how much milk a baby is receiving; 30 mL is 1 fluid ounce.

NICU   (neonatal intensive care unit): The part of a hospital for newborns with extra medical needs.

NPO   (*nil per os, which is a latin term*): No food or liquid given by mouth.

O_2 (oxygen): A gas in the air we breathe that is needed to sustain life. We breathe 21 per cent oxygen. Many preterm babies need extra oxygen to survive.

PDA   (patent ductus arteriosus): The ductus arteriosus is a normal connection between the aorta and the pulmonary artery (two main big blood vessels) in the fetus. At birth, because it is not useful anymore and the baby is breathing, it usually closes. It can stay patent (open) in preterm infants and cause babies some problems, such as breathing faster.

Peep   (positive end-expiratory pressure): Peep represents the pressure in the lungs at the end of the expiration. It can be intrinsic (what the body does naturally after expiration) or extrinsic (what the respirator does). The respirator gives pressure for every breath, but at the end of the breath peep is given to keep the lungs open.

PICC line (peripherally inserted central venous catheter): A type of tube that is put into a central (large) vein.

PO   (*per os*): By mouth (for example, "PO medication").

ROP   (retinopathy of prematurity): An eye condition that premature infants are at risk of. The retina is at the back of the eye and helps us see. There are four grades of ROP: grade 1 is usually not dangerous, but grade 3 is serious. Grade 4 is when the retina detaches, and this usually leads to blindness.

Stat   (not an abbreviation, but often written in capital letters and therfore mistaken as an abbreviation by many): From the Latin word *statim*, meaning immediately.

TPN   (total parenteral nutrition): Nutrition (proteins, fats, vitamins, sugars, etc.) fed into the veins.

UAC   (umbilical arterial catheter): A tube that is inserted in the artery of the umbilicus in the first days of life. This enables clinicians to draw blood without having to poke the baby.

UVC   (umbilical venous catheter): A tube that is inserted in the vein of the umbilicus in the first days of life. This is another kind of central line (like the PICC line) and enables the NICU to give intravenous nutrition and fluids without poking the baby for an IV.

Selected Bibliography

Charland, L. "Is Spock Mentally Competent? Competence to Consent and Emotion." *Philosophy, Psychiatry and Psychology* 5, no. 1 (March 1998): 67–81.

Haward, M.F., N. Gaucher, A. Payot, K. Robson, and A. Janvier. "Personalized Decision Making: Practical Recommendations for Antenatal Counseling for Fragile Neonates." *Clinics in Perinatology* 44, no. 2 (June 2017): 429–45.

Janvier, A. "How Much Emotion Is Enough?" *Journal of Clinical Ethics* 18 (2007): 362–5.

– "No Time for Death." *American Journal of Hospice and Palliative Medicine* 27, no. 2 (March 2010): 163–4.

Janvier, A., K. Barrington, K. Aziz, et al. "CPS Policy Statement for Prenatal Counselling before a Premature Birth: Simple Rules for Complicated Decisions." *Pediatrics and Child Health* 19, no. 1 (January 2014): 22–4.

Janvier, A., K. Barrington, and B. Farlow. "Communication with Parents Concerning Withholding or Withdrawing of Life Sustaining Interventions in Neonatology." *Seminars in Perinatology* 38, no. 1 (February 2014): 38–46.

Janvier, A., and S.R. Leuthner. "Chronic Patients, Burdensome Interventions and the Vietnam Analogy." *Acta Paediatrica* 102, no. 7 (July 2013): 669–70.

Janvier, A., J. Lorenz, and J. Lantos. "Antenatal Counselling for Parents Facing an Extremely Preterm Birth: Limitations of the Medical Evidence." *Acta Paediatrica* 101, no. 8 (August 2012): 800–4.

Janvier, A., and P. Shah. "The Premature Lottery in the Canadian Grey Zones." *Current Pediatric Reviews* 9, no. 1 (2013): 25–31.

Kahneman, D. *Thinking Fast and Slow*. New York: Farrar, Strauss and Giroux, 2011.

Kahneman, D., P. Slovic, and A. Tversky, eds. *Judgment under Uncertainty: Heuristics and Biases*. Cambridge: Cambridge University Press, 1982.

Nussbaum, M. *The Upheavals of Thought: The Intelligence of Emotions.* Cambridge: Cambridge University Press, 2001.

Shumacher, E.F. *A Guide for the Perplexed.* New York: Harper Perennial, 1977.

Staub, K., J. Baardsnes, N. Hébert, S. Newell, and R. Pearce. "Our Child Is Not Just a Gestational Age: A First-Hand Account of What Parents Want and Need to Know before Premature Birth." *Acta Paediatrica* 103, no. 1 (October 2014): 1035–8.

Resources and Further Reading

Books about Prematurity and/or Neonatal Intensive Care

Degl, J. *From Hope to Joy: A Memoir of a Mother's Determination and Her Micro Preemie's Struggle to Beat the Odds.* Mahopac Falls, NY: Lemon Tree Publishing, 2013.

Ewing, J.T. *Preemie Chronicles: Our NICU Experience.* Lulu.com, 14 December 2006.

Fei, D. *Girl in Glass: Dispatches from the Edge of Life.* New York: Bloomsbury, 2015.

Forman, V. *This Lovely Life: A Memoir of Premature Motherhood.* New York: Mariner Books, 2009.

French, Kelly, and Thomas French. *Juniper: The Girl Who Was Born Too Soon.* New York: Little, Brown, 2016.

Hopper, K. *Ready for Air: A Journey through Premature Motherhood.* Minneapolis: University of Minnesota Press, 2013.

Killilea, M. *Karen.* New York: Dell, 1967.

Mathews, M. *Preemie: Lessons in Love, Life, and Motherhood.* Hobart, NY: Hatherleigh Press, 2012.

Books about Bioethics and Neonatology

Lantos J. *The Lazarus Case.* Baltimore, MD: Johns Hopkins University Press, 2007.

Lantos, J.D., and W.L. Meadow. *Neonatal Bioethics: The Moral Challenges of Medical Innovation.* Baltimore, MD: Johns Hopkins University Press, 2008.

Verhagen, E., and A. Janvier. *Ethical Dilemmas for Critically Ill Babies.* Berlin: Springer, 2016.

Wilkinson, Dominic. *Death or Disability? The "Carmentis Machine" and Decision-Making for Critically Ill Children.* Oxford: Oxford University Press, 2013.

Basic Scientific Articles in Neonatology

This list is not exhaustive. It represents basic articles, and there are many more that are equally good. The blog neonatalresearch.org examines much of the neonatal literature and thousands of articles.

The Importance of Prenatal Steroids in Extremely Preterm Infants

Travers, C.P., et al. "Exposure to Any Antenatal Corticosteroids and Outcomes in Preterm Infants by Gestational Age: Prospective Cohort Study." *British Medical Journal* 356 (2017): 1–7.

Treating Pain in Neonatology

Ancora, G., et al. "Evidence-Based Clinical Guidelines on Analgesia and Sedation in Newborn Infants Undergoing Assisted Ventilation and Endotracheal Intubation." *Acta Paediatrica* 108, no. 2 (February 2018): 208–17. DOI: 10.1111/apa.14606.

Stevens, B., J. Yamada, G.Y. Lee, and A. Ohlsson. "Sucrose for Analgesia in Newborn Infants Undergoing Painful Procedures." *Cochrane Database of Systematic Reviews* 7 (2016). DOI:10.1002/14651858.Cd001069.

The Importance for Premedication before Intubation

Barrington, K. "Premedication for Endotracheal Intubation in the Newborn Infant." *Paediatrics and Child Health* 16, no. 3 (2011): 159–71.

Kangaroo Care

Jefferies, A.L., et al. "Kangaroo Care for the Preterm Infant and Family." *Paediatrics and Child Health* 17, no. 3 (2012): 141–6.

On the Importance of Probiotics to Decrease Necrotizing Entorocolitis

Janvier, A., et al. "The Politics of Probiotics: Probiotics, Necrotizing Enterocolitis and the Ethics of Neonatal Research." *Acta Paediatrica* 102, no. 2 (2013): 116–18.

Thomas, J.P., et al. "Probiotics for the Prevention of Necrotising Enterocolitis in Very Low-Birth-Weight Infants: A Meta-Analysis and Systematic Review." *Acta Paediatrica* 106, no. 11 (2017): 1729–41.

Interventions to Support Parents

Axelin, A., J. Outinen, K. Lainema, L. Lehtonen, and L.S. Franck. "Neonatologists Can Impede or Support Parents' Participation in Decision-Making during Medical Rounds in Neonatal Intensive Care Units." *Acta Paediatrica* 107, no. 12 (December 2018). DOI: 10.1111/apa.14386.

Brett, J., S. Staniszewska, M. Newburn, N. Jones, and L. Taylor. "A Systematic Mapping Review of Effective Interventions for Communicating with, Supporting and Providing Information to Parents of Preterm Infants." *BMJ Open* 1, no. 1 (June 2011). DOI: 10.1136/bmjopen-2010-000023.

Sabnis, A., S. Fojo, S.S. Nayak, E. Lopez, D.N. Tarn, and L. Zeltzer, "Reducing Parental Trauma and Stress in Neonatal Intensive Care: Systematic Review and Meta-analysis of Hospital Interventions." *Journal of Perinatology* 30, no. 3 (March 2019): 375–86. DOI: 10.1038/s41372-018-0310-9.

Umberger, E., et al. "Enhancing NICU Parent Engagement and Empowerment." *Seminars in Pediatric Surgery* 27, no. 1 (2018): 19–24.

Breastfeeding in Neonatology

Alves, E., et al. "Parents' Views on Factors That Help or Hinder Breast Milk Supply in Neonatal Care Units: Systematic Review." *Archive of Disease in Childhood Fetal and Neonatal Edition* 98, no. 6 (2013): F511–17.

Becker, G.E., et al. "Methods of Milk Expression for Lactating Women." *Cochrane Database of Systematic Reviews* 9 (2016). Cd006170. https://www.ncbi.nlm.nih.gov/pubmed/27684560

Cuttini, M., et al. "Breastfeeding Outcomes in European NICUs: Impact of Parental Visiting Policies." *Archive of Disease in Childhood: Fetal and Neonatal Edition* 104, no. (March 2019). doi: 10.1136/archdischild-2017-314723.

Grzeskowiak, L.E., et al. "Domperidone for Increasing Breast Milk Volume in Mothers Expressing Breast Milk for Their Preterm Infants: A Systematic Review and Meta-Analysis." *BJOG* 125, no. 11 (2018): 1371–8.

Romaine, A., et al. "Predictors of Prolonged Breast Milk Provision to Very Low Birth Weight Infants." *Journal of Pediatrics* 202 (November 2018). doi: 10.1016/j.jpeds.2018.07.001

On the Limitations of Routine Term Magnetic Resonance Imaging for Preterm Infants

Edwards, A.D., et al. "Effect of MRI on Preterm Infants and Their Families: A Randomised Trial with Nested Diagnostic and Economic Evaluation." *Archives of Disease in Childhood: Fetal and Neonatal Edition* 103, no. 1 (January 2018). DOI: 10.1136/archdischild-2017-313102.

Ho, T., et al. "Choosing Wisely in Newborn Medicine: Five Opportunities to Increase Value." *Pediatrics* 136, no. 2 (2015): e482–9.

Pearce, R., and J. Baardsnes. "Term MRI for Small Preterm Babies: Do Parents Really Want to Know and Why Has Nobody Asked Them?" *Acta Paediatrica* 101, no. 10 (2012): 1013–51.

The Importance of Not Using the Term "Doing Everything"

Feudtner, C., and W. Morrison. "The Darkening Veil of 'Do Everything'." *Archives of Pediatrics and Adolescent Medicine* 166 (2012): 694–5.

The Importance of Hope

Feudtner, C. "The Breadth of Hopes." *New England Journal of Medicine* 361 (2009): 2306–7.

Patient and Parental Perspectives

There is a lot of material in this category. I have included here a very limited number of important publications. These are those that were pointed to me as having changed the attitudes and behaviour of many providers.

Guon, J., et al. "Our Children Are Not a Diagnosis: The Experience of Parents Who Continue Their Pregnancy after a Prenatal Diagnosis of Trisomy 13 or 18." *American Journal of Medical Genetics A* 164A, no. 2 (2014): 308–18.

Miller, T. "Attack of the Redneck Mommy." http://www.tanismiller.com /redneckmommy-bestof

Parents of Elliot. "99 Balloons." https://www.youtube.com/watch?v=th6Njr-qkq0.

Taggart, T. "Two Conversations That Changed My Life." https://www.youtube.com /watch?v=vjRlFCgQ1e8.

Support Groups for Parents

This is a very limited list – it is impossible to include all the groups that exist for parents.

Canada and Quebec

CPBF/FBPC – Canadian Premature Babies Foundation / Fondation pour Bébés Prématurés Canadiens: http://cpbf-fbpc.org/ (prematurity)

Préma-Québec: http://www.premaquebec.ca/ (prematurity)

En cœur: http://en-coeur.org (cardiac malformation)

RT21: http://trisomie.qc.ca/ (trisomy 21)

International

CDH International: https://cdhi.org/ (congenital diaphragmatic hernia)

March of Dimes: https://www.marchofdimes.org/

Miracle Babies Foundation: https://www.miraclebabies.org.au/

SOFT – Support Organization for Trisomy 13 and 18: http://trisomy.org/

Milton Keynes UK
Ingram Content Group UK Ltd.
UKHW012228190424
441406UK00003B/260